W9-AMV-024

MANUAL
For
FUNCTIONAL
TRAINING

Edition 3

M. Lynn Palmer, Ph.D., P.T.
Professor
Graduate School for Health Studies
Program in Physical Therapy
Simmons College
Boston, Massachusetts

Janice E. Toms, M.Ed., P.T.
Director and Professor
Graduate School for Health Studies
Program in Physical Therapy
Simmons College
Boston, Massachusetts

With contributions by

Joan E. Edelstein, M.A., P.T.
Columbia University
New York, New York

Consultants

Charles Croteau, B.S.
Worcester, Massachusetts

Lynn Hammer, B.S., P.T.
Brighton, Massachusetts

F. A. DAVIS COMPANY • Philadelphia

F. A. Davis Company
1915 Arch Street
Philadelphia, PA 19103

Copyright © 1992 by F. A. Davis Company

Copyright © 1980, 1986 by F. A. Davis Company. All rights reserved. This book is protected by copyright. No part of it may be reproduced, stored in a retrieval system, or transmitted in any form or by any means, electronic, mechanical, photocopying, recording, or otherwise, without written permission from the publisher.

Printed in the United States of America

Last digit indicates print number: 10 9 8 7 6 5

NOTE: As new scientific information becomes available through basic and clinical research, recommended treatments and drug therapies undergo changes. The author(s) and publisher have done everything possible to make this book accurate, up to date, and in accord with accepted standards at the time of publication. The authors, editors, and publisher are not responsible for errors or omissions or for consequences from application of the book, and make no warranty, expressed or implied, in regard to the contents of the book. Any practice described in this book should be applied by the reader in accordance with professional standards of care used in regard to the unique circumstances that may apply in each situation. The reader is advised always to check product information (package inserts) for changes and new information regarding dose and contraindications before administering any drug. Caution is especially urged when using new or infrequently ordered drugs.

Library of Congress Cataloging-in-Publication Data

Palmer, M. Lynn.
    Manual for functional training / M. Lynn Palmer, Janice E. Toms, with contributions by Joan E. Edelstein ; consultants, Charles Croteau, Lynn Hammer. — Ed. 3.
        p. cm.
    Includes bibliographical references and index.
    ISBN 0-8036-6759-0 (softbound : alk. paper)
    1. Physically handicapped — Rehabilitation. 2. Physical therapy. 3. Patient education. I. Toms, Janice E. II. Edelstein, Joan E. III. Title.
    [DNLM: 1. Activities of Daily Living. 2. Handicapped. 3. Patient Education. 4. Physical Therapy. 5. Rehabilitation. WB 320 P175m]
    RD798.P34 1991
    617.1'03 — dc20
    DNLM/DLC
    for Library of Congress   91-34541
                                                                                         CIP

Authorization to photocopy items for internal or personal use, or the internal or personal use of specific clients, is granted by F. A. Davis Company for users registered with the Copyright Clearance Center (CCC) Transactional Reporting Service, provided that the fee of $.10 per copy is paid directly to CCC, 222 Rosewood Drive, Danvers, MA 01923. For those organizations that have been granted a photocopy license by CCC, a separate system of payment has been arranged. The fee code for users of the Transactional Reporting Service is 8036-6759 / 92 0 + $.10.

MANUAL
For
FUNCTIONAL TRAINING

EDITION 3

DEDICATED TO OUR STUDENTS: PAST, PRESENT, AND FUTURE

PREFACE TO THE THIRD EDITION

We are pleased that the *Manual for Functional Training* continues to meet the needs of students and practitioners. This third edition of the book addresses some of the many changes that have occurred in the last decade both in scientific knowledge and equipment technology for the enhancement of individuals with handicaps. It is important for handicapped individuals to become and remain as functionally independent as possible and to be active members of the community in everyday activities, including work and recreation. Also, significant improvements in medical and surgical technology have given individuals an opportunity to survive severe traumatic injuries or nervous system problems. Advancements in wheelchair technology and orthotic and prosthetic devices have allowed more of these individuals to become functionally independent. Therapists need to be aware of the new technology and recent methods of improving the level of independence for the most severely involved person. For example, not long ago people with a C-2 or C-3 spinal cord lesion did not survive.

We have responded to the comments and critiques of the second edition of the *Manual for Functional Training* by incorporating many of the suggestions made and adding some changes. We collaborated with experts in the various fields to provide up-to-date information and greater depth in specific areas, such as amputations and traumatic brain injuries. Significant modifications were made in the area of the functional activities for wheelchair users.

The text was also greatly reformatted. For instance, the functional activities are now in chapters that have been designated by disability. The text begins with chapters giving the basic information on major disabilities that is, disabilities involving the lower limbs and trunk. These include spinal cord injury or meningocele; disabilities involving all four limbs and trunk such as spinal cord injury, multiple sclerosis, or Guillain-Barré; and disabilities involving one side of the body such as cerebral vascular accidents or traumatic brain injury. The chapters on functional activities for the various levels of involvement are divided into subsegments according to the levels of independence. For example, the chapter on involvement of lower limbs and trunk includes bed mobility, dressing, mat activities, wheelchair mobility, transfers, and upright activities.

Photographs of individuals with the actual disabilities performing the activities have been added. The addition of these photographs will allow the reader to better visualize the activities being performed.

We have expanded the wheelchair mobility section, particularly in the area of activities for individuals with lower limb and trunk involvement and with involvement of all four limbs and trunk. Also, we have added a chapter on orthotics, and expanded and updated the chapter on amputation and prosthetics. The chapter on wheelchairs, assistive devices, and home modifications now includes suggestions for designing or remodeling a home to make it more accessible for wheelchair users. Some of the information for the chapter was gathered from the Office of the Secretary of State, the Commonwealth of Massachusetts, Architectural Barriers Board. Also, the home improvement section includes an evaluation form developed by the therapists at the Greenery Rehabilitation and Skilled Nursing Center in Brighton, Massachusetts.

M. Lynn Palmer
Janice E. Toms

PREFACE TO THE SECOND EDITION

This second edition of the *Manual for Functional Training* has been generated in part because of the success of the first edition, and because of the need to update some of the material.

The book has been an important reference for practicing therapists, students, and many other health science personnel who are involved with helping others reach their highest level of functional independence.

This edition reflects changes that were suggested by those who have used the book. We felt a responsibility to respond to the many suggestions and have collaborated with others to add new material and provide greater detail in specific areas. The most significant modifications are in the "Spinal Cord Injuries," "Cerebral Vascular Disorders," and "Amputations" chapters. These chapters present more current information, greater detail, and clarification of the existing material. The number of illustrations has also been increased to help clarify the text.

The format of this book has remained the same because it is practical and easy to use.

This new edition of the *Manual for Functional Training* surpasses the scope of the original text. We trust that it will provide a lasting benefit to future generations of health personnel, clinicians, instructors of health science students, patients, and anyone involved with the management of individuals requiring physical rehabilitation.

A special expression of appreciation goes to the Physical Therapy Department at Rancho Los Amigos Hospital, Downey, California for many of the ideas and suggestions that have been incorporated into this book.

One of the outstanding features of this book is the number and quality of the illustrations. We are very grateful to Regina Bean and Cheryl Piperberg, B.F.A. for providing these excellent drawings.

We also would like to express our appreciation to Althier Pino for the many hours she spent putting this text on the word processor and the clinical facilities and authors that gave us permission to use samples of their evaluation forms, illustrations, and other material that helped us develop a complete functional training manual.

M. Lynn Palmer
Janice E. Toms

ACKNOWLEDGMENTS

We want to thank Diane U. Jette, P.T., of the Department of Physical Therapy, Simmons College, Boston, Massachusetts, for her constructive critique and helpful suggestions for improvement of the third edition. We also thank Jeffrey Medeiros, M.D. of the Department of Clinical Pathology, New England Deconess Hospital, Boston, Massachusetts, and Sharon Marich, B.S., P.T. of Dedham, Massachusetts, for their input on CVA and amputee management, respectively, in the second edition.

In addition, we want to express our sincere appreciation to Charles Croteau and Lynn Hammer, who provided valuable input into the chapters on wheelchair mobility and traumatic brain injury, respectively. We are also grateful to Peter R. Lorange and the patients and therapists at Cushing Hospital in Framingham, Massachusetts and the Greenery Rehabilitation and Skilled Nursing Center in Brighton, Massachusetts for allowing us to take photographs of them performing functional activities.

CONTENTS

Introduction

Functional training consists of evaluating the functional independence level of a physically handicapped individual and assisting the individual in gaining the highest practical level of independence in daily living activities. Planning a treatment program for patients requires the selection of activities that they can perform, as well as the selection of skills that may advance them to a higher functional level.

When teaching functional activities it is necessary to analyze the component motions of a given activity and to practice each component as an exercise; finally, the activity can be practiced in its entirety. Careful observation of the patient during the performance of activities will be necessary to determine the methods that will allow the person to perform safely, with the least expenditure of energy.

In planning treatment programs the therapist should take into consideration the physical and motivational readiness of the learner and should plan for goal-directed activities. Goal-directed activities are performed and practiced in an environment similar to that in which the motor skill will be used. Goal-directed functional activities will provide motor learning that has meaning and significance for the learner. Many common functional activities involve eccentric and concentric types of muscle contractions, yet few of our therapeutic techniques incorporate this principle into the exercise program. It is also important to recognize and allow for the physiologic response of the nervous system, which allows the learner to think through the activity prior to performing it.

Teaching functional activities includes providing opportunities for the learner to visualize the activity and to practice the activity in the appropriate goal-directed environment. Practice should continue until the actions become automatic. In an attempt to allow for some individual problem solving in the situation and activities, repetitions should not be performed in exactly the same manner each time. Assistance, both verbal and physical, should be withdrawn as soon as this is safely possible. This provides the necessary security while avoiding an undesirable dependency on the therapist.

This manual focuses on how to teach patients to perform independently. In the early stages of learning, guarding and assistance may be desirable until the activity is performed independently and safely.

Factors that influence the success of a treatment plan but are sometimes difficult to measure are (1) the motivation of the patient; (2) the attitudes of the family, friends, and hospital staff; (3) the availability and quality of technical and financial resources; and (4) the continuity of medical care.

The ability to function independently in daily life does not depend on the ability to walk. Many individuals are independent in a wheelchair and will never be functional walkers. It is understood that an individual's goals may vary according to his or her disability, age, occupation, and home and work situations.

This manual is designed to be used as a textbook for all levels of health science students and as a reference book for practicing clinicians. It describes functional activities for patients with involvement of one side, of lower limbs and trunk, and of all four limbs and trunk, as well as for those who have experienced lower limb amputations. The activities for each chapter progress sequentially from lying and sitting activities through ambulation.

The chapters on the functional significance of spinal cord lesions, brain trauma, and level of limb amputations provide a brief overview of the clinical picture, prognosis, and problems related to the disabilities. The intention is to help the reader understand the activities and objectives of functional training. If more detail regarding the clinical significance of any of the disabilities is desired, numerous textbooks are available on those subjects.

For each general category of physical handicap, the material is presented sequentially from the lowest level of function, with emphasis on the clinical application of assisting, guarding, and teaching techniques. Each activity has been thoroughly analyzed and each component of the activity is presented in its logical sequence. When instructing patients it is important to be cognizant of each sequential step necessary to perform the activity. To avoid being bombarded with commands for each step, the patient should be given the goal of the activity and allowed to perform it. If the activity is not being performed safely or the patient is experiencing difficulty accomplishing it, then appropriate instructions should be conveyed to assist in the safe performance. Consciously directed movements interfere with performance. It is the therapist's responsibility to identify the appropriate time for corrections and allow for adequate repetitions to develop automatic (subcortical) motor activities.

Individuals who have suffered a head injury may have to relearn functional motor skills in much the same way that the skills were learned as children. Three broad stages of motor learning are (1) understanding of the task, (2) establishing sensory and motor associations, and (3) integrating movement patterns at an automatic level. During the first stage the patient must be motivated and able to comprehend the task. Simple step-by-step instructions are necessary if short-term memory is impaired. Active patient participation in the activity is required for learning to occur. Sensory input and feedback is essential so that meaningful information is received by the central nervous system (CNS) for adequate learning to occur. Practicing the activity helps neuronal integration and leads to automaticity of motor behavior. Because brain plasticity may allow the formation of new and modified synapses during learning, practice may be required for months or years before new synapses develop and become functional.

Motor learning rechannels impulses to produce new spatial and temporal relationships among neurons. During the early stages, when learning is difficult, one has to concentrate on individual parts of a pattern. Consciously directed movement interferes with smooth operation of the subcortical mechanisms. Attempted performance usually includes a number of movements that serve no useful purpose. As learning progresses there is a gradual reduction in the amount of cortical involvement. Finally, a simple thought may be sufficient to initiate a whole train of motor events. Smooth coordinated movements are at a subcortical level. Development of motor control needs underlying normal postural muscles. Therapeutic techniques incorporated into the treatment plan should include establishing a program to develop appropriate muscle tone in the postural muscles to enhance the functional activities.

Individuals with CNS lesions may need to develop a new motor program. A motor program will store a set of commands that, when executed, will produce a movement. Such a program may also be modified to produce a variation of a movement. Learning a motor skill requires feedback for accuracy of movement. Motor learning is a set of processes associated with practice of motor experiences leading to relatively permanent changes in the capability for responding. Feedback strengthens the motor scheme. Highly practiced and skilled activity is automatic through motor learning. Changes can occur through practice and feedback within the CNS to establish skilled actions. These changes are developed through lowering synaptic thresholds, increasing the number of dendritic processes, which increases the synaptic regions, and collateral sprouting of adjacent neurons.

Carolee J. Winstein, P.T., Ph.D., summarizes motor learning as follows:

1. The therapeutic strategies used to effect temporary changes in motor performance may not be those that effect relatively permanent changes associated with motor learning and the retention of motor skills.
2. Practice schedules with a high frequency of augmented feedback have been shown to benefit motor performance, but the intelligent scheduling of feedback presentations during practice, in which lower frequencies of feedback are used, can enhance the learning and retention of motor skills.
3. Structuring the treatment session to reduce contextual variety leads to improved motor performance, but the intelligent implementation of increased contextual variety during practice can enhance the learning and retention of motor skills.

Chapter 12 includes some samples of functional training evaluation forms, assessment forms for amputees and prosthetics, and a home evaluation tool.

Although the authors have limited this text to the procedures that are necessary to teach the patient functional activities, they are very much aware of and committed to the concept that the goal of functional independence includes more than the teaching of functional activities. Therapeutic techniques such as facilitation, inhibition, and muscle strengthening and stretching are a few examples of the treatment procedures that would be included in the plan of care for the total rehabilitation of a patient with a physical disability.

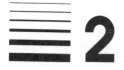 **2**

Spinal Cord Injuries

Trauma is one of the most common causes of spinal cord injury. Trauma to the spinal cord, either by compression or by contusion, is most common in young adult men. Spinal cord injury may be from a penetrating wound from a bullet or knife; a fracture dislocation resulting in transection of cord; compression from a tumor; and osteophytes, arachnoiditis, extradural abscess, herniated disc, or collapsed vertebrae. Another common cause of injury to the spinal cord is vascular malfunction, which results from thrombosis of the cord vessels, an embolus, or hemorrhage. There are also congenital causes such as meningomyelocele, infections such as transverse myelitis and syphilis, diseases such as multiple sclerosis, and finally hysterical paralysis.

Injuries to the spinal cord may result in complete, partial, or mixed somatic sensory, motor, and autonomic nervous system involvement. Although rare, a complete lesion is caused by a complete transection or compression of the spinal cord; no sensation or voluntary motor function is noted below the level of injury. An incomplete lesion may be the result of partial transection or cord contusion; some evidence of sensation or motor function is preserved below the level of injury. With a contusion of the spinal cord there is edema, hemorrhage, and diaschisis (spinal shock) at and below the level of the injury, resulting in failure of the spinal cord to function for a variable period of time. Diaschisis usually lasts from 3 to 6 weeks; however, complications may prolong it.

A lesion of the spinal cord at or above the T-1 spinal cord level will result in quadraplegia in which all four limbs and the trunk are involved. A spinal cord lesion below T-1 usually spares the upper limbs and results in a classification of paraplegia in which there is involvement of the trunk and lower limbs.

The spinal cord begins as an extension from the medulla oblongata of the brain stem at the level of the foramen magnum and in the adult extends to the level of the second lumbar vertebra, ending as the conus medullaris. Early in fetal life the cord fills the entire length of the vertebral canal. As the fetus develops, the rate of growth of the vertebral column is greater than that of the spinal cord. Therefore, the adult spinal cord is shorter than the length of the vertebra column; as a result the spinal cord segments are not aligned with the corresponding vertebra. The approximate corresponding vertebral levels to the conus medullaris are shown here.

Vertebral Level	Conus Medullaris
1st coccygeal	2 months prenatal
1st sacral	3 months prenatal
4th lumbar	4 months prenatal
3rd lumbar	5 months prenatal to birth
2nd lumbar	Postnatal

Although somewhat variable, the diameter of the spinal cord in the widest portions at the cervical and lumbar enlargements is no larger than an individual's index finger. The cord is protected by three layers of tough connective tissues—the meninges—and is encased within the bony vertebral canal, which is reinforced by strong, long and short ligaments, and muscles.

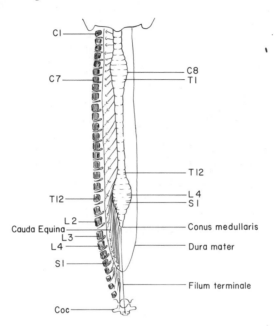

The spinal cord is anatomically and physiologically divided into 31 segments. Each segment gives rise to a pair of spinal nerves that contribute to the formation of the peripheral nervous system. As a consequence of growth, the spinal cord segments move upward in relation to the vertebra, and the nerve roots that were originally horizontal assume an increasingly oblique and downward direction.

Spinal nerves emerge below their corresponding vertebra, except at the cervical vertebral level where the first cervical spinal nerves emerge between the occiput and the atlas (first cervical vertebra). The second pair of cervical spinal nerves emerges below the atlas to enter the periphery. The spinal nerves continue to emerge from the vertebral canal through the intervertebral foramen above the corresponding vertebra throughout the cervical area. The eighth pair of cervical spinal nerves emerges between the seventh cervical and first thoracic vertebra. Each pair of spinal nerves has a corresponding spinal cord segment and vertebra.

The relationship between spinal cord segments and the vertebrae is important when identifying the level of spinal cord lesions. The cervical spinal cord segments correspond in location with the numbered vertebrae. In the upper thoracic area, the corresponding vertebrae are approximately two spinal cord segments lower; in the lower thoracic region, three segments lower. For example, the fourth thoracic vertebra is approximately level with the sixth thoracic spinal cord segment. The lumbar and sacral spinal cord segments occupy a space approximately opposite the ninth thoracic through the second lumbar vertebra. This fact is of clinical importance for two reasons: (1) traumatic spinal cord lesions may be classified according to the vertebral level of the injury, which may or may not correspond to the spinal cord segment; and (2) dermatomes, the cutaneous areas supplied by the sensory component of each spinal cord segment, are used clinically in diagnosing the level of spinal cord lesions.

In the trunk, the somatic sensory portion of the spinal nerves and the dermis of the skin are arranged in consecutive circling bands. The bands are schematic representations of sensory innervation. The ventral primary rami of the first thoracic nerve divide into a large and a small branch. The large branch enters the brachial plexus to supply the skin of the medial arm. The small branch is the first intercostal nerve supplying the intercostal space. The second thoracic nerve frequently gives branches to the first. This situation will account for a lack of T-1 dermatome representation on the anterior chest wall. In the limbs, owing to the formation of the plexuses, the segmental distribution becomes obscured. As a result of the growth of the lower limbs during development the proximal lumbosacral spinal nerve segments are aligned in elongated strips along the medial aspect of each limb; the distal portions are distributed posterolaterally. The upper limbs are rotated in a lateral direction during development; therefore, the spinal cord segments are represented on the upper limbs in the following manner: C-5 and C-6 are on the lateral aspect; C-7 is in the midline of the hand; and C-8 and T-1 are on the medial aspect of the limb. The nerves supplying adjacent dermatomes overlap; therefore, one dorsal nerve root produces a decrease in sensation rather than a complete loss.

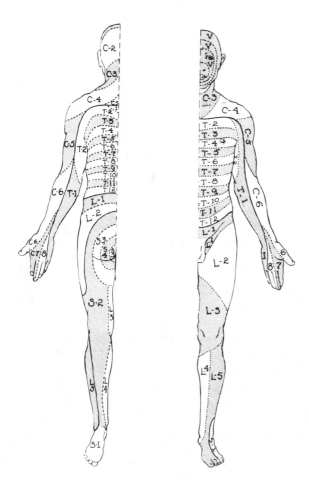

(Adapted from Chusid, J: Correlative Neuroanatomy and Functional Neurology, ed 18. Lange Medical Publications, Los Altos, California, with permission.)

The most common site for a lesion is the T-12–L-1 vertebra, which is the most mobile area of the back. A complete lesion occurring between T-2 and T-12–L-1 results in bilateral paralysis of the lower limbs. Complete lesions at T-1 and above result in involvement of all four limbs and trunk. Cauda equina injuries occur at the first lumbar vertebra and below, damaging the lumbar and sacral roots before they leave the neural canal. The prognosis for this lesion is good because the nerves injured are peripheral. Peripheral nerves have a better prognosis for regeneration than neuronal damage within the central nervous system (CNS).

A flexion-rotation injury of the thoracolumbar spine usually results in a fracture dislocation of the vertebra. This injury is the most common cause of paraplegia.

The most common injury to occur in the cervical area is caused by excessive extension, often resulting in quadriparesis. Extension and dislocation injuries rarely occur in the thoracolumbar spine because of bony structures and the support offered by the longitudinal ligaments.

Compression injuries may result in a fracture of the vertebral disk or body, with or without any neurologic deficit. Healing of the bone requires 4 to 6 weeks. While the bone is healing, the anterior and posterior longitudinal ligaments offer stability.

Another possibility with a spinal cord injury is root escape. A patient with root escape has suffered spinal cord damage, but the peripheral nerve roots at the level of the lesion have escaped injury.

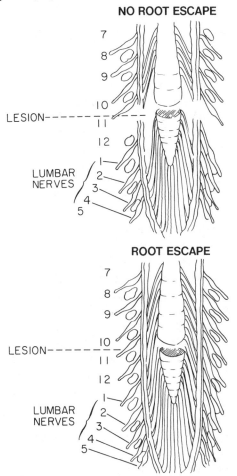

The Brown-Séquard syndrome results from a hemisection of the cord. Because the descending motor fibers cross in the medulla and the ascending sensory fibers cross in the spinal cord and in the medulla, the site of injury is on the same side as the motor paralysis. The patient will exhibit signs and symptoms of contralateral loss of pain and temperature sense below the level of lesion and ipsilateral spastic paralysis and loss of deep sense below the level of lesion.

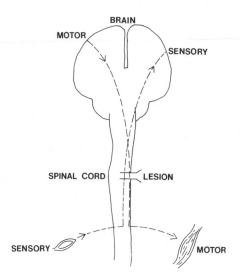

The CNS goes through a process of degeneration and recovery subsequent to an insult similar to the degeneration of the myelinated peripheral nervous system. At the lesion site, traumatic degeneration occurs immediately, which causes the axoplasm to leak out from both the proximal and distal cut ends. Therefore, the ends of the neuronal processes are set back to a distance of one or two nodes of Ranvier (about 2 mm) from the cut ends, both proximally and distally. Retrograde degeneration occurs in the cell bodies of the neurons in which all presynaptic terminals contacting the dendrites and cell bodies of the injured neurons will withdraw, thus decreasing synaptic effectiveness. Also, there is degeneration of the distal segment of each neuron including the myelin sheath.

In the CNS regeneration lasts only for 1 or 2 weeks and then is aborted. The regeneration attempt begins about 2 mμ proximal to the injured neurons. The axonal ends are swollen and contain numerous axoplasmic organelles; this is referred to as the terminal club. The terminal club advances within the microcyst. The microcyst is formed by remaining myelin, which is plugged by the aggregation of organelles and provides a small cavity to house the terminal club. The terminal club continues to expand and eventually will rupture, presumably because there is no basement membrane tube (neurolemma) as in the peripheral nervous system to limit the excessive expansion of the club. With the rupture of the terminal club, the organelles are dispersed into the extracellular spaces and the end of the axons are further set back from the initial region. Digestive enzymes (lyzosomes) contained within the neurons are released, causing tissue autolysis. This process is repeated several times until the axons end at a collateral or the process is self-limiting with the entire regenerative process terminating. The cavity formed from the microcysts will eventually fill in with astrocytic scarring.

One of the many research attempts at regeneration of the spinal cord has been implantation of peripheral nerve grafts for the purpose of constructing nerve cell relay bridges at the site of the injury in order to reestablish connections from the proximal to distal portions. Also, discovery of nerve growth factors in the CNS may make it possible to inject the factor into the nervous system in an attempt to influence regeneration immediately prior to the occurrence of scarring. Another project in process is the application of a direct electrical current, over a period of weeks, to induce regeneration of the neuronal processes in the spinal cord. In addition, cold lasers and induction of drugs are being studied as a direct mechanism for spinal cord regeneration.

The CNS, failing in its attempt to regenerate, goes through a process of recovery. Remaining nervous tissue will develop denervation supersensitivity, which tends to stimulate collateral sprouting and an unmasking of previously ineffective synapses. Synaptic restoration will occur after the initial depression of the nervous system following diaschisis, but the arrangement of the neuronal circuitry is far from its original normal development. This rewiring process is an attempt made by the CNS to regenerate; however, it is not normal and may be one explanation for the development of spasticity following a spinal cord lesion.

The study of regeneration of the spinal cord is still in its infancy; however, there is enormous potential for this to occur, which provides hope for those suffering from quadriplegia or paraplegia.

One of the techniques currently used in the management of spinal cord injuries is functional electrical stimulation. The purpose of this approach is to maintain muscle integrity until proper innervation can occur. Experiments are also being conducted using functional electrical stimulation to simulate ambulation for paraplegics.

Certain steroid drugs, administered within 8 hours after spinal injury, have provided increased pinprick and light touch sensations and improved muscle strength in some persons with spinal cord injury. These drugs benefit the patient by reducing swelling caused by the release of chemicals from the injured neurons, which in turn results in damage to the adjacent cells and neurons.

CLINICAL PICTURE

The immediate emotional response after injury depends on the speed of onset. Any life-threatening complications associated with an injury may affect the patient's adjustment to paralysis. Associated injuries such as shock, acute blood loss, and chest trauma often accompany a spinal cord injury. Depression must be expected and is manifested in various ways—for example, refusal of treatment, lateness for appointments, and hostility toward personnel.

The respiratory capacity, which depends on the number of remaining abdominal and intercostal muscles, is dependent on the level of the injury, which will affect the extent to which these muscles can function to ventilate the lungs.

During the period of diaschisis, flaccid paralysis (loss of motor function with loss of muscle tone, absent reflexes, and loss of sensory function) exists below the level of the lesion; complete loss of bowel and bladder control also occurs. Diaschisis is usually followed by the development of spasticity, which favors extensor muscles but sometimes involves the flexor group. Spasticity is defined as an increased resistance to passive stretch and seldom occurs in lesions below the second lumbar vertebral level. The degree of spasticity seems to vary from patient to patient. The autonomic and the somatic nervous systems may become disrupted. For example, if the lesion is above the level of the first thoracic spinal cord segment, then sweating (a result of autonomic function) is lost.

Vague feelings of discomfort in the lower limbs often occur after the spinal cord recovers from shock. This does not mean that muscle and sensory return are occurring unless the individual can differentiate light touch and sharp and dull sensation. The prognosis is poor for muscle and sensory return if the lesion is complete. If the lesion is incomplete, some return of function is noted within 24 hours after injury. Maximum return will occur in 3 to 6 months.

Spinal cord injury results in a neurogenic bladder. A neurogenic bladder is not under voluntary control and may either be spastic or flaccid. This condition occurs when there is an interruption of the sympathetic or parasympathetic portion of the nervous system. Individuals with injuries above the level of the second lumbar vertebra develop a spastic (upper motor neuron) bladder. Similar to the bladder of an infant, the spastic bladder reflexively empties when the bladder is full.

Because the patient has lost bowel and bladder function, immediate catheterization is required after injury to prevent bladder distention and hydronephroses. The patients usually receive straight drainage using an internal Foley catheter.

During the rehabilitation program patients are often concerned about sexual ability. Men with complete spinal cord lesions may have either reflexive erections set off spontaneously or by stimulation but are not capable of ejaculation.

Drugs may now be injected into the base of the penis that will dilate the corpus cavernosus for maintenance of an erection. Men with incomplete lesions may have varied sexual abilities. The level of sexual function depends on the presence or absence of reflex activity primarily associated with the degree to which the autonomic nervous systems (ANS) remains intact.

If there has not been prolonged disturbance of their hormonal balance, women will have a return of menses usually within a year of spinal cord injury; some may not even miss a cycle. Women may experience orgasms, depending on the level of the lesion and sensation. Women who were previously fertile can still conceive, regardless of whether a lesion is complete or incomplete. They may have a normal pregnancy but usually require a cesarean delivery. These women will be able to breast-feed if desired.

No one can tell these patients definitely what their sexual function will be. This is usually determined by the urologist 6 months after injury.

PRECAUTIONS AND COMPLICATIONS

Without proper nursing care, patients confined to the bed are apt to develop deformities and pressure sores. Early range of motion and proper positioning help to prevent hip, knee, and plantarflexion contractures.

Contractures must be avoided at all costs, with the exception of the tenodesis contracture of the finger flexors and wrist extensors in quadriplegics.

Pressure sores can be prevented. If not prevented, they lead to prolonged hospitalization and a delay in the rehabilitation program. One method of prevention is turning the patient every 2 hours by qualified hospital personnel. If a reddened area occurs, the patient's position is immediately changed to relieve pressure until the redness disappears completely. The patient is instructed in skin inspection and assumes the responsibility for skin care. The therapist's responsibility is to be constantly aware of the condition of the patients' skin, to react to red areas on the skin as an emergency situation, and to see that pressure is removed. The therapist must also help educate the patient about the importance of skin inspection and frequent change of position to avoid pressure sores. Areas of the body that seem to be the most frequently involved are ischial tuberosities, malleoli, heels, greater trochanters, and elbows. Also, new growth of skin over areas previously injured will break down more quickly and easily.

When bones are not subjected to weight bearing, they lose calcium, resulting in brittle bones (osteoporosis) and an increased tendency to fractures. The urinary system attempts to rid the body of excess calcium, the accumulation of which often leads to kidney and bladder stones. A program of standing using a tilt table or a standing frame, with or without braces, should be implemented to help alleviate these complications.

Paraplegics and quadriplegics may have a tendency for an unstable spine. These patients may be admitted for rehabilitation 1 to 2 weeks after injury. To avoid possible reinjury to the cord, new patients must be examined by roentgenograms or magnetic resonance imaging (MRI) before upright activities are begun.

Ligamentous and soft tissue healing usually occur in 6 weeks; during this time, log roll the patient in bed if the spine is unstable. If a cast or brace is applied while the spine is unstable, rehabilitation activities can be started earlier. If sensation is not intact precautions must be taken to avoid skin breakdown around the iliac crests. Flexion-extension roentgenograms are taken to determine stability at the fracture site. Bone usually ossifies in 3 months; a spinal fusion may be indicated to protect the lumbar roots if the bone does not solidify. Upright activities are started when roentgenograms indicate a stable back.

The following symptoms of instability should be reported immediately to the patient's physician:

1. Pain and tenderness at the fracture site
2. Increased radiating pain
3. Increased neurologic signs and decrease in muscle power

Owing to lack of sensation, pressure sores are a complication common in patients with spinal cord injury. Pressure sores are necrotic areas of soft tissue, skin, or subcutaneous tissue caused by prolonged pressure. They are subject to infection that could migrate to bone.

Neurogenic bladder complications are not the same from one person to another. During normal micturation, the bladder empties by voluntarily relaxing the skeletal muscle sphincter with contraction of the bladder. With a spinal cord injury the sphincter either fails to close properly causing leaking or does not open sufficiently causing retrograde pressure into the ureters and kidneys. Residual urine may remain in the bladder, rendering it a prime target for infection and kidney stones. Bladder problems, such as urinary tract infections, may be a critical threat to the patient's life and health.

With decreased function of the intercostal and abdominal musculature, the spinal cord injured patient is at increased risk of respiratory tract infection.

There is also a danger of blood pooling in the lower limbs during upright activities owing to the lack of muscle contractions to pump the venous blood back to the heart. Wrapping the lower limbs with elastic bandages or wearing elastic stockings will help decrease the pooling of the blood and the resulting orthostatic hypertension that often accompanies prolonged bedrest. Patients with spinal cord lesions involving the sympathetic outflow to the heart and lungs may experience a situation in which the heart and respiratory rate may not be able to increase sufficiently to provide for adequate oxygenation of the blood. A conditioning program that gradually increases the demands on the heart and lungs is appropriate for individuals with spinal cord injuries.

Certain complications are more commonly seen in quadriplegics than in paraplegics. Among these complications is autonomic dysreflexia. This condition is apparently related to release of norepinephrine at ganglia of the sympathetic nervous system no longer under effective spinal cord control. This release may be triggered by a visceral stimulus to the ANS caused by bladder distention, pressure sores, kidney malfunction, catheter irritation, abnormal positioning of a body part or changing of body position, or infections. This state may occur with a varying degree of symptoms ranging from headache, chills, flushing, and restlessness, to a severe pounding headache, excessive perspiration, elevated blood pressure, and increased spasticity. It can produce intracerebral hemorrhage and death.

Autonomic dysreflexia is an emergency situation. *Return the patient to the room and notify the head nurse immediately.*

FUNCTIONAL SIGNIFICANCE OF SPINAL CORD LESION LEVEL*

The purpose of this section is to discuss the correlation that exists between the level of spinal cord lesions and the eventual functional potential of the patient. In the absence of medical complications, the most important factor in this relationship is the amount of muscle power remaining to the individual. This power is determined by the levels of innervation of the critical muscle groups. Because these levels are fairly well documented, it should be possible to estimate the functional potential of a given patient if the level of the lesion is known. Such an estimation has value for all members of the rehabilitation team. At the outset, it serves to delineate a possible goal for the patient and later functions as a yardstick to the success of therapy.

Although this goal may be carefully delineated on the basis of muscle distribution, many factors can prevent the patient from reaching it. The most limiting factors are spasms, decubiti, insufficient motivation, deformity, sensory loss, urinary infection, stones, and incontinence. One or a combination of these problems may be present. It cannot be emphasized too strongly that the patient will be able to use remaining muscle power fully only if these complications can be minimized or resolved (Table 2–1).

TABLE 2–1. Critical Levels of Function*

Deltoid, biceps	C-5
Lastissimus, serratus, pectoralis, radial wrist extensors	C-6
Triceps, wrist and finger extensors and flexors	C-7
Hand intrinsics, ulnar side of wrist and fingers	T-1
Upper intercostals, upper back	T-6
Abdominals, thoracic extensors and flexors	T-12
Hip flexors, quadriceps	L-4

*The critical muscle groups are innervated predominantly at or above the illustrated level.

*Modified from Long, C and Lawton, EB: The functional significance of spinal cord lesion level. Arch Phys Med Rehabil 36(4):249, 1955.

TABLE 2-2. Functional Significance of Spinal Cord Lesion Level

Activities	C-5	C-6	C-7	T-1	T-6	T-12	L-4
Self-care: Eating	−	±	+	+	+	+	+
Dressing	−	−	±	+	+	+	+
Toileting	−	−	±	+	+	+	+
Bed independence: Rolling over; sitting up	−	±	+	+	+	+	+
Moving about in bed: Supine or sitting	−	−	±	+	+	+	+
Wheelchair independence: Transfer from/to wheelchair	−	±	±	+	+	+	+
Ambulation: Functional (includes to standing position)	−	−	−	−	±	+	+
Attendant: Lifting	+	+	±	−	−	−	−
Assisting	+	+	+	±	±	−	−
Homebound work with hands	−	−	+	+	+	+	+
Outside job	−	−	−	±	±	+	+
Private car	−	−	−	−	+	+	+
Public transportation	−	−	−	−	±	±	+
Braces or devices	H	H	BLH PS	BL PS	±BLS	±BLP	SI

Devices: H—hand (e.g., splints, slings)
Braces: BL—bilateral long-leg brace
        P—pelvic band
        S—spinal attachment
        SI—short-leg brace

\+ achievable by all patients
± achievable by some patients
− not achievable by any patients or not applicable

For the purpose of discussion, seven critical levels of spinal cord severance will be described. Beginning with the C-5 segment, the addition of each successive critical segment adds an important increment to the muscle power of the patient. Table 2-1 summarizes the major muscle groups added at each critical level. Table 2-2 summarizes the estimated relationship between spinal cord lesion level and the functional capacity of the patient.

This section is limited to a survey of the average patient—one who is young, well-motivated, strong, and without intercurrent disease, and who has thorough training and constant practice in functional activities. All lesions are considered to be complete and sharply delineated to the discussed level. When a patient is listed as having a lesion at a given level, this is the lowest level in which all musculature remains functional. Levels will be discussed from C-5 caudal to demonstrate the functional significance of each critical increment (Table 2-2).

FUNCTIONAL CAPACITY

C-5

The patient with a lesion just below C-5 has full innervation of the trapezius, sternocleidomastoid muscles, and the upper cervical paraspinal musculature. This combined musculature enables the patient to stabilize and rotate the neck and to elevate and upwardly rotate the scapulae. The patient also has use of rhomboids, deltoids, and all the major muscles of the rotator cuff, although these are only partially innervated because they share their nerve supply with C-6. These muscles provide scapular adduction, glenohumeral abduction, medial and lateral rotation, and weak shoulder flexion and extension. The functions of strong depression, flexion, protraction, and adduction are absent at the shoulder joint. Elbow flexion is possible as the biceps and brachioradialis muscles both remain partially innervated. There is no muscular function in the wrist or hand. Unfortunately, experience has shown that the absence of shoulder prime movers (latissimus dorsi, pectoralis major, serratus anterior) and the incomplete innervation of the stabilizers prevent the remaining musculature from being functional. The patient may have difficulty rolling over or coming to a sitting position in bed. Only the exceptional patient may manage some eating activities without special hand devices. Patients may be able to propel an electric wheelchair with adaptive equipment. The patient's endurance is low because of reduced respiratory reserve. Ambulation is, of course, out of the question; patients are necessarily confined to a wheelchair. An attendant is usually necessary for these patients for a lifetime to assist them in all self-care activities and to lift them to and from the wheelchair. To make lifting easier for the attendant, the bed should be the same height as the wheelchair. The wheelchair is equipped with many adaptations, allowing it to be brought closer to bed, toilet, or car. These adaptations include removable deskarms and swingaway footrests. An adjustable bed is used to facilitate bed care. To compensate for the inability to stand, a tilt table is used daily for at least 1 hour to maintain vascular tone and bone density.

Patients with C-5 level injury usually cannot make a living by the use of their upper limbs. In some instances, it may be possible to use an electric typewriter or a computer terminal with the use of a mouthstick or hand splints, with a sling or rocker splint supporting the forearm.

C-6

A substantial functional increment is added at C-6. The rotator cuff musculature becomes fully innervated, and the serratus anterior, latissimus dorsi, and pectoralis major muscles receive partial but significant innervation. Nerve supply to the biceps brachii muscle is now complete. Muscles appear at the wrist, nearly always the extensor carpi radialis, and sometimes the flexor carpi radialis.

The strong rotator cuff musculature now permits good use of rotation and abduction of the glenohumeral joint. The prime movers give true adduction, flexion, extension, and scapular protraction. These functions of the prime movers are not fully developed at C-6 because of incomplete innervation, the variability of the individual levels of major nerve supply, and the absence of good stabilization of the prime movers. Respiratory reserve is still low.

The biceps muscle, of course, provides strong elbow flexion, assisted by the brachioradialis muscle, which has gained another segment of innervation. The radial wrist extensors and flexors primarily extend and flex the wrist, but the extensor has an important secondary function. The extensor can use the remaining elasticity of the finger flexors to produce a weak closure of the hand—tenodesis contracture. Therefore, in some instances, large-handled, lightweight objects can be grasped actively. However, in most cases, the object can be grasped, the forearm supinated, and the object will be balanced in the palm of the hand.

Even with absent grasp, the patient may take advantage of elbow flexors to sit up independently in bed or at least to assist in this activity. This may be performed by pulling on a rope that is looped about the forearm and firmly attached to the foot of the bed.

The shoulder strength of patients with C-6 level injury permits them to assist in rolling over in bed. They cannot independently move about in bed while recumbent because they cannot lift their body weight with existing musculature. However, an occasional patient may be able to assist in lifting for transfers to the wheelchair. The patient does this by pressing the hands firmly against the supporting surface, taking full advantage of the forcible substitution of shoulder adduction for elbow extension.

Patients may be able to feed themselves without specific hand devices and perform part of their toilet and dressing activities by using the grasp and balance technique. A great deal of assistance is still needed. Patients may not be regarded as independent in self-care. An adjustable bed is advisable to facilitate bed care. A tilt table is used to maintain conditioning.

As ambulation is impossible, the patient is confined to a wheelchair. During transfer activities it is easier for the attendant if the bed is at the same height as the wheelchair, and the wheelchair is equipped with the aforementioned adaptations to permit a closer approach to bed, toilet, or car. Patients with lesions at the C-6 level can propel their own wheelchair on smooth, level surfaces. Wheelchair propulsion is possible through the use of elbow flexors and shoulder adductors and flexors. To perform this activity, the thenar eminences are pushed tightly against the wheel handrim for traction, to compensate for the lack of grasp. To improve traction, handrims are plastic coated or may be wrapped with surgical tubing. The rims may also have projections for ease of handling for a low quadriplegic individual. Gloves are recommended not only for traction but also for protection and cleanliness, but they will be difficult to don.

Although possible, a homebound job involving use of the hands is difficult for most of these patients; however, some individuals develop sufficient skill to use specially adapted machinery such as used in monographing or addressing. Some high quadriplegic individuals learn to type well with sticks on a computer or word processor, but complications arise in folding stationery and inserting materials into the machine. If individuals with lesions at the C-6 level wish to become active outside the home, public buildings and transportation must be accessible.

C-7

The patient with sparing of the C-7 segment of the spinal cord has three important functional additions: triceps, common finger extensors, and long finger flexor muscles. Primary innervation for each of these groups varies between C-7 and C-8 in individual cases; however, significant function is usually present in each of these if C-7 is spared. The triceps muscle is consistently stronger, as it obtains some innervation as high as C-6. A strong triceps muscle enables patients to stabilize the elbows in extension, so that the shoulder depressors, now fully innervated, can act through the elbow in lifting the body weight. The advantages of grasp and release, afforded by finger extensors and flexors, need not be emphasized. However, this grasp and release is not powerful. The intrinsic muscles of the hand are not yet significantly innervated, and the hands lack their flexion strength and extension dexterity.

The patient with a C-7 lesion is able to become more independent in bed and wheelchair activities. At this level individual skill and coordination may allow exceptional patients to make the transition to complete wheelchair independence. All patients can roll over and sit up in bed and can move about in the sitting position. Patients may need assistance in lifting or turning the pelvis while recumbent—a motion used in putting on pants. Although some patients require help in transferring to and from the wheelchair, this help consists now of an assistive push instead of a lift. Little assistance is required for toileting and dressing activities; eating can be done independently. To facilitate the transfer from the wheelchair, the wheelchair must be adapted for close approach and the bed should be at the same height as the chair seat. Patients can propel their own wheelchair independently for long distances on smooth surfaces but may require help on rough terrain.

Some patients with C-7 lesions are able to ambulate to some extent with crutches if adequately braced. Generally this is not a very practical goal. The finger flexor muscles permit grasping the crutches, and the triceps muscles provide stability of the elbow. To maintain the upright posture, the patient needs lower limb, pelvic, and back orthotics. The only independent gait possible is the drag-to gait.

Applying the external orthosis and attaining the erect posture cannot be done without a great deal of assistance. Therefore, ambulation with these restrictions, although achieved by some patients, cannot be considered functional. However, in some instances standing in parallel bars may be prescribed instead of standing on the tilt table.

Patients with a lesion at the C-7 level are still essentially confined to a wheelchair. They need a part-time, and in many cases a full-time, assistant. The endurance of the C-7 patient is limited by low respiratory reserve.

Occupations requiring use of the hands are more feasible because finger flexors and extensors muscles are functional. The type of work is limited by weakness of grasp; therefore, activities involving tight grasp such as leather tooling or metal work are not recommended. Also, activities requiring firm finger dexterity such as watchmaking are not feasible. Possible vocations include bookkeeping, telephone services, computer programming, typing, and use of office machines.

Low quadriplegic individuals have the ability to drive an automatic shift automobile when it is adapted with hand controls. Most are able to maneuver the wheelchair into and out of the car.

T-1

The patient with a T-1 lesion has full innervation of the upper limb musculature, including the essential intrinsic muscles of the hand. These patients have strength and dexterity in grasp and release, as well as fully innervated proximal musculature. The ulnar side of the wrist now has its full nerve supply, and crutch walking benefits from this addition. The patient still lacks trunk stability, respiratory reserve of intercostal origin, and trunk fixation of the origins of the upper limb prime movers. Patients with lesions at T-1 are independent in bed activities and they are also able to transfer independently to and from the wheelchair. Occasionally a patient may still need some assistance in this procedure. The patient is independent in all activities of self-care, except in those requiring lifting the body while recumbent.

With functional upper limbs and orthoses, the patient at the T-1 level can perform a drag-to gait independently. Because of full body bracing, attaining the erect position is a very laborious procedure requiring a great deal of help. Therefore, ambulation usually cannot be considered functional but is prescribed for exercise purposes. A well-adapted wheelchair allowing close approach to the bed, which is the same height as the chair, is still essential.

Jobs outside the home and jobs involving use of the hands are practical. There is no limit to sedentary jobs for the T-1 patient or for any patient with a lesion below this level. Most patients develop sufficient sitting balance to drive a hand-controlled car and experience little difficulty with the transfer or in lifting the chair into and out of the car.

T-6

Patients with a lesion at the T-6 level present one major functional gain over T-1 patients: they have a complete, strong chain of upper limb and thoracic musculature, stabilized against a well-coordinated pectoral girdle. Innervation is now supplied to the long muscles of the upper back and to the upper intercostals and transversus thoracis. Thus the patient has a tight grasp, supported by proximal musculature that in turn is stabilized against a thorax that can be fixed for heavy lifting. Added innervated intercostals give these patients an increment of respiratory reserve that increases their endurance.

These functional additions are enough to provide independence in all phases of self-care. Even the application of full-body bracing becomes possible. Patients can stabilize their upper limbs adequately to use them to lift the pelvis in applying braces while recumbent. Transferring to and from a wheelchair becomes easily possible independently by using the strong pectoral girdle and triceps muscles. Consequently, the patient usually needs no attendant. The wheelchair should still be adjusted as described earlier.

The patient is braced with a low spinal attachment and bilateral long leg orthoses. With this bracing patients can stand erect for indefinite periods. They are also able to ambulate once they have reached the erect standing position. Because of their strong, stabilized upper limbs, they are capable of performing an independent swing-through gait. However, the safer and more practical gait remains the swing-to gait. Unfortunately, the use of ambulation is restricted by the slowness and laboriousness of attaining the erect position; therefore, only the exceptional patient, who develops unusually strong upper limbs, with good balance and coordination, will use ambulation functionally on level ground or inside the house.

To assist the patient in attaining the standing position, and thus encourage ambulation, such aides as door bars, parallel bars, or stall bars are prescribed for the home. Even if ambulation is not used functionally, the patient is encouraged to stand for at least an hour daily. Some patients report that they feel more comfortable standing than sitting and prefer to do some of their work in a standing position. For these patients special standing adaptations of work equipment are encouraged.

Elevation activities are markedly impaired. Because hips and knees are locked with the orthoses, all elevation must be accomplished by pure push-up in the shoulder girdle. This push-up is adequate in most patients only for the ascent of very low stairs with a handrail. The patient cannot ascend standard stairs even with a handrail and cannot climb curbs. Public transportation is therefore impossible. An outside job can be reached by private hand-controlled or chauffeured car. Patients are able to transfer independently from wheelchair to car. Most patients with T-6 lesions have sufficient sitting balance to drive a hand-controlled car, and some learn to place their wheelchair in and out of the car. Jobs must still be essentially of a sedentary nature with the possible standing modifications previously described.

T-12

The patient with a lesion at the T-12 level has full innervation of the rectus abdominus, the oblique muscles of the abdomen, the transversus abdominus, and all muscles of the thorax. There is still weakness of the lower back where lumbar musculature is not innervated. The patient does not have innervation of the primary hip hikers, quadratus lumborum, and lower erector spinae muscles. Hip hiking can be accomplished with relative ease by the secondary hip hikers, including the internal and external obliques and the latissimus dorsi muscles. With this musculature, the patient becomes independent in self-care, wheelchair, and ambulation.

Patients are braced with bilateral knee, ankle, foot orthoses (KAFO) for ambulation. They can use a two-point alternate, a four-point, or a swing-through gait. The four-point and the two-point alternate gaits are achieved through the use of the secondary hip hikers. Using all these gaits, the patients are usually independent in ambulation. They can ambulate freely on reasonably rough surfaces, inside and outside. They can also negotiate curbs, either backward by swinging the legs up (the hip joint now being free anteroposteriorly) or forward by swinging up, as part of a continuous swing-through gait.

With the ability to tilt the pelvis, these patients can negotiate standard stairs (8 inches) easily with a handrail. The formidable bus step can be climbed laboriously. This enables the patient to take public transportation, but use of a private car is more practical. Of course, rush hour travel presents special problems for paraplegics who are using public transportation.

There are very few vocational limitations in sedentary or nonsedentary jobs away from home for a patient with a lesion at T-12. Even ramps or stairs into the place of employment are no longer contraindications to placement. The patient needs no attendant, and often needs no wheelchair during the course of the day's work. However, for convenience in moving about the home (for instance, to and from the bathroom) a wheelchair is usually prescribed. The adaptations of the chair are determined by the demands of the home. For convenience some patients also take their wheelchair to and from work.

L-4

The patient with a lesion just below L-4 has the added functional assistance of the quadratus lumborum, lower erector spinae, quadriceps, and primary hip flexor muscles. The major stabilizers of the hips are absent, and the ankle remains flaccid. These factors predetermine the patient's gait and orthotics. The knee is supported in extension by the quadriceps muscles so that KAFOs are no longer necessary. The flail ankles must still be supported; a foot and ankle orthosis (AFO) is used for this purpose. It is advisable in most cases to use a limited motion stop allowing about 15 degrees of motion in dorsiflexion. The limited motion serves as a support to prevent footdrop during the swing phase of the gait. The patients' gait is a bilateral maximus-medius gait, with the added disability of absent hamstring muscles and flail ankles. This produces a number of deforming factors. The lack of the gluteus maximus and hamstring muscles causes the hips to snap back sharply against the anterior hip ligaments shortly after heelstrike. To do this, they must maintain the knee in extension. This extension of the knee in the absence of the hamstring muscles tends to produce genu recurvatum. Also, the necessity to keep the pelvis extended against the anterior hip ligament produces a compensatory lumbar lordosis that is eventually deforming in nature.

A patient with the previously described musculature and gait could be completely independent without crutches or canes. However, because of the long-term deforming effects of the unsupported gait, bilateral canes or crutches are usually prescribed prophylactically. By minimizing the extremes of lateral and posterior swings of the pelvis and through careful gait training the lumbar lordosis and genu recurvatum can both be reduced. This reduction of deforming forces serves as protection against the later development of lumbar lordosis compression or traumatic arthritis of the knee.

The patient with a lesion at L-4 is completely independent in all phases of self-care and ambulation. The major limitations are in elevation. Because of absent gluteus maximus and hamstring muscles, elevation must be accomplished with the quadriceps muscles. This is difficult but can be accomplished with the assistance of a hand firmly applied to the anterior thigh, or with a handrail, crutch, or cane. Canes with support above the wrist (such as the Lofstrand) are advisable, as the standard wooden cane does not provide enough upper limb stability. A wheelchair may still be convenient at home and in certain job situations. Job limitations are still present. The patient cannot be expected to stand for long periods or perform a job requiring constant rising from a chair or a great amount of elevation activities.

Summary

The correlation between spinal cord lesion level and functional capacity has been discussed. In the absence of medical and psychiatric complications, the most important factor in this relationship is the distribution of the remaining muscle power. Early in the course of rehabilitation, general functional goals can be outlined on the basis of the remaining muscle power. However, individual differences cannot be overlooked. Spasm, urinary infection, lack of coordination, and lack of motivation are some of the most common restricting factors that may occur. A patient having one or more of these complications may reach a more limited goal than another patient with loss of muscle power but no complications. Thorough training and constant practice in functional activities are essential for all patients.

Patients with a cervical lesion have partial strength in their upper limbs. They may groom and feed themselves but usually require a full-time attendant for all other activities. They are confined to a wheelchair and to homebound jobs. Table 2–3 provides a summary of upper-limb spinal cord innervation.

Patients with a high thoracic lesion have full upper limb strength and are independent in transfers to and from the wheelchair and in self-care activities. They may be able to ambulate with help of an orthosis but in most instances cannot ambulate functionally. They are still primarily wheelchair patients and may require a part-time attendant. A homebound job is most practical. Table 2–4 provides a summary of lower-limb spinal cord innervation.

Patients with midthoracic lesions have good upper limb and thoracic stabilization. They are independent in self-care and wheelchair activities. Although they can ambulate on level ground, use of a wheelchair may be more practical for work away from home.

Table 2-3. Cervical Segmental Innervation

MUSCLE	C-5	C-6	C-7	C-8	T-1
Diaphragm					
Trapezius					
Levator Scapula	▓				
Supraspinatous	▓				
Teres Minor	▓				
Deltoid	▓	▓			
Subscapularis	▓	▓			
Infraspinatus	▓	▓			
Rhomboids	▓	▓			
Brachialis	▓	▓			
Brachioradialis	▓	▓			
Biceps	▓	▓			
Supinator		▓			
Extensor Carpi Radialis		▓			
Teres Major		▓			
Serratus Anterior		▓	▓	▓	
Pronator Teres		▓	▓		
Pectoralis Major—Clav.		▓	▓		
Pectoralis Major—Sternal			▓	▓	
Latissimus Dorsi			▓	▓	
Abductor Poll. Longus			▓	▓	
Extensor Poll. Longus			▓	▓	
Extensor Dig. Communis			▓	▓	
Extensor Carpi Ulnaris			▓	▓	
Triceps			▓	▓	
Flexor Carpi Radialis			▓	▓	
Palmaris Longus			▓	▓	
Flexor Carpi Ulnaris				▓	
Flexor Dig. Superficialis				▓	▓
Flexor Dig. Profundus				▓	▓
Flexor Poll. Longus				▓	▓
Abductor Poll. Brevis				▓	▓
Opponens Poll.				▓	▓
Adductor Poll.					▓
Lumbricales					▓
Interossei					▓

This is just a guide; individual differences occur.

Key: Shaded area indicates the segmental level of innervation. White area above the shaded area indicates innervated muscles.

POTENTIAL LEVEL OF FUNCTION

The potential level of function can be fairly well correlated with the level of spinal cord injury. However, other factors must be considered, including age, weight, motivation, presence of spasticity or respiratory insufficiency, length of time since onset, and diseases. See table on page 22.

PATIENT MANAGEMENT

The immediate concern with a spinal cord injury is the prevention of further damage to the spinal cord. Proper first aid care is essential at this point. The initial medical management of the person with a spinal cord injury is immobilization of the involved

Table 2–4. Lumbar and Sacral Segmental Innervation

MUSCLE	L-1	L-2	L-3	L-4	L-5	S-1	S-2	S-3
Iliopsoas		▓	▓					
Sartorius		▓	▓					
Pectineus		▓	▓					
Gracilis			▓	▓				
Adductor Longus			▓	▓				
Adductor Brevis			▓	▓				
Adductor Magnus			▓	▓	▓			
Quadriceps Femoris			▓	▓				
Obturator Externus			▓	▓				
Semimembranosus				▓	▓	▓		
Semitendinosus				▓	▓	▓		
Anterior Tibialis				▓	▓			
Tensor Fascia Lata				▓	▓			
Gluteus Medius				▓	▓	▓		
Gluteus Minimus				▓	▓	▓		
Posterior Tibialis				▓	▓			
Biceps Femoris					▓	▓	▓	▓
Extensor Hall. Longus					▓	▓		
Extensor Dig. Longus					▓	▓		
Peroneus Tertius					▓	▓		
Peroneus Brevis					▓	▓		
Peroneus Longus					▓	▓	▓	
Gastrocnemius						▓	▓	
Soleus					▓	▓	▓	
Plantaris					▓	▓	▓	
Gluteus Maximus					▓	▓	▓	
Flexor Hall.						▓	▓	
Flexor Dig.						▓	▓	
Foot Intrinsics						▓	▓	▓

Key: Shaded area indicates the segmental level of innervation.
   White area above the shaded area indicates innervated muscles.

area with body and neck splints before any transportation occurs. Medically, immobilization may include surgery. Immediately, most patients receive indwelling catheters. Good nursing care and pain control are also important throughout the acute phase.

Most patients feel they will have complete return of function. This makes them reluctant to accept treatment. Generally the potential for successful rehabilitation is greatest when there is a large homogenous group of patients. All persons involved must encourage the patients to work with what they have at the time, while reassuring them that as changes occur the program goals will be altered. (Refer to Table 2–2 for realistic long-term goals.)

One aspect of patient management that necessitates the involvement and understanding of the entire health care team is the bowel and bladder program. The goals of the bowel and bladder program are to establish a routine bowel movement time that does not interfere with daily activities and to make the patient catheter free. The latter is easier for men, who can eventually use an external catheter. Because an adequate external collecting device has not yet been found for women, they must wear pads and plastic pants for protection. This lack of adequate protection often leads to hesitancy to ambulate in female patients.

The integrating center for micturition is in the conus medullaris of the spinal cord. The type of bladder depends on the location of the lesion, whether it is at, above, or below the conus medullaris. A flaccid or lower motor neuron bladder results from a lesion at the level of the conus medullaris and can be emptied by pressure on the abdomen, by straining, or by Credé's maneuver (the patient doubles

Level	Key Muscle Control	Functional Goals
C-4	Neck Upper trapezius	Independently propel electric wheelchair using tongue switches Limited self-care (feeding, applying makeup) using arm supports and externally powered hand splints
C-5	Shoulder Elbow flexors	Independently propel wheelchair with plasticized handrims or projections Assist in wheelchair transfer to bed and from bed to wheelchair Assist in turning self in bed Light hygiene and self-feeding using externally powered hand splints.
C-6	Clavicular portion of pectoralis major Wrist extensors	Independently propel wheelchair with plasticized handrims Independently turn self in bed Independently relieve ischial pressure while sitting in wheelchair Independently perform range of motion to limbs including lower limbs except straight leg raising Independently transfer to and from bed, toilet, and auto using a transfer board and possibly overhead loops Some may independently put wheelchair into car May independently drive a car with hand controls Assist in self-feeding, hygiene (shaving, grooming hair), dressing, writing, and skin inspection, using wrist-driven flexor hinge hand splints when prehension is required
C-7 to C-8	Elbow extensors Wrist flexors Weak hand	Independently transfer to and from bed, toilet, and auto with or without a transfer board Independently put wheelchair into car Independent in all self-care except catheter without hand splints or adaptive equipment Some household activities from wheelchair Assist in standing with posterior leg splints and pelvic support
T-1 to T-7	Upper limb	Some may independently transfer to and from bathtub and ground Some may independently ascend and descend curbs Independently perform full range of motion to all limbs Independently stand with posterior leg splints and pelvic support Complete self-care including catheter
T-8 to T-12	Trunk	Independently ambulate with extensive bracing (Owing to high energy consumption used and difficulty in putting on braces with a pelvic band, patients usually do not functionally ambulate and therefore need a wheelchair)
L-1 to L-3	All trunk Hip flexors Hip adductors	Independently ambulate using long-leg braces and forearm crutches, include stairs and getting up from wheelchair and ground to standing. Most still use wheelchair part time
L-4 to S-2	Quadriceps (no spasticity)	Independently ambulate with short leg braces and forearm crutches *Should* be completely free of wheelchair

up the fists and exerts pressure above the bladder). This technique usually gets rid of the urine without leaving significant residual. Another method of management is the superpubic catheter. This technique, which allows continual draining, helps to prevent a buildup of residuals but tends to shrink the size of the bladder.

Following clearance from the urology department the nursing staff starts the patient on a bladder training program. The catheter is clamped off on the hour; the patient drinks one glass of fluid; the catheter is unclamped 5 minutes before the hour and allowed to drain for approximately 5 minutes or until the bladder is empty. The catheter is then clamped and this cycle is repeated during the waking hours. The patient is on straight drainage at night.

Bladder training continues until a balanced bladder function is attained. This is determined by performing a residual urine test. At a designated time the catheter is removed. After 1 hour, if the patient voids either reflexively or by straining, the residual volume in the bladder is checked by reintroducing the catheter and draining the bladder. Bladder function is determined to be balanced or unbalanced with regard to the residual/capacity ratio. One method used is the ratio of residual over capacity as a percentage: 0 to 20 percent for an upper motor neuron bladder, and 0 to 10 percent for a lower motor neuron bladder. When this balance is reached, the catheter may be removed.

Catheters should be removed as soon as safety permits to control or prevent infection from an indwelling catheter. Some patients, usually paraplegics because they have control over the intrinsic muscles of the hands, are able to learn to perform self-catheterization. The individual is taught to insert a clean catheter and every 2 to 3 hours to drain the bladder. They are encouraged to have a consistent fluid intake of 1500 to 3000 ml of fluid per day, depending on their size. If the bladder is spastic, which is usually the case when the lesion is above the level of the conus medullaris, drugs may be used for relaxation of the detrussor muscle. Timeliness and cleanliness are crucial for minimizing infections and developing a successful program.

Some clinicians have used electrical stimulation for bladder control. This technique, which involves the implanting of electrodes into the nerve roots supplying the bladder, has been used on a limited basis but has met with considerable success.

Some patients may require surgical intervention for bladder control. One method, the transurethral resection (TUR) of the prostate, bypasses the urinary bladder. This technique relaxes the bladder to allow for greater filling. Other methods used to control a spastic bladder, which affect the autonomic nerves to the bladder or severance of the sphincter muscles, are considered last resort techniques because they are irreversible.

Kidney and bladder stones are a continual problem for the spinal cord injured person. Currently, the use of ultrasound to break up the stones has been successful and eliminates the need for surgery. Drugs have also proved successful in breaking up stones.

The bowel training program is initiated on admission to a rehabilitation program. The nurse discusses with the patient bowel habits prior to the injury and establishes a schedule plan for bowel movements. It is important to eat balanced meals and maintain proper fluid intake. Enemas and laxatives are not recommended because they interfere with the development of rectal tone.

To establish a satisfactory routine for bowel movements, glycerine suppositories are used. Once they are inserted, bowel movements usually occur 15 to 20 minutes later. Once the patient has achieved 1-hour sitting tolerance, a commode chair is used. If no movement occurs, digital stimulation of the rectum is done to start the reflex. The goal of bowel training is to encourage patients to have a bowel movement at regular intervals and to maintain muscle tone of the bowel.

The therapist's responsibility is to know if the patient is on a bladder and bowel program and to cooperate with the schedule. Arrangements should be made for the patient to continue the bladder program during the day. If bowel movements occur during treatment, the therapist should discuss with the nurse the possibility of a change of time for giving the suppository.

Individuals with spinal cord injuries will be spending variable amounts of time in a wheelchair. Proper positioning and use of cushions are essential to control posture and relieve pressure. The technique for positioning and seating systems is described in Chapter 3 under patient management.

The overall goals in the rehabilitation of a patient with a spinal cord injury are to teach the patient to perform at the maximum level of functional independence, prevent contractual deformities, and prevent pressure sores. To reach these goals, specific programs must be designed for the individual patient. Details on teaching the patient function activities are presented in Chapters 8–11.

Brain Injuries

Injuries to the brain may be a result of failure of proper fetal development, problems during the birthing process, high fevers, cerebral vascular accidents, degenerative disorders, or trauma. Among the most frequently treated by therapists are individuals who have had cerebral vascular accidents (CVAs) and traumatic brain injuries (TBIs).

Head trauma, which results in brain injury, may be caused by a blow to the head from a projectile missile, a motor vehicle or bicycle accident, or a fall. Head gear offers some protection, as do seatbelts. Since the advent of automobile seatbelts, more individuals receiving head injuries have survived the accidents. Motor vehicle accidents are the single most common cause of TBIs. Twice as many men as women sustain head injuries, and the majority of them are between the ages of 15 and 24 years old. The nature of traumatic brain injuries are as variable as the individual. Disabilities may result in one-sided weakness, weakness of the lower limbs and trunk, or involvement of all four limbs. The areas affected within the central nervous system (CNS) and the extent of the injuries will determine the mental, emotional, behavioral, and physical outcome of the individual's rehabilitation. In planning the management of individuals who have suffered TBIs it is necessary to take into account all facets of the physical and psychosocial aspects of the individual for optimal results during rehabilitation.

Stroke, CVA, apoplexy, and shock are general terms used to describe a sudden deterioration of cerebral function secondary to vascular compromise. Strokes account for more than half of all neurologic problems seen in a hospital setting and are the third most common cause of death in the United States. More importantly, many more patients who suffer a stroke survive and must learn to live with neurologic defects.

Any pathologic process involving the vessels of the brain can cause a stroke. The causes of stroke are many and include cerebral infarct, hypertensive intracerebral hemorrhage, ruptured saccular (berry) aneurysm, ruptured arteriovenous malformation (AVM), arteritis, trauma, and other miscellaneous conditions. Cerebral infarcts are overwhelmingly the most common cause of stroke and therefore will be emphasized.

An infarct is a site of localized necrosis (cell death) precipitated by deprivation of blood (ischemia) and therefore oxygen to that tissue. Usually total occlusion of a cerebral vessel is the cause of ischemia and will lead to a cerebral infarct. However, not all vessel occlusions produce an infarct, nor is total occlusion a prerequisite to an infarct. Rapidity of occlusion, adequacy of collateral circulation, and systemic blood pressure also play a role. Rapid total occlusion of a cerebral vessel favors the development of a cerebral infarct. However, if collateral blood vessels also supply the same tissue (as supplied by the occluded vessel) or if the occlusion occurs slowly allowing collateral circulation to develop, an infarct may not result. Partial occlusion (stenosis) of a cerebral vessel usually will not produce a cerebral infarct. If systemic hypotension is also present, however, the combination of decreased blood pressure and stenosis may deprive brain tissue of blood and cause infarction.

Two pathologic processes account for virtually all cerebral infarcts: thrombosis and embolism. A thrombus is a blood clot that forms within the living vascular system (as opposed to coagulated blood in a test tube, which is not a thrombus). An embolus is a detached fragment of thrombus that is carried by the bloodstream to a site distal from its origin.

The risk factors for stroke are primarily the risk factors of atherosclerosis. These factors include hypertension, diabetes mellitus, hyperlipidemia, tobacco use, and possibly obesity and a sedentary lifestyle. Atherosclerosis is a predisposition to the development of cerebral thrombi and emboli by at least two mechanisms:

1. Thrombi are more likely to form in a cerebral vessel stenosed by atherosclerotic plaques because blood flow is slowed and the vessel's tunica intima is injured (exposing underlying collagen that is thrombogenic).
2. Atherosclerosis of the coronary arteries is often the cause of thrombi within the left side of the heart from which fragments detach and embolize to the cerebral arteries.

A period of diaschisis (cerebral shock) resulting from trauma or an infarct lasts for varying lengths of time and immediately follows the insult. After this period of diaschisis the brain will begin a recovery phase in those areas remote from the primary site of the lesion. This recovery produces an entire series of structural and functional changes within circumscribed areas of the CNS. This process, which occurs in response to a lesion, does not necessarily lead to normal function. Traditionally it has been stated that the CNS does not regenerate, as does the peripheral nervous system. The CNS attempts regeneration but it becomes aborted (see Chapter 1). Perhaps a more appropriate term for what is taking place in the CNS is recovery rather than regeneration. Appropriate input into the system during this phase influences the final outcome for the patient. This is a critical time for all persons involved with the rehabilitation of the patient to apply techniques that will have the highest potential for achieving near normal function.

The following description of the events that will occur after damage to a single neuron, as it occurs in experimental situations, is given to aid in the understanding of the process and the selection of appropriate techniques for the patient's rehabilitation program.

1. *Denervation supersensitivity:* This is a period of hyperirritability of the postsynaptic membrane receptor sites. This same phenomenon occurs in the peripheral system, causing a dispersion of the acetylcholine receptor sites on the muscle membrane from the region of the end plate. It results in widespread chemical sensitivity resembling an immature muscle fiber. The receptor sites on the postsynaptic neuron are left naked or vacated.
2. *Collateral sprouting:* Adjacent intact neurons, which also synapse on the postsynaptic neuron, are stimulated by the hypersensitivity of the postsynaptic membrane, sending out collateral branches from their axons to synapse on the vacated receptor site. The vacated synaptic receptor sites are reinnervated by the adjacent neurons that have developed collateral sprouts, which are called synaptic reclamation.

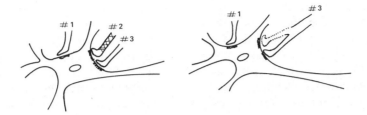

3. *Bouton stripping:* When the postsynaptic neurons are damaged, the presynaptic terminals withdraw and lose contact with the dendrites or cell body. The dendritic process on the damaged neuron will shrink and lose its functional connection. In the peripheral nervous system this bouton stripping is followed by the process in which the motor neuron regenerates and reinnervates its muscle fibers and the afferent boutons are restored.
4. *Unmasking ineffective synapses:* There appear to be unused or dormant synapses within the CNS. With injury to the naturally functioning neurons the postsynaptic membrane will be enhanced to activate the dormant synapses, which have existed since development.
5. *Structural changes in preexisting interneurons:* Following onset of a lesion the adjacent interneurons tend to alter themselves by increasing the length of their processes, which extend into a new area, and increasing the size of their synaptic terminal. This change in the interneurons may be one of the causes for spasticity. It is an example of CNS reorganization, plasticity, or remodeling.

The CNS has the capability to make use of unused pathways or establish new routes. The establishment of synaptic connections is the mechanism that the CNS has for the process of recovery. Bouton stripping and collateral sprouting with synaptic reclamation and changes in the presynaptic interneurons are three examples of ways in which rewiring occurs within the CNS following an infarct. The amount of recovery is dependent on the extent of the damage plus the amount and type of remodeling that occurs. The remodeling is a reorganization within the network of the CNS. Direction and guidance of the remodeling is dependent of the level of understanding and capabilities of the health care team providing the rehabilitation services to the patient.

The CNS has many centers to control motor behavior extending from the cerebral cortex to the spinal cord. Recovery depends not only on the extent of the lesion and damage to the CNS but also on the level of the individual's activities and motor patterns within the CNS prior to the infarct. The greater the memory of normal movement, the greater the chances for recovery of those movements.

CLINICAL PICTURE

Traumatic brain injuries or cerebral infarcts tend to occur in different characteristic clinical manifestations, which often allow differentiation if a careful history is obtained. Thrombi occur almost exclusively in elderly patients with severe atherosclerosis (and often hypertension). Thrombi tend to form in large vessels at sites of previous local damage to the vessel wall (e.g., atherosclerotic plaques). As a result, thrombi occur most commonly at the sites most severely and commonly involved by athero-sclerosis (e.g., bifurcation sites). Thrombi usually occur singly and therefore all neurologic deficits can be explained by occlusion of one artery. Thrombi often occur during sleep and patients awaken unaware of a deficit until they attempt movement. Most patients experience transient ischemic attacks (TIAs), short periods of neuro-logic dysfunction that completely resolve, prior to the occlusive thrombus and cere-bral infarct. A thrombus forms slowly, accounting for the steplike development of deficits that occur over the course of hours or even days.

Emboli, though occurring most frequently in elderly patients with atherosclero-sis, can cause cerebral infarcts in children and young adults. Emboli are usually smaller than thrombi and therefore travel more distally in the circulation, occluding smaller arteries. Emboli do not tend to occlude vessels at sites of previous local damage. Emboli are often multiple and lodge in different cerebral arteries, often causing neurologic deficits that cannot be explained by occlusion of one vessel. Cerebral infarcts due to emboli most often occur when the patient is awake. The infarct occurs suddenly without the warnings of preceding TIAs. The neurologic deficits develop rapidly. Because thrombi in the left heart are the most common source of cerebral emboli, most patients with cerebral embolic infarcts have evidence of heart disease—usually atrial fibrillation of a myocardial infarct in adults or congenital heart disease in children.

The neurologic deficits caused by cerebral infarct or trauma are determined exclusively by the size and location of the infarct or damage. It is only with an extensive knowledge of neuroanatomy that the neurologist can deduce the site of damage by the neurologic deficits observed. Because only a few simple concepts are outlined here, the reader is urged to consult a reference textbook on neuroanatomy.

There are four primary categories of deficit that will affect the rehabilitation outcomes of a head-injured individual. The categories are behavior, cognition, com-munication, and sensory-motor functions. The problems often interface with one another. Most adults with severe head injury have deficits in two or more of these areas. Each problem can be at a different level of severity.

Behavioral problems may result in changes in personality such as anger, anxiety, impulsiveness, and socially inhibited responses. These changes in behavior must be considered and modified at the onset of the individual's rehabilitation. Agitation is a common problem. Deficits in cognition and communication, such as memory loss and aphasia are some factors that may increase agitation.

Behavioral problems also may be a result of cognitive difficulties. Some of the cognitive deficits demonstrated with TBIs are memory impairment, decreased atten-tion span, altered state of awareness, and loss of higher cortical function of abstract reasoning.

Expressive aphasia and dysarthria are communication problems that may require using communication boards. Also, certain deficits such as the inability to produce the volume necessary for effective communication may be the result of insufficient respiratory patterns.

Dysfunction of the motor and sensory systems is a major problem limiting the level of functional independence for patients. Following a head injury, patients have difficulty transmitting and coding sensory information. According to Rinehart (see bibliography), sensory impairment may result in visual disturbances such as diplopia, in taste disturbances such as hypogeusia, and in touch-pressure disturbances such as hypersensitivity. Arousal may be decreased by inadequate stimulation reaching the reticular activating system. Impairment of filtering and selectively processing sensory information may be impaired. This will cause a decrease in attention span, which leads to difficulties in motor learning. Damage to the posterior parietal lobe produces perceptual disturbances that affect motor performance. Changes occur in the perception of body image and its orientation in space through touch and visual sensory inputs. A unilateral deficit will result in difficulties with dressing, eating, and other motor activities.

After a TBI, individuals have associated difficulties with motor control and learning. Identified problems include muscle weakness and a lack of synergy and timing. Lesions of the motor cortex produce muscle weakness and changes in muscle tone. Although spasticity has been thought to interfere with posture and voluntary motor movements, the loss of cortical command signal to the muscles that results in muscle weakness may have a more profound effect on motor behavior. Loss of patterned muscle responses for automatic postural adjustments and movement patterns also may occur after a traumatic head injury and contribute to poor equilibrium responses and motor behavior during upright activities. Patients with cerebellar dysfunction will display motor disorders such as dysmetria, adiadochokinesia, ataxia, and intention tremors. Movement disorders of timing are also evident with damage to the basal ganglia and associated pathways. These individuals would demonstrate poverty of movement or bradykinesia.

Arterial Supply

The vascular supply of the brain is derived from two major systems, the internal carotid arteries and vertebral-basilar arteries, which anastomose at the base of the brain to form the circle of Willis.

Basal View of Cerebral Blood Vessels

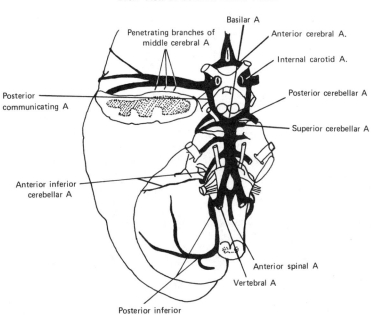

(Adapted from Adams, RD and Victor, M: Principles of Neurology, ed 2. McGraw-Hill, New York, 1981, with permission.)

The anterior cerebral arteries originate from the internal carotid arteries and supply the anterior frontal lobes, the medial and inferior posterior frontal and parietal lobes, and contribute to the anterior internal capsule and basal ganglia.

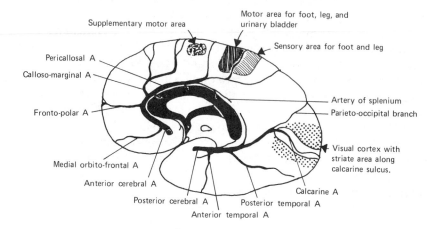

Medial Aspect of Cerebral Hemisphere

(Adapted from Adams, RD and Victor, M: Principles of Neurology, ed 2. McGraw-Hill, New York, 1981, with permission.)

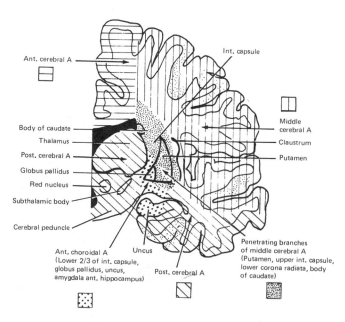

Coronal Section of Cerebral Hemisphere. (From Adams, RD and Victor, M: Principles of Neurology, ed 2. McGraw-Hill, New York, 1981, with permission.)

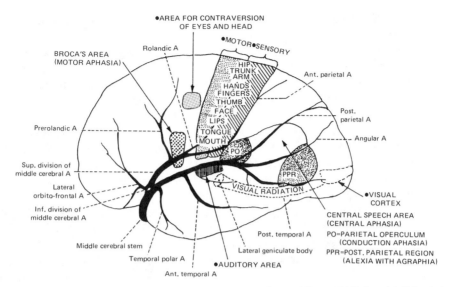

Lateral aspect of cerebral hemisphere. (From Adams, RD and Victor, M: Principles of Neurology, ed 2. McGraw-Hill, New York, 1981, with permission.)

The middle cerebral arteries originate from the internal carotids and supply the entire lateral cerebral hemisphere excluding the anterior frontal and posterior occipital lobes and contribute to the internal capsule and basal ganglia. The posterior cerebral arteries originate from the basilar artery and supply the midbrain, inferior and medial temporal lobes, and posterior occipital lobes, and contribute to the posterior basal ganglia. The vertebral and basilar arteries supply the brain stem, spinal cord, and cerebellum.

Changes in activity in various regions of the brain appear to be reflected in the relative amount of blood flowing through those regions. This discovery has made it possible to identify and study the interaction of various areas of the brain during ongoing human behavior by measuring the regional changes in blood flow.

Patterns of electrical activity can be recorded from electrodes placed at various points on the scalp, called electroencephalogram (EEG). Different wave forms are indicative of different forms of hemispheric activity. A link can be shown between the amount of EEG activity in the hemispheres and the type of task performed by the subject to allow a continuous measure over time and can be used to study ongoing activity in the brain while the subject performs long, complex tasks; however, it is difficult to see changes that relate to the occurrence of specific stimulus events.

CNS PATHWAYS AND CORTICAL SPECIALIZATION

The motor cortex, situated in the precentral gyrus (see figure above), aggregates into two corticospinal tracts that decussate (cross) in the medulla oblongata. Some sensory tracts cross in the spinal cord (e.g., spinothalamic tract, which transmits pain and temperature), and some cross in the medulla oblongata (e.g., posterior columns, which transmit proprioception); others do not cross (e.g., spinocerebellar tracts, which are involved in the coordination of movement).

The cerebral hemisphere that controls speech, known as the dominant hemisphere, is the left cerebral hemisphere for all right-handed and many left-handed people. An infarct in the dominant hemisphere results in aphasia (inability to express or understand the spoken word), agraphia (inability to write), and alexia (inability to read). The left hemisphere controls verbal and written communication and the understanding of written communication in 85 to 92 percent of all humans. Often accompanied by some aphasic deficits is the difficulty in word finding and naming. Expressive (Broca's) aphasia involves the premotor area of the frontal lobe adjacent to the lateral fissure. This region controls the motor aspects of speech. Patients with expressive aphasia speak very little and have an absence of grammatical parts of speech and proper inflections. Comprehension of the spoken word is intact, and they seem to be aware of most of their speaking errors.

Receptive aphasia (Wernicke's) involves the posterior temporal gyrus. This region is functionally designated for the interpretation of written language and speech. Speech may vary from being slightly odd to completely meaningless.

Conduction aphasia is caused by a lesion in the tracts that connect Broca's and Wernicke's regions. Patients with conduction aphasia are unable to repeat what is heard. Spontaneous speech is often meaningless fluent jargon. Comprehension of the spoken and written word is largely intact.

Global aphasia is a severe impairment of all language-related functions.

The right hemisphere is often capable of comprehending certain simple noun words such as house, chair, and cup. The right hemisphere contributes more conceptual aspects of language communication. It complements the left hemisphere speech and language processing through more subtle communication skills such as emotional intonation, aspects of metaphors, and some qualities of humor.

The inability to read is the result of a disconnection between certain visual processing areas in the occipital lobe and the angular gyrus in the parietal lobe.

The area adjacent to the calcarine fissure is the primary visual cortex; a lesion here will result in cortical blindness. The association visual cortex is involved in recognition and identification and processing of visual input, which enables one to decide how to use the visual input. Constructional apraxia involves a loss in the ability to reproduce or construct figures by drawing or assembling. There seems to be a loss of visual guidance or an impairment in forming visual images although basic visual and motor functions appear intact. The optic tracts and optic radiations transmit visual impulses from the contralateral visual fields of each eye. See figure on page 33.

The right hemisphere seems to be dominant for perception and spatial localization. Some forms of perceptual deficits such as agnosia seem to implicate involvement of both hemispheres. Agnosia, the failure to recognize objects, cannot be attributed to a defect of vision or to intellectual or language impairment. It occurs with a bilateral lesion to the parietal-occipital regions or damage to these areas on the left coupled with damage to the commissural pathways that connect each hemisphere. Astereognosis, the inability to recognize familiar objects through palpation, even though sensation in normal, occurs with a right posterior parietal lesion. Visual perception disorders such as depth and figure-ground perception are primarily right hemisphere functions.

Hearing is functionally located in the superior temporal gyrus of both hemispheres. Bilateral lesions will result in cortical deafness. The association cortex adjacent to the superior temporal gyrus functions in recognition and identification of auditory input, processes auditory inflow, and enables a person to decide how to use

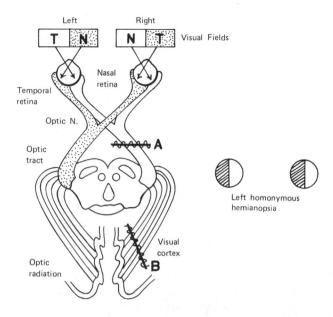

auditory input. A person who has more accuracy in identifying words presented to the right ear than the left is called a dichotic listener. This is influenced by attention (which ear is reported on first) and a memory component (because the right hemisphere does not hold information well). The aspects of musical processing that require judgments about duration, temporal order, sequencing, and rhythm differentially involve the left hemisphere, whereas the right hemisphere is differentially involved when judgments about tonal memory, timbre, melody recognition, and intensity are required.

The precentral gyrus is the functional area for skilled voluntary movement. Lesions in this region result in flaccid paralysis for voluntary movements, loss of fine skilled movements contralaterally, and motor apraxia. Apraxia is the inability to perform certain learned or purposeful movements on command despite the absence of paralysis or sensory loss. The motor association cortex in the premotor region of the frontal lobe functions in postural control, generalized body movements, directional movements, and general orientation movements.

The postcentral gyrus of the parietal lobe is the primary sensory areas for touch, pain, temperature, and proprioceptive sensory input. The association cortex involves fine discrimination and interpretation of tactile, sensorimotor, and proprioceptive stimuli such as stereognosis, body image, and self-awareness.

The prefrontal regions of the cortex are the association areas for emotional perception. Associated with the prefrontal region is the limbic system, which functions to represent feelings, affect, and state of mind. In general, persons with left hemisphere lesions display feelings of despair, hopelessness, and anger, whereas right hemisphere damage is associated with an indifferent euphoric reaction, in which minimization of symptoms, emotional placidity, and elation are common.

Memory, a function of both hemispheres, combines language information (retained best by the left hemisphere) and visual-spatial information (retained by the right hemisphere).

Attention is primarily a right hemispheric function. A lesion results in anosogno-

to recognize or acknowledge bodily defect. Individuals with this defect demonstrate neglect of the left side of the body and the areas surrounding the left side of the body.

The ability to recognize people, places, and time, and to be logical and artistic, may be related to the function of the right hemisphere. The left hemisphere tends to be more scientific and calculating in its processing.

With this basic outline of anatomy, one can predict by the neurologic deficits produced which artery has been occluded or which regions have been subjected to traumatic brain injury. However, these predictions are not necessarily realistic because (1) many cerebral infarcts result from occlusion of smaller arteries or branches from main arteries and therefore cause more limited neurologic deficits, and (2) large vessel occlusion often results in death.

With time, cerebral healing occurs as the dead brain tissue is replaced by scar (gliosis). If the lesion was small, the patient may completely recover or have only minimal residual disability. If the lesion was large, substantial residual neurologic deficits remain.

When evaluating and treating patients who have suffered from a cerebral vascular accident or trauma, it is important to understand that the cerebral hemispheres are not identical or mirror images of one another. A patient who may dress only one side of the body or put clothes on upside down is demonstrating what can happen when specialization within a hemisphere has been disrupted.

The functional distinctions (cerebral specializations) of the cerebral hemispheres follow.

HEMISPHERIC LATERALIZATION

Dominant Hemisphere (Left 85%)	Nondominant Hemisphere (Right 15%)
Motor	
1. Controls voluntary movements for right side of body 2. Coordinates bilateral movements 3. Controls rapid and complex motor skills	1. Controls voluntary movements for left side of body 2. Coordinates contralateral movements 3. Controls fine (figure designs) movement patterns
Somatic Sensation	
1. Superficial and deep for right side of body	1. Superficial and deep for left side of body
Vision	
1. Receives input from right visual field first 2. Letter discrimination	1. Receives input from left visual field first 2. Spatial processing, seeing things in three dimensions; manipulates objects in space 3. Sense of direction and following maps 4. Remembers shapes and faces
Hearing	
Hears vowels, consonants, and rhythms	Hears music, melodies, and tones
Tactile	
Nontactile	Recognizes objects by touch (stereognosis) bilaterally

HEMISPHERIC LATERALIZATION *Continued*

Dominant Hemisphere (Left 85%)	Nondominant Hemisphere (Right 15%)
Language	
1. Controls verbal and written communication 2. Understands written communication 3. Talks with hands	1. Nonverbal
Nonverbal Functions	
1. Reasons Performs calculations 3. Symbolic thinking 4. Formulates sentence structure and grammar 5. Scientific thinking	1. Creative 2. Artistic and musical abilities 3. Imaginative
Perception	
	1. Body image awareness 2. Sensory interpretation
Emotion	
	1. Controls emotional response 2. Perceives emotions in others
Handedness	
Right	Left, true in approximately 3% of population

Generally speaking, the right (nondominant) cerebral hemisphere is developed for visual-spatial activities and the left (dominant) hemisphere for verbal-analytical activities. Language is controlled in the dominant hemisphere in 98 percent of the right-handed population and 60 percent of the left-handed population. The mix of hemispheric functions is said to be highly variable. Some individuals have both language and some visual-spatial functions crowded onto the same side. It is believed that stuttering is caused by language being controlled by both hemispheres. Men have a greater tendency than women to have visual-spatial abilities, lateralized to the right hemisphere. Dyslexia, identified as the failure to develop lateralization of visual-spatial abilities, is more common in men than in women. Age and genes are also factors influencing hemispheric lateralization. A child under 5 years old shows less evidence of lateralization and has the ability to relocate specific functions following injury to a hemisphere. After age 5 this flexibility is lost. It has been observed that left hemiplegics have a tendency to deny their stroke.

As stated earlier, an understanding of the functional areas associated with each cerebral hemisphere will influence patient management. The treatment should be specifically designed to take into account all aspects of the deficit rather than treating only the obvious motor and sensory deficits.

Summary

Patients who have suffered traumatic head injuries involving the brain may demonstrate one-sided weakness or weakness of all four limbs and trunk. Retrograde amnesia or posttraumatic amnesia (a memory impairment) may result as a clinical manifestation of a traumatic head injury.

Cerebral vascular diseases and traumatic brain injuries produce not only profound physical changes but also emotional and psychologic changes in patients. Loss of control of the body may be overwhelming. Emotional and behavioral reactions to the trauma often present obstacles to learning. Depression, anxiety, fear, frustration, anger, hostility, or denial may prevent patients from cooperating with those attempting to work with them. The patient's reaction to this damage and the current situation must be understood so that steps may be taken to resolve obstacles that prohibit optimal functioning.

The prognosis in the early stages is usually difficult to determine; however, a residual sensory-motor disability is common.

COMPLICATIONS

Bowel control is regained in most patients within a few days following their insult, particularly if they are able to use a bedpan. Patients with persistent bowel incontinence may develop fecal impaction. A rigid bowel program should be implemented as soon as possible.

Initially a patient may require an indwelling catheter to prevent distention of the flaccid bladder. As the patient leaves the flaccid stage, the bladder tone returns and the catheter should be removed; otherwise incontinency may continue to be a problem. Normal bladder control is usually regained within 4 to 5 days.

Many hemiplegic patients will have accompanying hypertension, which may adversely affect the outcome of the individual's treatment plan. It may be necessary to discuss the problem of hypertension with the patient's physician.

The hemiplegic patient's lower limb may have a tendency to develop osteoarthritis owing to inadequate sensation and malalignment during ambulation. Also, immobilized joints on the involved side may become painful; the most commonly involved are the shoulder, wrist, and hip. Hemiplegic patients are also more prone to falling. Fractures of the involved hip are common, requiring immediate orthopedic care.

Certainly, psychologic reactions may complicate the recovery program. Anxiety is a common reaction to cerebral damage. Anger, aggression, and frustration are characteristic attitudes and are often directed toward the hospital personnel or family. It is important to be sympathetic, patient, and understanding. Psychologic reactions may lead to depression. Patients may cry easily and frequently. Psychologic support and management are important to the individual and are necessary for a successful rehabilitation program.

PATIENT MANAGEMENT

Rehabilitation of the patient with one-sided involvement caused by a cerebral vascular accident or trauma should start early and should be intensive. The need for a rehabilitation program arises from the functional deficits that follow cerebral damage. Varying degrees of functional impairment remain, ranging from total inability to leave the bed to almost complete self-sufficiency, with some residual difficulties in the use of the involved upper limb or in standing and ambulation.

The goal of rehabilitation is to provide an opportunity for the patient to lead as fulfilling a life as physical, emotional, and socioeconomic resources permit. All personnel involved in the management of the patient must be aware of the neuromuscular, emotional, social, and vocational problems associated with brain injuries.

The initial step in the rehabilitation program is a thorough evaluation and the establishment of realistic goals. A comprehensive approach to patient management includes many rehabilitation services such as physical therapy, speech and hearing, occupational therapy, psychologic counseling and social service, vocational counseling, and recreational services.

Initial management involves the development of an atmosphere of trust and confidence for the patient and the patient's family. A subjective evaluation, which would be part of the initial management, should include patient interview, health, social, and medical history. The subjective assessment should be followed by the objective physical assessment.

During the acute phase, when medical lifesaving management takes priority, care must be taken to prevent contractures and decubiti through correct bed positioning and range of motion activities.

As spasticity can often develop rapidly, external devices such as splints, bivalve casts, or orthotics can be used to prevent contractures. In the supine position the involved upper limb should be positioned to prevent tightness of shoulder adductors and medial rotators, with the forearm and hand supported. A patient with involvement of the lower limb usually demonstrates a footdrop and lateral rotation at the hip. Support to the ankle and hip may be achieved by using a pillow or rolled towels.

In the acute phase following a head injury it is important to pay close attention to positioning and skin integrity. Patients should be repositioned a minimum of every 2 hours to prevent the development of decubiti. Any prominent area must be viewed as a potential area for breakdown (e.g., ears, occiput, scapula, greater trochanter). Pressure on the heel and lateral malleolus is particularly important. If the patient lies on the involved side for a long time the greater trochanter will be vulnerable to skin breakdown. The same holds true for the sacrum with extended periods of time in the supine position.

Spasticity often causes soft tissue contractures for patients with TBIs. Progressive serial casting can be used to manage deformities resulting from spasticity. Casting is recommended in the early stages of rehabilitation so immobilization occurs while the patient is in the lowest level of consciousness. Casting is a skill that must be developed to be effective and to prevent complications.

As soon as the patient is medically stable, active treatment should begin. Weight-bearing may be helpful in normalizing tone and maintaining joint range of motion, especially ankle dorsiflexion and hip and knee extension. Getting patients into the upright position as soon as possible may also help excite the reticular activating system, resulting in an increase in the patient's level of arousal.

Positioning and seating is an important aspect of rehabilitation for those individuals who will be spending time in a wheelchair. When assessing sitting position, therapists should always begin at the pelvis. Optimal position is in a slight anterior pelvic tilt with no rotation in the horizontal plane. The thighs should be fully supported to distribute forces equally, with the hip joints as close to a 90-degree angle as possible and in neutral rotation. The knee joints should also be as close to a 90-degree angle as possible with both feet fully supported in a neutral dorsiflexion/plantarflexion and in slight eversion position. Maintaining the pelvis in a level position optimizes the trunk, neck, and head position, which should also be in a neutral midline position. The lumbar and cervical vertebrae should be in a slight lordosis.

If the pelvis, trunk, and limbs are not optimally positioned, the seating system should be adapted to facilitate an optimal position. If the patient is assessed and found to have a fixed pelvic obliquity, this should be supported by the seating system. If the obliquity is flexible, the seating system should facilitate a weight shift off the weight-bearing side. Once the pelvis is as level as possible, trunk posture should be observed. If the trunk is not in midline, a three-point system should be used to facilitate proper trunk control. This system would have a trunk support at the apex of the curve with lateral support on the opposite side above and below the concavity of the curve.

When head control is not normal, a head support should be used that facilitates midline positions and active control. The upper limbs should not be used to aid in support for the trunk. The seating system should facilitate and support the trunk well enough so that the upper limbs can be used for functional activities.

If the lower limbs are involved, they should be in a position close to 90 degrees of hip and knee flexion with neutral foot position. Hip guide pads can be used to keep the hip joints out of rotation. For those with adductor tone an abductor wedge can be used. Individuals with excessive extensor tone may find it helpful to inhibit the tone by maintaining the feet in a weight-bearing position on the footplate. Also, maintaining the hip and knee joints in flexion with the pelvis in a slight anterior tilt will help moderate the extensor tone. The optimal seat-to-back angle is 90 degrees. If hip joint range of motion does not allow this, the seat may need to be wedged in either direction. Again it is important to try and keep the pelvis level; therefore, to accommodate an asymmetric hip joint deformity, the seat should be split. For example, if the right hip-to-back angle can be 90 degrees and the left hip-to-back angle only 80 degrees, then the left side of the seat supporting the thigh should be wedged 10 degrees. By splitting the seat to support the thighs separately, the pelvis position stays level with equal weight-bearing at each ischium. This can also be accomplished with foam under the thigh to support the deformity or facilitate a weight shift.

A tilt-in-space mechanism is helpful for patients who do not exhibit enough head control when the wheelchair is upright, or who require frequent pressure relief, or exhibit a forward head, forward shoulders, and kyphotic posture. In all of these cases the patient's seat-to-back angle can remain unchanged and the patient can be easily tilted in space.

Some important factors to remember when designing a patient's seating system are as follows:

1. Facilitate proper alignment.
2. Do not oversupport; allow the patient to use what active control is available.
3. Support fixed obliquities.
4. Do not support flexible obliquity; facilitate a better alignment by adding support under or on the weight-bearing side.
5. Reassess the seating system often; patients' changes should be reflected in their seating system. As the individual improves, less support may be needed.

Treatment of the individual is essentially the same, regardless of the person's age. Being young may be a beneficial factor in time spent for recovery and also the extent of the involvement. As the nervous system matures, its ability to change or modify is reduced. As a result, children usually have a better prognosis than older patients.

The physical therapy treatment plan should include neurophysiologic principles of therapeutic exercise and activities that will lead to the highest level of functional independence for the patient.

As the transition from a controlled environment (such as the rehabilitation center) may be different than the transition to home and the community, it is important to assimilate that environment in the treatment setting. Community integration programs may be appropriate prior to an ultimate independent or home discharge.

Evaluation of the brain-injured patient and neurophysiologic principles of exercise are not included in this book. The intent is to cover the activities that would assist patients in reaching their highest level of functional independence.

BEHAVIORAL MANAGEMENT

Behavior may be the result of mental or cognitive activity. Adequate cognitive function involves goal-directed processing of an activity. Neurobehavioral changes in the brain-injured population have a relationship to the structural changes in CNS tissue that are a consequence of the impact of the force on the cranium and the secondary, pathologic processes that further destroy tissue. Although each head-injured individual and each injury are unique, the neurobehavioral changes that occur subsequent to cerebral trauma have many common characteristics.

Recovery of cognitive function usually follows a pathway that is predictable and may be described in behavioral terms. Observation and assessment of the brain-injured patient responses are especially important during the early phases of recovery when the individual lacks the cognitive ability to cooperate with the testing. One available method of categorizing behaviors is the Levels of Cognitive Function, a behavioral scale representing the progression of cognitive recovery demonstrated through behavioral changes. (The assessment form shown in Chapter 12 was developed by Rancho Los Amigos Hospital, Downey, CA, and adapted by the Greenery Rehabilitation and Skilled Nursing Center, Boston, MA.)

The patient who presents in a confused stage and exhibits inappropriate behaviors may benefit from behavioral management techniques. This approach requires a small quiet treatment area with few distractions rather than a large, busy, or noisy treatment room. Sessions may need to be short (i.e., 10 to 15 minutes or less), depending on how much information the individual can comprehend and retain in a given amount of time. A reward system may help motivate patients to work toward their goals. During this time, head-injured patients may require anger control therapy. This involves helping the patient, each time a different task is attempted, gain or regain control over anger so that the task can be continued and the goal achieved. It is important to help the confused and agitated patient achieve success with functional tasks. If patients feel positive about their abilities, they will more likely be willing to continue working toward a goal of greater independence.

When working with the patient who displays a lack of insight and reasoning abilities, it is necessary to have concrete goals for the patient and break functional tasks into their components. For example, when the long-term goal is ambulation its component parts must be discussed and worked on in a concrete fashion. The person may be unable to understand that working on lower limb strength and control in positions other than walking will lead to improved lower limb control in walking. The patients may not have the insight to understand that they are at present unable to walk or even stand. They are therefore unable to recognize the need to address lower limb strengthening and motor control activities. Carry-over of learned information for functional tasks is more likely if that information is presented concretely, avoiding vague and abstract instructions.

4

Amputations and Prosthetics

MEDICAL CONSIDERATIONS

Etiologies of Amputations

Amputations are either congenital limb deficiencies or acquired as the result of disease or trauma. Amputation of the lower limb is at least 10 times more common than that of the upper limb. Acquired (surgical) amputations are indicated when the patient's welfare will be significantly improved by the removal of an irreparably diseased, damaged, deformed, dangerous, or dysfunctional part of the body. The most common reasons for amputation are as follows:

1. *Vascular Disease:* The major cause of lower limb amputation is peripheral vascular disease, especially arteriosclerosis, in which the blood supply to the lower limbs is compromised. The presence of diabetes accelerates the circulatory disturbance. A limb with faulty circulation is vulnerable to infection, which may culminate in gangrene, endangering life by extending proximally. Other vascular disorders that may lead to amputation are Buerger's and Raynaud's diseases.
2. *Tumor:* Neoplastic disease in the limb, such as osteogenic sarcoma, may necessitate amputation to prevent metastasis to vital organs.
3. *Trauma:* This includes crushing and traction injuries and burns that are so severe that the blood supply is irreparably damaged and gangrene or chronic infection is inevitable. When multiple tissues are injured, reconstruction is no longer feasible. Amputation may also be elected in the presence of intractable pain.
4. *Congenital Anomaly:* Some congenital deformities are revised surgically to enable the patient to achieve greater function and more acceptable appearance by subsequent prosthetic fitting.

Other Surgical Considerations

An acquired amputation in which the sutures are not closed is termed an open amputation. This is a temporary condition that allows drainage of infectious material and is followed by a surgical closure. The more common closed amputation is one in which the skin has been sutured.

Amputation limbs may be categorized as end-bearing or non–end-bearing. Prosthetic use is facilitated if the patient can tolerate full loading through the distal end of the limb, as in the case of ankle or knee joint disarticulation. End-bearing offers maximum comfort and leverage to control the prosthesis. Comfort results from supporting all weight on the horizontal bottom of the limb. Non–end-bearing amputations through the bony shaft predominate; the individual bears weight primarily on the steeply sloped sides of the limb.

Assuming that the amputation limb is healthy with adequate circulation, the longer the limb, the greater the function realized by the patient. Although circulatory status is the primary determinant of the amputation site, appearance is a consideration; amputation at the end of the thigh or leg may result in distal bulbousness unacceptable to some individuals.

Common Complications

Amputation limbs are subject to various complications, resulting from surgical or prosthetic factors or from recognized, but unpreventable, causes.

Ulceration

Ulceration may be associated with local ischemia along the surgical scar. Abrasion or compression by an improperly fitting postsurgical dressing or prosthesis can cause ulceration anywhere on the amputation limb.

Local Pain

All severe nerve ends form a neuroma. If a neuroma becomes entangled in scar tissue or is subjected to tension and pressure from the prosthesis, it may produce pain. The neuroma may be treated surgically or by various electrical modalities. Infections are another source of pain; they usually respond to medication.

Phantom Sensation and Pain

Almost all patients, except those with congenital anomalies, feel the missing body parts. Phantom limb sensation is a painless feeling that the severed limb is still attached. The perception can be constant, intermittent, or temporary and may involve the entire severed limb or only a distal segment. Phantom limb pain is an uncomfortable feeling of the missing limb perceived by relatively few individuals. The pain is often described as "knife jabs" or "electrical shocks." It may be sharp or crampy, steady or fleeting, mildly annoying or incapacitating. Medications, surgery, electrotherapy, and various relaxation techniques are used to decrease phantom limb sensations and pain, yielding varying results. Pain usually ceases eventually, although some patients are troubled indefinitely.

PROSTHETIC PRESCRIPTION

The type of prosthesis should be compatible with the individual's level of amputation and predicted functional activity. The patient should be able to don the prosthesis independently as well as transfer and ambulate safely. The prosthesis should be durable enough to withstand the patient's anticipated activity and must be financially acceptable to the funding source, whether public, private, or personal. Occasionally, several prostheses are required to meet all the individual's vocational or athletic needs.

Clinic Team

Optimum management of the person with an amputation is provided by the clinic team, key members of which are the physician, prosthetist, and physical therapist. These workers should formulate the prosthetic prescription and agree as to the adequacy of the prosthesis and the patient's performance with it. The clinic team should address the experiences and preferences of the patient and family. Clinics also call on the services of a social worker, psychologist, vocational counselor, and other personnel to meet the needs of individual patients.

Physician

Overall management of the patient is the responsibility of a physician. Although an amputation is performed by a vascular, general, or orthopedic surgeon, subsequent care usually is supervised by a specialist in physical medicine and rehabilitation, an orthopedist, or, in some children's clinics, a pediatrician. Physicians who lead clinic teams usually have completed postgraduate education in prosthetics.

Prosthetist

The prosthetist constructs the definitive prosthesis and may also provide immediate, early, temporary, and recreational appliances. Prosthetists are college graduates who are certified by the American Board for Certification in Prosthetics and Orthotics.

Physical Therapist

Preoperative, postoperative, and prosthetic training is provided by physical therapists, sometimes aided by physical therapist assistants. In some clinics, therapists fabricate immediate, early, or temporary prostheses. Because therapists work on a regular basis with the patient, their recommendations regarding prosthetic components and performance standards are important to optimum patient management.

Types of Prostheses

The major categories of prostheses are immediate, early, temporary, permanent, and recreational. A given patient may be fitted with one or more of these devices.

Immediate Prosthesis

An immediate prosthesis is applied at the time of surgery and consists of a plaster dressing or similar encasement, to which is attached a pylon and foot-ankle assembly. The individual with an amputation at or above the knee may also have a knee unit in the prosthesis. See figure on page 44.

Early Prosthesis

An early prosthesis is a similar appliance applied after surgery, but before sutures have been removed. Both the immediate and early prostheses are designed to control postoperative edema and thereby reduce pain and foster healing. The socket may or

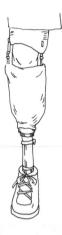

Immediate postsurgical fitting.

may not be removable: in the latter case, the pylon is detached whenever the user is not standing or walking. Weight-bearing on the amputated side must be minimized until sutures are removed. The psychologic benefits from early mobility are vast.

Temporary Prosthesis

After sutures have been removed, the patient should be fitted with a temporary prosthesis, which aids in maturation of the amputation limb, improves the user's overall physical condition, enables the individual to engage in gait and transfer training, and helps the clinic team to evaluate the patient's requirements for a permanent prosthesis. It includes a plaster or plastic socket, pylon, and foot-ankle assembly, and for knee disarticulation and higher amputations, a knee unit.

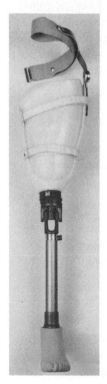

Temporary above-knee prosthesis with the solid ankle cushion heel (SACH) foot, aluminum pylon, locked knee unit, plastic adjustable socket, and pelvic belt suspension. (From Edelstein, JE: Prosthetic assessment and management. In O'Sullivan, SB and Schmitz, TJ (eds): Physical Rehabilitation: Assessment and Treatment, ed 2. FA Davis, Philadelphia, 1988, p 417, with permission.)

Permanent Prosthesis

A permanent or definitive prosthesis is a replacement for the missing limb, that should provide excellent fit, alignment, appearance, and construction.

Recreational Prostheses

Special prostheses can facilitate the client's performance in various sports. For example, a waterproof prosthesis is appropriate for swimming. Recreational prostheses augment the permanent appliance, enabling the individual to achieve greater ambulatory performance.

CURRENT PROSTHETIC OPTIONS

Partial Foot Prostheses

Prostheses for partial foot amputations may consist of a simple foam shoe filler to compensate for absent toes. The foot with transmetatarsal or more proximal amputation may be encased in a custom-made plastic socket mounted on a shoe insert.

Syme's Prostheses

Syme's amputation, named for Dr. James Syme, involves transection of the tibia and the fibula just above their articular surfaces: the tough calcaneal pad is placed distally to enhance end-bearing. This amputation provides the patient with a long bony lever to control the prosthesis, and the ability to ambulate when not wearing a prosthesis. Some individuals object to the bulbous end of the amputation limb. The prosthesis consists of a foot-ankle assembly and a socket that encases the amputation limb and suspends the prosthesis on the limb.

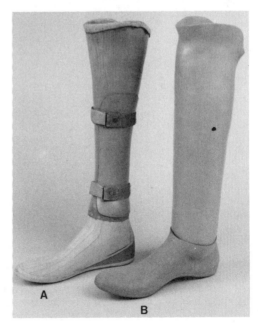

Syme's prostheses. A. Socket with removable medial door. B. Socket with expandable liner. (From Edelstein, JE: Prosthetic assessment and management. In O'Sullivan, SB and Schmitz, TJ (eds): Physical Rehabilitation: Assessment and Treatment, ed 2. FA Davis, Philadelphia, 1988, p 412, with permission.)

Foot-Ankle Assemblies

A Syme's version of the solid ankle cushion heel (SACH) foot is most commonly used. It has a rubber heel wedge that compresses during heel contact to absorb shock and facilitate plantar flexion. The heel also allows inversion and eversion. A wooden keel mounted above the heel provides stability. The junction between the heel and the rubber toe permits toe hyperextension in late stance. The SACH foot is reasonably cosmetic, because there is no crease between the top of the foot and the socket. It is quiet, inexpensive, and has low maintenance, but does not contribute springiness to the gait.

Newer feet suitable for Syme's prostheses are special models of some of the energy storing/releasing feet designed for below-knee prostheses.

Sockets

Custom molded over a plaster cast of the patient's limb, the socket is made of rigid plastic, usually polyester laminate, which can be shaped and colored to match the individual's sound leg.

The socket for the patient with a bulbous end usually has a removable medial door to facilitate donning the prosthesis. After the limb is lodged in the socket, the patient straps the door to the socket.

A more attractive socket incorporates an expandable inner liner. It can be used when there is minimal difference in circumference between the mid and distal portions of the amputation limb.

Below-Knee Prostheses

The below-knee prosthesis is composed of a foot-ankle assembly, shank, socket, and provision for suspension.

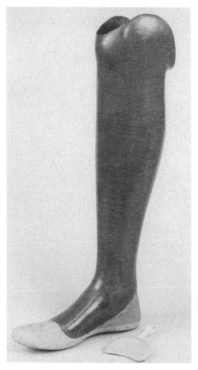

Below-knee prosthesis with SACH foot, exoskeletal shank, patellar-tendon-bearing socket, and supracondylar suspension. Note the removable wedge to be inserted medially. (From Edelstein, JE: Prosthetic assessment and management. In O'Sullivan, SB and Schmitz, TJ (eds): Physical Rehabilitation: Assessment and Treatment, ed 2. FA Davis, Philadelphia, 1988, p 409, with permission.)

Foot-Ankle Assemblies

All prosthetic feet provide plantar flexion and absorb shock in early stance and permit toe hyperextension in late stance. Although they are manufactured to suit most adults, some designs are also made in children's sizes. Most feet are available in high- and low-heeled models to fit into various styles of shoes. Many have simulated toes for individuals who wear sandals.

Nonarticulated Feet

Most frequently prescribed is the SACH foot. It is nonarticulated, with no mechanical joint at the point corresponding to the anatomic ankle. The prosthesis presents a smooth contour from foot to shank, without any cleft. The version for prostheses for below-knee and higher amputations has a wooden keel somewhat smaller than that needed for the Syme's prosthesis. Newer feet differ in keel design and materials, having a synthetic keel that bends during early and mid stance to store energy and recoils in late stance, thereby releasing some of the stored energy. They enable the wearer to walk, run, and jump more easily but are more expensive than the SACH foot; some are also less durable.

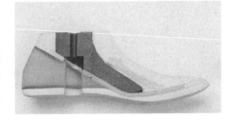

SACH nonarticulated foot-ankle assembly. (From Edelstein, JE: Prosthetic assessment and management. In O'Sullivan, SB and Schmitz, TJ (eds): Physical Rehabilitation: Assessment and Treatment, ed 2. FA Davis, Philadelphia, 1988, p 408, with permission.)

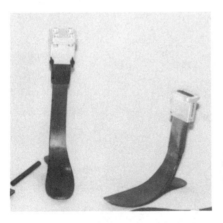

Springlite nonarticulated foot-ankle assemblies designed to store and release energy during stance phase. The rod can be inserted in a hole in the posterior portion of the foot to alter the wearer's gait.

Articulated Feet

Occasionally, a single-axis foot is required. The articulated assembly is a wooden foot hinged to an ankle section. Plantarflexion and dorsiflexion are controlled by posterior and anterior rubber bumpers, respectively. The foot portion has provision for toe hyperextension. The single-axis foot promotes knee stability in early stance by allowing the sole to contact the floor quickly, placing an extension torque on the knee joint. It lacks provision for inversion and eversion and requires more maintenance than do nonarticulated assemblies. More complex articulated feet provide triplanar motion, but are heavy.

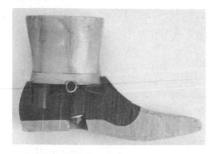

Single-axis articulated foot-ankle assembly. (From Edelstein, JE: Prosthetic assessment and management. In O'Sullivan, SB and Schmitz, TJ (eds): Physical Rehabilitation: Assessment and Treatment, ed 2. FA Davis, Philadelphia, 1988, p 408, with permission.)

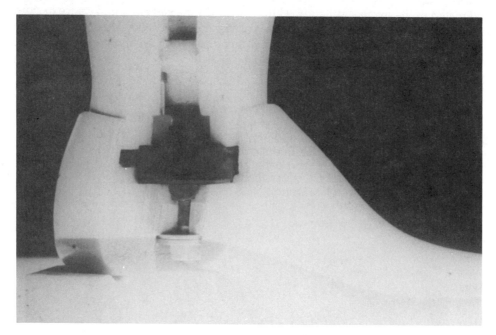

Articulated foot-ankle assembly providing triplanar motion.

Shanks

The shank, mounted between the foot and the socket, must be rigid enough to withstand the force exerted by the wearer during all ambulatory activities. Most shanks also enhance the cosmetic appeal of the prosthesis by the use of anatomically shaped and colored materials. Shanks may be either exoskeletal or endoskeletal.

Exoskeletal Shanks

The standard model is exoskeletal, with the support on the outside of the shank. It is usually made of wood carved to match the contour of the contralateral limb, and coated with polyester laminate tinted to the patient's skin color. The interior of the shank is hollowed to reduce weight without much diminution of structural rigidity.

The exoskeletal shank is relatively inexpensive to fabricate and impervious to damage from fluids.

Endoskeletal Shanks

An endoskeletal or "modular" shank has a rigid central supporting member, the pylon, and a synthetic foam cover shaped like the opposite leg. A heavy stocking is pulled over the foam. Modular prostheses are more attractive because they resemble the texture of the sound limb. They also subject clothing to less abrasion. In addition, the pylon has screws that facilitate minor angular adjustments. Although the endoskeletal shank does not save appreciable weight when used in the below-knee prosthesis, the prosthesis for a patient with knee joint disarticulation or higher amputation is lighter if it includes an endoskeletal shank.

The resilient covering requires periodic replacement when the outer stocking becomes soiled or torn or when the foam plastic has deteriorated. The cover does not withstand the abrasion of frequent kneeling.

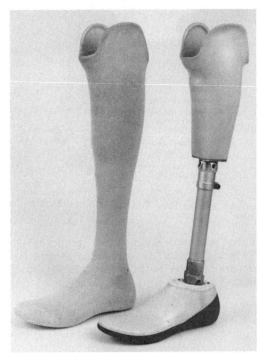

Below-knee prosthesis with SACH foot, endoskeletal shank, patellar-tendon-bearing socket, and supracondylar suspension. A, Prosthesis with synthetic foam cover. B, Prosthesis with cover removed to expose the pylon. (From Edelstein, JE: Prosthetic assessment and management. In O'Sullivan, SB and Schmitz, TJ (eds): Physical Rehabilitation: Assessment and Treatment, ed 2. FA Davis, Philadelphia, 1988, p 410, with permission.)

Sockets

The socket most frequently prescribed for the below-knee prosthesis is the patellar tendon–bearing (PTB) design. It is a total contact socket that derives its name from its use of the patellar tendon (patellar ligament) for some weight-bearing and rotational control. Weight is borne throughout the amputation limb, particularly on the patellar tendon, gastrocnemius muscle belly, medial tibia, and shaft of the fibula. Total contact decreases edema and maximizes the weight-bearing area and sensory feedback for the wearer. When fabricating the socket, the prosthetist takes special care to minimize pressure over bony prominences in the areas of the tibial condyles, crest and distal end, and fibular head and distal end.

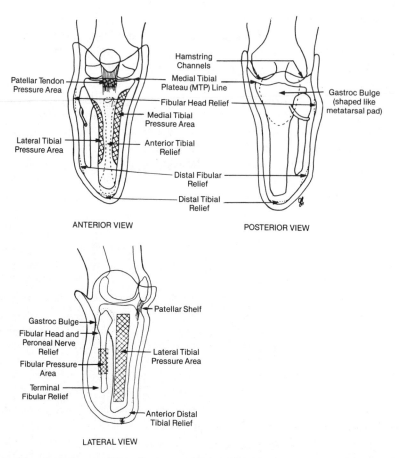

Patellar tendon-bearing socket diagrams. (From Edelstein, JE: Prosthetic assessment and management. In O'Sullivan, SB and Schmitz, TJ (eds): Physical Rehabilitation: Assessment and Treatment, ed 2. FA Davis, Philadelphia, 1988, p 411, with permission.)

Lined Socket

Most sockets are made of rigid polyester laminate with a resilient polyethylene foam liner which conforms to the amputation limb. The liner facilitates adjusting socket fit to accommodate atrophy of the amputation limb: patches of leather can be glued to the exterior of the liner to reduce the interior volume. The liner, however, acts as a heat insulator and adds to the bulkiness of the prosthesis.

Unlined Socket

The socket may be made to be worn without a liner. The patient is shielded from the rigid surface by a medium-weight wool sock.

Suspensions

Some component or design feature of the below-knee prosthesis is needed to enable the device to stay on the wearer's leg, particularly in the swing phase of walking.

Supracondylar Cuff

The most economic suspension is the supracondylar cuff, a strap attached to the medial and lateral walls of the socket and passing over the femoral epicondyles. The wearer can tighten or loosen the cuff easily. Some individuals, however, do not like the silhouette created by the cuff when the knee is flexed during sitting.

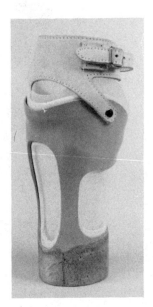

Leather supracondylar cuff attached to a rigid plastic frame supporting a flexible plastic patellar-tendon-bearing socket. (From Edelstein, JE: Prosthetic assessment and management. In O'Sullivan, SB and Schmitz, TJ (eds): Physical Rehabilitation: Assessment and Treatment, ed 2. FA Davis, Philadelphia, 1988, p 410, with permission.)

Supracondylar Brim

The medial and lateral margins of the socket may terminate above the femoral epicondyles. Suspension is achieved with the addition of a wedge inserted medially inside the socket after the patient dons it. The wedge reduces the proximal circumference, thus preventing the prosthesis from dislodging. The sitting silhouette is generally satisfactory. A major drawback to supracondylar suspension is its lack of adjustability. It is also more difficult to fabricate, thus accounting for a more costly prosthesis.

A variant is supracondylar/suprapatellar suspension, in which the anterior, medial, and lateral walls terminate higher than in the prosthesis suspended by a cuff. The higher anterior wall is indicated for the patient with a very short amputation limb. When the wearer sits, the rigid anterior wall is quite conspicuous.

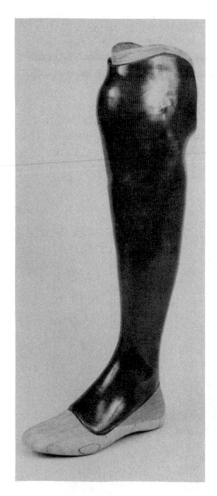

Below-knee prosthesis with SACH foot, exoskeletal shank, patellar tendon-bearing socket, and supracondylar/suprapatellar suspension. (From Edelstein, JE: Prosthetic assessment and management. In O'Sullivan, SB and Schmitz, TJ (eds): Physical Rehabilitation: Assessment and Treatment, ed 2. FA Davis, Philadelphia, 1988, p 413, with permission.)

Thigh Corset

Addition of metal hinges to the socket maximizes mediolateral stability. The associated leather thigh corset provides a large surface to support the wearer's weight. The corset is easily adjusted. It is used infrequently because it takes more time to don, it increases the weight of the prosthesis, and its mechanical knee joints do not articulate along the same axis as those of the anatomic knee. See figure on page 53.

Suspension Accessories

Some patients wear a rubber sleeve in place of the cuff or in addition to supracondylar suspension. The sleeve fits snugly over the distal thigh and proximal socket to create a smooth silhouette. It provides very snug suspension. Donning, however, requires two strong hands.

A waist belt with an anterior elastic strap, known as a fork strap, may be added to the cuff or the thigh corset for additional suspension. Many individuals, however, do not like being encumbered around the torso.

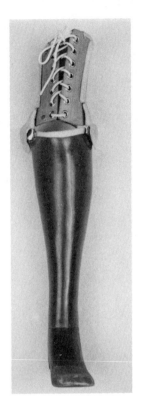

Below-knee prosthesis with SACH foot, exoskeletal shank, patellar tendon-bearing socket, and a thigh corset. (From Edelstein, JE: Prosthetic assessment and management. In O'Sullivan, SB and Schmitz, TJ (eds): Physical Rehabilitation: Assessment and Treatment, ed 2. FA Davis, Philadelphia, 1988, p 413, with permission.)

Knee Disarticulation Prostheses

A knee disarticulation prosthesis is worn by individuals whose tibia has been removed from the femur, as well as by those having amputation through the femoral condyles. In all instances, the patient retains end-bearing and has excellent femoral leverage to control the prosthesis, as well as rotary stability by means of the femoral epicondyles. See figure on page 54.

Infrastructure

Any type of foot-ankle assembly may be included in the knee disarticulation prosthesis. The shank may be exoskeletal or endoskeletal, depending on the individual's cosmetic, financial, and functional needs.

Knee Assemblies

The preferred knee unit has a thin proximal plate for attachment to the socket to minimize protrusion of the prosthetic knee when the patient sits. A specially designed hydraulic knee unit is often included to provide best control of the swing of the shank.

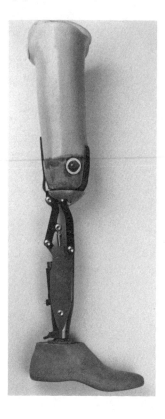

Knee disarticulation prosthesis with SACH foot, endo-skeletal shank, hydraulic polycentric knee unit, and quadrilateral suction socket. (From Edelstein, JE: Prosthetic assessment and management. In O'Sullivan, SB and Schmitz, TJ (eds): Physical Rehabilitation: Assessment and Treatment, ed 2. FA Davis, Philadelphia, 1988, p 418, with permission.)

Sockets and Suspensions

The patient who retains the full width of the femoral epicondyles is usually fitted with a socket having an anterior opening to facilitate donning. The socket terminates in the proximal thigh, if the amputation limb tolerates full end-bearing. The proximal margin of the socket may extend to the pelvis to reduce distal loading and to augment rotary control and suspension. If the circumference of the distal thigh is similar to that of the midthigh, then a socket having no anterior opening may be worn; this socket usually has a removable resilient liner to aid donning.

Above-Knee Prostheses

Patients with amputations through the femur above the epicondyles and below the greater trochanter are fitted with an above-knee prosthesis. As with below-knee amputations, the longer the bony lever arm, the easier it will be to control the prosthesis.

Infrastructure

The SACH foot is typically used for above-knee prostheses; however, any type of foot can be prescribed. The single-axis foot may benefit a frail patient or one with bilateral amputations because the assembly can be adjusted to plantarflex as easily as the user requires.

Exoskeletal shanks predominate because of their lesser cost; however, the weight savings and cosmetic appeal of the endoskeletal shank should be considered for people with above-knee amputations.

Knee Assemblies

Most knee units have a friction mechanism to dampen the motion of the shank during swing phase. Some assemblies include an extension aid to bias the knee toward extension during the latter portion of swing phase. A few components have a stabilizing device.

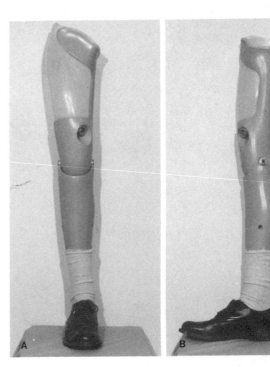

Above-knee prosthesis with SACH foot, exoskeletal shank, single-axis constant friction knee unit, and quadrilateral flexible socket with suction suspension. A, Anterior view. B, Medial view.

Hinges

Most assemblies have a single-axis hinge, which is simple and offers satisfactory function. More complex, polycentric units have a linkage system that causes the center of rotation to change as the knee is moved. At extension the axis is relatively posterior and superior, contributing to the stability of the prosthesis. See figures on page 56.

Friction Mechanisms

The shank of an above-knee prosthesis behaves much like a pendulum during swing phase, with the arc of motion determined by the acceleration imparted by the patient in early swing. To imitate the swing of the sound limb, most knee units have a friction mechanism.

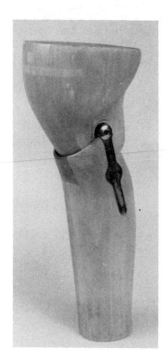

Single-axis knee unit. (From Edelstein, JE: Prosthetic assessment and management. In O'Sullivan, SB and Schmitz, TJ (eds): Physical Rehabilitation: Assessment and Treatment, ed 2. FA Davis, Philadelphia, 1988, p 414, with permission.)

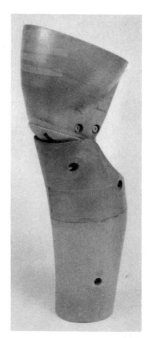

Polycentric knee unit. (From Edelstein, JE: Prosthetic assessment and management. In O'Sullivan, SB and Schmitz, TJ (eds): Physical Rehabilitation: Assessment and Treatment, ed 2. FA Davis, Philadelphia, 1988, p 414, with permission.)

Constant Friction

The typical constant friction unit has a knee bolt with a clamp that can be adjusted easily to change the resistance to knee motion. It is inexpensive and lightweight but does not compensate for changes in walking speed. Constant friction also resists knee motion during midswing when rapid movement is preferred.

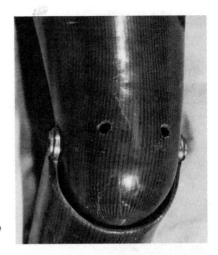

Single-axis, constant friction knee unit. Note the two screws that permit adjusting the friction.

Variable Friction

A more sophisticated type of mechanism damps knee movement during early and late swing but offers minimal resistance to midswing. This concept is incorporated in most fluid-controlled knee units.

Fluid-Controlled Friction

Fluid-controlled units offer patients a smoother, more normal-looking gait because they adjust the amount of friction according to the user's pace. The assembly has a cylinder linked to the knee hinge. The cylinder may be filled with oil (hydraulic unit) or air (pneumatic unit). These components are more expensive than those with sliding (mechanical) friction, such as the basic knee bolt and clamp unit. The patient who is too weak to walk rapidly does not benefit from the hydraulic or pneumatic swing phase control.

Extension Aids

Some knee units have an anterior elastic strap, which is stretched during knee flexion in early swing and recoils to help extend the knee in late swing. An alternate model has a strap or spring inside the unit. Extension aids help to ensure that the prosthetic knee will be extended when the patient initiates stance phase.

Stabilizers

Most individuals derive adequate stability from the alignment of the prosthesis. Some frail patients, however, require mechanical stabilization.

Manual Lock

This feature provides maximum stability found useful by the person who does not have reliable muscular control or by some individuals who climb ladders or stand for prolonged periods—especially on lurching trains or buses. The lock interferes with prosthetic clearance during swing phase; consequently, these prostheses should be shortened 1 cm. The manual lock must be disengaged when the wearer sits.

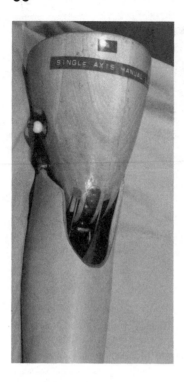

Single-axis knee unit with manual lock. Note the white knob that the wearer uses to disengage the lock.

Brake

A brake resists knee flexion in early stance, then releases automatically during late stance so that swing phase is not impeded. Such units are relatively heavy and mechanically complex. They are available with constant, sliding friction, as well as with hydraulic friction.

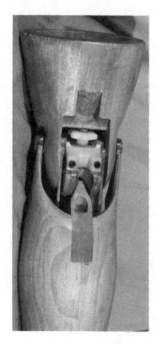

Single-axis knee unit with constant friction, internal spring extension aid, and brake.

The Henschke-Mauch Swing 'N Stance unit is a popular hydraulic mechanism for elderly patients who rely on the braking action during early stance phase, even though they do not take advantage of the swing phase control. The unit offers the additional options of a manual lock and a means of disconnecting the stabilizer.

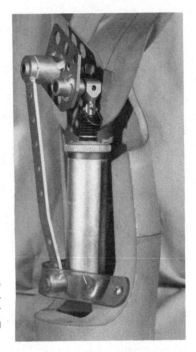

Mauch Swing 'N Stance single-axis, hydraulic knee unit, which provides both brake and lock options depending on the position of the ''U'' shaped fixture at the back of the unit. The unit is attached to half a thigh-shank component to expose the knee bolt.

Sockets

The above-knee socket fits the relatively fleshy thigh. Two socket configurations are in current use. Both contact the limb totally and subject the sides and bottom of the amputation limb to varying amounts of load. Either type of socket may be made entirely of rigid plastic or may be a combination of a flexible socket nested in a rigid frame. The latter model is usually more comfortable because heat dissipates through its thin walls, the flexible plastic conforms to the contour of the chair when the wearer sits, and the plastic yields to changing limb contour during the various phases of gait. The flexible material is more apt to crack than the rigid plastic.

Quadrilateral Socket

The posterior socket wall provides a horizontal seat for weight-bearing on the ischial tuberosity and gluteal muscle mass. The anterior wall is approximately 6 cm higher than the posterior wall and directs pressure posteriorly to retain the tuberosity on its seat. The anterior wall features a convexity along its medial two thirds, providing maximum contact over Scarpa's femoral triangle. The medial wall has a channel for the tough adductor longus tendon, which should be used as a guide when donning the prosthesis. The posteromedial corner has a relief for the hamstring tendons. The posterolateral corner has a concavity to afford room for the gluteus maximus muscle to contract. The anterolateral corner has a relief for the rectus femoris. The lateral wall terminates slightly above the greater trochanter, with a concavity allowing for this bony prominence.

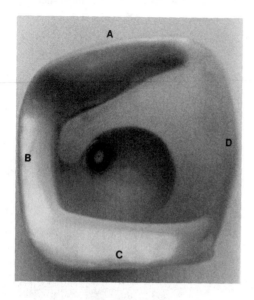

Quadrilateral flexible above-knee socket in a rigid frame. A, Anterior brim. B, Medial brim. C, Posterior brim. D, Lateral brim. (From Edelstein, JE: Prosthetic assessment and management. In O'Sullivan, SB and Schmitz, TJ (eds): Physical Rehabilitation: Assessment and Treatment, ed 2. FA Davis, Philadelphia, 1988, p 416, with permission.)

Ischial Containment Socket

The walls cover the ischial tuberosity and part of the ischiopubic ramus to augment socket stability. The mediolateral width of the socket is narrower than that of the quadrilateral socket for maximum frontal plane stability and minimum bulk between the legs. The anterior wall is somewhat lower than in the quadrilateral socket, while the lateral wall extends above the greater trochanter. The relative advantages and clinical indications of the designs remain controversial. Most patients achieve similar function with either type if properly fitted.

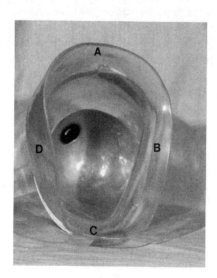

Ischial containment flexible above-knee socket in a rigid frame. Note the relatively narrow mediolateral dimension. A, Anterior brim. B, Medial brim. C, Posterior brim. D, Lateral brim.

Suspensions

Types of suspension for the above-knee prosthesis are total suction, partial suction with aid of a Silesian bandage or a pelvic belt, or nonsuction using pelvic belt suspension.

Total Suction

Suction suspension requires a snug socket equipped with a one-way valve to allow air to be expelled during stance phase. No sock is worn. This type of suspension maximizes sensory feedback and prosthetic control, minimizes edema, and offers good appearance inasmuch as no straps are worn around the torso. A prosthesis with suction suspension demands considerable skill to apply. Because a sock is not worn, the patient cannot accommodate volume changes. A prosthesis for a short amputation limb may be difficult to suspend by total suction.

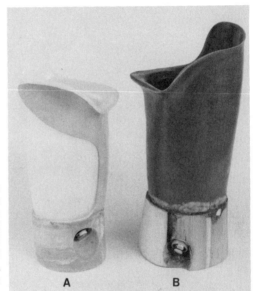

Quadrilateral above-knee sockets with suction suspension. A, Flexible socket in a rigid frame. B, Rigid socket. (From Edelstein, JE: Prosthetic assessment and management. In O'Sullivan, SB and Schmitz, TJ (eds): Physical Rehabilitation: Assessment and Treatment, ed 2. FA Davis, Philadelphia, 1988, p 416, with permission.)

Partial Suction

Partial suction suspension is achieved with a fairly snug socket having a valve and a Silesian bandage or pelvic belt. Partial suction suspension enables the individual to enjoy moderate control of the prosthesis and permits adjusting socket fit by adding or subtracting socks. Auxiliary suspension also augments rotary control of the prosthesis and increases the wearer's security when performing vigorous activities.

Silesian Bandage. This is a fabric band that attaches to the socket laterally, circles the trunk, and is buckled anteriorly on the socket. See figure at top of page 62.

Pelvic Belt. The pelvic belt offers maximum mediolateral and rotary stability. It is used particularly for those with very short or weak amputation limbs. A belt enclosing a rigid metal or polypropylene band is joined to a hinge joint on the lateral socket wall. This suspension is heavy, expensive, apt to become noisy, and creates a bulky appearance. The leather belt absorbs perspiration. See figure at bottom of page 62.

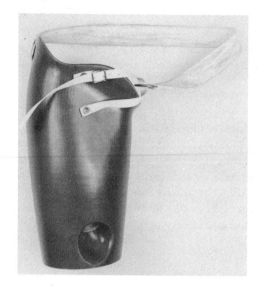

Quadrilateral rigid above-knee socket with Silesian bandage and partial suction suspension. (From Edelstein, JE: Prosthetic assessment and management. In O'Sullivan, SB and Schmitz, TJ (eds): Physical Rehabilitation: Assessment and Treatment, ed 2. FA Davis, Philadelphia, 1988, p 416, with permission.)

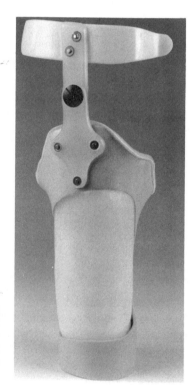

Quadrilateral flexible socket in a rigid frame with plastic pelvic belt suspension. (From Edelstein, JE: Prosthetic assessment and management. In O'Sullivan, SB and Schmitz, TJ (eds): Physical Rehabilitation: Assessment and Treatment, ed 2. FA Davis, Philadelphia, 1988, p 417, with permission.)

Nonsuction

The few patients who cannot tolerate a reasonably snug socket have their prostheses suspended solely by a pelvic belt. In place of a valve, the socket has a ventilation hole.

Hip Disarticulation and Hemipelvectomy Prostheses

Unlike more distal amputations, the major cause of hip disarticulation and hemipelvectomy amputation is cancer. In hip disarticulation, the femur is separated from the acetabulum, while hemipelvectomy involves removal of some or all of the pelvis. Individuals whose femur has been amputated at the greater trochanter or above are also fitted with a hip disarticulation prosthesis.

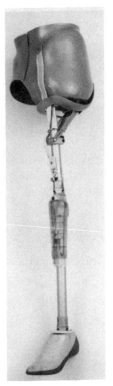

Hip disarticulation prosthesis with SACH foot, endoskeletal shank and thigh section, single-axis constant friction knee with an extension aid, single-axis hip joint with an extension aid, and rigid plastic socket. (From Edelstein, JE: Prosthetic assessment and management. In O'Sullivan, SB and Schmitz, TJ (eds): Physical Rehabilitation: Assessment and Treatment, ed 2. FA Davis, Philadelphia, 1988, p 418, with permission.)

Infrastructure

The prosthesis can incorporate any type of prosthetic foot. An endoskeletal shank is customary to reduce weight. Any model knee unit can be used, provided it has an extension aid. It is unusual to require a locking mechanism.

Hip Assemblies

The hip hinge is placed on the socket in such a position that stability during standing and walking is achieved without the use of a hip lock. The prosthesis includes a hip extension strap to limit step length.

Sockets and Suspensions

A socket made of rigid plastic laminate or flexible plastic in a frame encompasses the entire pelvis. The hip disarticulation prosthesis is suspended from both iliac crests and the ipsilateral ischial tuberosity. Most hemipelvectomy prostheses are suspended from the contralateral iliac crest, abdomen, and lower ribs.

PREPROSTHETIC MANAGEMENT

A program for care should begin prior to surgery. If the patient's physical condition permits, the program should include instruction in the use of crutches and conditioning exercises. An explanation of the postsurgical routine should be given.

Following surgery, exercises are initiated that will maintain motor power and prevent contractures. Stabilizing the volume and shape of the amputation limb and fostering the patient's independence in daily activities are major goals.

Flexibility

Flexibility exercises and positioning combat knee and hip flexion, abduction, and lateral rotation contractures, which would interfere with standing and walking with the prosthesis.

Positioning

The therapist should instruct the patient in proper positioning.

Supine

1. Avoid using pillows under the amputation limb.
2. Keep the hip (and knee) joints extended.
3. Keep the lower limbs close together.

Prone

1. Select the prone position as much as possible, assuming that the patient does not experience difficulty breathing while lying in that position.
2. Keep the hip (and knee) joints extended.
3. Avoid excessive hip lateral rotation.

Sitting

1. Keep the knee joint extended, with the limb supported on a firm surface.
2. Sit with the hips level.
3. Avoid prolonged sitting.

Standing

1. Use a tilt table with or without an immediate or early prosthesis for limited weight-bearing.
2. Stand with or without an immediate or early prosthesis, bearing most weight on a walker or parallel bars.

Motor Power and Coordination

Exercise Principles

Preoperatively, patients should be instructed in the types of exercises that will be important after surgery. Gentle isometrics can be initiated as early as the first postoperative day. The goals of postoperative exercises are as follows:

1. To maintain and increase joint range of motion.
2. To enhance coordination and strength.
3. To improve endurance and vital capacity.

Typical Exercise Program

The following exercises are suitable for most individuals with lower limb amputation at any level.

Postoperative Days 1 to 3

1. Deep breathing and relaxation exercises, to increase vital capacity and decrease anxiety.
2. Isometric exercises for the gluteal, adductor, and medial rotator muscles; patients with below-knee amputation should also perform quadriceps muscle setting.
3. Assistive range of motion of the amputation limb, unless the postsurgical dressing restricts motion.
4. Progressive resistive exercise to the contralateral joints as tolerated.
5. Standing and transfer training if the patient's physical status permits; weight-bearing should be limited to 10 kg while sutures are in place.

Postoperative Days 3 to 10

1. Active exercise of the amputation limb.
2. General conditioning exercise for the shoulders, trunk, and contralateral lower limb to prepare patients for the demands of ambulating with a prosthesis and for engaging in wheelchair activities.
3. For patients with below-knee amputation, gentle resistance to the hip on the operated side as tolerated.
4. Transfer and gait training.

Postoperative Days 10 to 14

1. Resistive exercise to the amputation limb when healing has occurred (exercise should emphasize hip extension, abduction, adduction, medial rotation, and, for those with below-knee amputation, knee extension).
2. General body conditioning.

Edema Control

Following surgery, most amputation limbs exhibit edema, which is partly due to the trauma of surgery. Reducing edema lessens postoperative pain, fosters healing, and, when a prosthesis is provided, helps the patient to retain fit. Except for open amputations, edema is controlled by compressive dressings and elevation of the amputation limbs.

Compressive dressings may be rigid, semirigid, or elastic. They may be applied as early as the time of surgery or introduced later. Some form of dressing should be worn until the amputation limb is no longer edematous. The limb will continue to shrink until the patient wears the prosthesis on a regular basis. If compressive dressings are not used consistently prior to the delivery of the definitive prosthesis, the limb will shrink drastically, so that the socket will soon become too loose, subjecting the skin to abrasion. Consequently, a new socket will have to be made earlier than usual, a costly and time-consuming procedure during which the patient is deprived of the prosthesis.

Compression should be used in any of the following conditions:

1. If permanent prosthesis has not yet been received.
2. If the prosthesis is not being worn daily (swelling could make it impossible to don the prosthesis).
3. If donning is impossible (compress and elevate the amputation limb for 1 hour, then attempt donning).
4. If the patient has received a permanent prosthesis but the limb has not yet stabilized (continue compression nightly; some individuals need to compress indefinitely because of persistent volume fluctuation).
5. If pain occurs at night (compression may reduce the discomfort).

The duration of compression varies. Some limbs stabilize within 8 weeks from the time the prosthesis is first worn. To determine whether the limb has stabilized, have the patient omit compression overnight. If donning the prosthesis is not difficult the next morning, routine compression may be discontinued.

Rigid Dressing

A rigid dressing is a compressive plaster cast applied at the time of surgery or soon after and removed when the wound has healed, approximately 2 weeks later. A second rigid dressing may then be applied if the amputation limb is flabby. The patient may require a bivalved plaster dressing after the temporary or definitive prosthesis is delivered.

Plaster may form the proximal portion of an immediate postoperative prosthesis. It fosters early partial weight-bearing, maintenance of postural reflexes, and the psychologic benefit of having two lower limbs. Patients fitted with a rigid dressing generally spend less time in the hospital and can be fitted with a definitive prosthesis earlier than those who have other dressings. The opaque dressing prevents wound inspection, unless a window has been cut in the plaster or a removable version is used; however, general body signs usually indicate whether healing is progressing.

Semirigid Dressing

Two forms of semirigid dressing are the Unna dressing and air splints. Both are self-suspending, eliminating the need for waist or shoulder straps used with the rigid dressing. Both are easy to apply and remove, are nonextensible, and are lightweight. The below-knee versions permit the patient to flex the knee slightly, reducing the stiffness associated with a plaster cast. As with the rigid dressing, the semirigid ones prevent knee flexion contracture.

Semirigid dressings may be applied at the time of surgery or any time thereafter and used until the volume of the amputation limb stabilizes.

Unna Dressing
Unna bandage is fabric saturated with a mixture of zinc oxide, calamine, and glycerine. It creates a thin dressing, ideal for the above-knee amputation limb because there is minimal medial bulk. As with a plaster dressing, an Unna bandage is applied professionally, obviating problems of patient compliance. If an immediate or early prosthesis is desired, a plaster or plastic socket will have to be made to support the pylon assembly.

Air Splints
The most common type of air splint consists of two layers of flexible plastic joined at the edges; donning is aided with an anterior zipper. The clinician inserts the amputation limb into the plastic, then inflates the splint. Because air is fluid, pressure in the splint is always uniform. One may supplement the splint with an aluminum frame to permit bipedal ambulation. The bulkiness of the splint compels the wearer to stand and walk with a moderately wide base. The thin plastic is subject to punctures.

Elastic Fabric

The least compression is provided by elastic fabric, whether in bandage or sock form. Both types tend to dislodge when the patient moves, requiring that they be reapplied frequently. The dressing may be an elastic "shrinker" sock or elastic bandage.

Elastic Socks
Socks are manufactured in various lengths and widths, in cylindrical and conical models to suit below- and above-knee amputation limbs. The fabric provides maximum compression distally with progressively less compression proximally. They are relatively easy to apply; however, the sock is difficult to suspend, even with a garter belt, on flabby above-knee amputation limbs. Successively smaller socks must be worn to maintain effective compression.

Sock selection is based on specific measurements.

Below-Knee

1. *Distal circumference:* 5 cm from the medial end of the amputation limb.
2. *Proximal circumference:* 10 cm above the medial tibial plateau.
3. *Length:* Medial end of the amputation limb to the medial tibial plateau, plus 10 cm.

Above-Knee

1. *Distal circumference:* 5 cm above the medial end of amputation limb.
2. *Proximal circumference:* Groin at the level of the adductor tendon.
3. *Length:* Medial end to the adductor tendon.

Elastic Bandage
An inexpensive material, elastic bandage must be removed and reapplied every 4 hours during the day, particularly before upright activities and at bedtime, or when it bunches or is no longer snug. Bandage should never remain on the limb for more

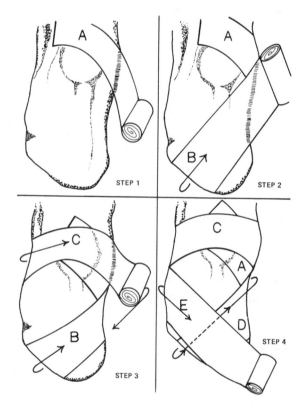

than 24 hours without rewrapping. If the patient complains of throbbing in the amputation limb, the bandage should be removed and reapplied with less tension. It should be washed in warm sudsy water, rinsed thoroughly, and dried on a flat surface. A bandage that has lost its elasticity or is wrinkled should be discarded.

Tension in the bandage should be about two thirds of its maximum stretch. Compression should be greater distally, with layers overlapping about half of the bandage width on each turn. Safety pins are the most effective anchor.

Below-Knee. 8 to 10 cm wide bandage

1. Patient should be supine or sitting, with the knee extended.
2. Start with an oblique turn (step 1).
3. Proceed posteriorly to the lateral distal aspect of the limb, gently pulling the bandage obliquely to lift the tissues, over the anterodistal aspect (step 2).
4. Run the bandage posteriorly to the knee, then anteriorly, and superiorly to the patella (step 3).

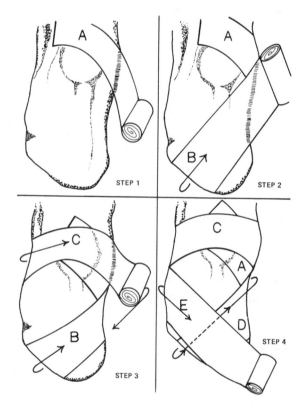

5. Repeat steps 2 and 3 until most of the bandage is used.
6. Make oblique and figure 8 turns to finish the bandage (step 4).

Long Above-Knee. Two or three 10 to 15 cm wide bandages

1. Patient should be supine with the thigh extended; or lying on the intact side with that knee and hip flexed for stability, and the thigh extended; or sitting on the edge of the bed or chair.
2. Begin with an oblique turn on the anterior aspect of the amputation limb (step 1).

3. Combine figure 8 and oblique turns until firm compression is obtained distally (steps 2 and 3).
4. Return to step 1. Bandage should be high in the groin to prevent adductor roll, medial redundant tissue.
5. Make oblique and modified figure of 8 turns on the amputation limb to finish the bandage.

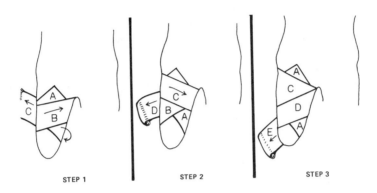

STEP 1   STEP 2   STEP 3

Short or Flabby Above-Knee

1. Patient should be supine with the thigh extended; or lying on the intact side with that knee and hip flexed for stability, and the thigh extended; or sitting on the edge of the bed or chair.
2. Begin with a hip spica (step 1). Place the bandage on the sound side between the iliac crest and the waist. Roll the bandage around the pelvis. Pass over the contralateral iliac crest, obliquely across the midline of the body and over the ipsilateral greater trochanter. Run the bandage posteroproximally, pulling the limb into adduction. Continue to the proximomedial aspect, keeping the bandage high in the groin to avoid adductor roll. Pull the bandage up and out to the proximolateral aspect.
3. Continue wrapping the bandage obliquely from the posteroproximal medial aspect of the thigh anteriorly to cover the lateral end of the amputation limb (step 2).
4. Combine oblique and modified figure 8 turns until firm compression is obtained and the bandage is entirely used (step 3).

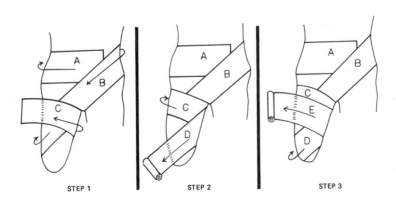

STEP 1   STEP 2   STEP 3

Massage and Hygiene

The therapist should instruct the patient in procedures to decrease hypersensitivity of the limb. Gentle touching and patting of the amputation limb can progress to vigorous massage. When the suture line is healed, deep friction massage can be initiated to lessen adhesions. A compressive dressing also decreases skin hypersensitivity. The patient should not get the dressing wet, nor put anything inside the dressing. Articles used for scratching can injure delicate skin.

The amputation limb should be washed with mild soap, rinsed, and allowed to dry thoroughly prior to prosthetic wear. Bathing at night ensures that the skin will be dry in the morning. Soaking for long periods promotes edema. Safety devices in the bathroom, such as grab bars and a shower chair, may be required. Powder should be used sparingly and lotions, moisturizers, and creams avoided because they may cause dermatitis.

Mobility

The wheelchair designed for individuals with lower limb amputations has a longer base of support, which prevents the chair from tipping backward. It should include swing-out footrests to support the sound leg and to reduce pressure on the posterior thigh from the above-knee socket or the thigh corset on a below-knee prosthesis. Footrests are not necessary for the patient with bilateral amputation who does not wear prostheses. The wheelchair may be needed temporarily until the individual masters prosthetic use or may be a permanent adjunct. Agile persons with unilateral amputation may be taught to hop or use crutches with a prosthesis.

PROSTHETIC MANAGEMENT

To derive the maximum benefit from a prosthesis, a patient must understand how the prosthesis functions, how to don it, and how to control it. Without sound training, few people achieve optimum function from the prosthesis. Individuals must learn efficient control of the amputation limb and prosthesis in daily, occupational, and recreational pursuits. Improper fit or malfunction of the prosthesis impedes training. Consequently, the assessment procedures outlined in Chapter 12 are a prerequisite to prosthetic training.

The time required for training depends on the complexity of the prosthesis and the physical and mental condition of the patient. Cardiac disease, diabetes, multiple amputations, and skin disorders prolong training. Training can be terminated when the following criteria are met:

1. The patient has reached the highest functional level consistent with the individual's physical, mental, and prosthetic status.
2. The patient tolerates wearing the prosthesis long enough to achieve maximum function.
3. The patient feels confident with the prosthesis.
4. The amputation limb presents no open or irritated areas.

Donning

Independent donning is essential if the patient is to wear the prosthesis on a regular basis following discharge from the training program.

Partial Foot, Syme's, Below-Knee, and Knee-Disarticulation Prostheses

The amputation limb should be protected with a sock of appropriate material and thickness. The prosthesis should be worn with a pair of shoes in good repair—particularly the heels, which should be of a height that suits the specific prosthetic foot. These prostheses may be donned by the seated patient; however, the thigh corset should be fastened when the user stands in order to lodge the amputation limb completely in the socket. If the prosthesis has a removable liner, it should be donned prior to inserting the limb into the socket.

Above-Knee Prostheses

Donning the prosthesis with total suction suspension is usually done while the person stands. A pull sock, elastic bandage, or nylon stocking is applied so that it reaches the groin on the amputated side. The patient inserts the distal end of the pulling fabric through the valve hole, then alternately shifts weight from the prosthesis to the sound limb while pulling the fabric entirely out of the valve hole. When the limb is firmly seated, the individual replaces the valve. Alternatively, one may lubricate the thigh with lotion or powder, then push into the socket.

If the prosthesis has partial suction suspension, the patient dons a sock, inserts the limb into the socket, draws the end of the sock through the valve hole, and pulls until the thigh is lodged properly. The sock end is then tucked into the socket, the valve installed, and the Silesian bandage or pelvic belt fastened.

A prosthesis suspended without suction merely requires that the sock-covered thigh be placed in the socket and the pelvic belt buckled.

Hip-Disarticulation and Hemipelvectomy Prostheses

These devices may be donned in the standing or sitting position. The patient wears a sock or an undershirt tailored to cover the amputation limb, which is inserted into the socket, after which the socket may be fastened.

Ambulation

Chapter 11, Functional Activities for One-Sided Involvement, details procedures for training the patient with unilateral amputation to transfer, balance, walk, and climb stairs and curbs.

Tables 4–1 and 4–2 indicate prosthetic and anatomic causes for gait deviations exhibited by individuals wearing below- and above-knee prostheses. Refer to Chapter 12 for comprehensive evaluation of above- and below-knee checkout forms.

TABLE 4–1. Below-knee Prosthetic Gait Analysis

Deviation	Prosthetic Causes	Anatomic Causes
Excessive knee flexion in early stance	Insufficient plantarflexion Stiff heel cushion or plantar bumper Excessive socket flexion Socket malaligned too far anteriorly Excessive posterior placement of cuff tabs.	Knee flexion contracture Weak Quadriceps
Insufficient knee flexion in early stance	Excessive plantarflexion Soft heel cushion or plantar bumper Insufficient socket flexion Socket malaligned too far posteriorly	Pain at anterodistal aspect of amputation limb Weak quadriceps Extensor spasticity Knee arthritis
Excessive lateral thrust	Excessive inset of foot Excessive socket adduction	
Medial thrust	Outset of foot Insufficient socket adduction	
Early knee flexion in late stance "drop off"	Insufficient plantarflexion Distal end of keel or toe break misplaced posteriorly Soft dorsiflexion stop Excessive socket flexion Socket malaligned too far anteriorly Excessive posterior placement of cuff tabs	Knee flexion contracture
Delayed knee flexion in late stance "walking uphill"	Excessive plantarflexion Distal end of keel or toe break misplaced anteriorly Stiff dorsiflexion stop Insufficient socket flexion Socket malaligned too far posteriorly	Extensor spasticity Knee arthritis

From Edelstein, JE: Prosthetic assessment and management. In O'Sullivan, SB and Schmitz, TJ (eds): Physical Rehabilitation: Assessment and Treatment, ed 2. FA Davis, Philadelphia, 1988, p 423, with permission.

TABLE 4–2. Above-knee Prosthetic Gait Analysis

Deviation	Prosthetic Causes	Anatomic Causes
Lateral trunk bending	Short prosthesis Inadequate lateral wall adduction Sharp or excessively high medial wall Malalignment in abduction	Weak abductors Abduction contracture Hip pain Very short amputation limb Instability
Wide walking base (abducted gait)	Long prosthesis Excessive abduction of hip joint Inadequate lateral wall adduction Sharp or excessively high medial wall Malalignment in abduction	Abduction contracture Adductor tissue roll Instability
Circumduction	Long prosthesis Excessive stiffness of knee unit Inadequate suspension Small socket Excessive plantarflexion	Abduction contracture Poor knee control
Medial (lateral) whip	Faulty socket contour Malrotation of knee unit	
Rotation of foot on heel strike	Stiff heel cushion or plantar bumper Malrotation of foot	
Uneven heel rise	Inadequate knee friction Lax or taut extension aid	
Terminal swing impact	Insufficient knee friction Taut extension aid	Excessively forceful hip flexion

TABLE 4-2. Above-knee Prosthetic Gait Analysis *Continued*

Deviation	Prosthetic Causes	Anatomic Causes
Foot slap	Soft heel cushion or plantar bumper	
Uneven step length	Faulty socket contour	Weak hip musculature
	Inadequate knee friction	Hip flexion contracture
	Lax or taut extension aid	Instability
Lordosis	Inadequate support from posterior brim	Hip flexion contracture
		Weak hip extensors
	Inadequate socket flexion	
Vaulting	Long prosthesis	Walking speed exceeding that
	Inadequate suspension	for which friction in a
	Inadequate knee friction	sliding friction knee unit
	Excessive plantarflexion	was adjusted
	Small socket	

From Edelstein, JE: Prosthetic assessment and management. In O'Sullivan, SB and Schmitz, TJ (eds): Physical Rehabilitation: Assessment and Treatment, ed 2. FA Davis, Philadelphia, 1988, p 424, with permission.

Care of the Prosthesis

The prosthesis requires conscientious maintenance to provide satisfactory performance. The socket should be washed with mild soap and water, rinsed, and dried nightly. The patient should avoid contacting any portion of the prosthesis with sharp objects. The foot-ankle assembly and the shoe should be kept clean and dry. The above-knee prosthesis that has a fluid-controlled knee unit should be stored upright. The suction valve should be removed at night to allow air to circulate through the socket. The valve and its receptacle should be brushed clean. The prosthesis should be refurbished by the prosthetist annually or whenever any of its components does not function optimally.

Clean, dry socks should be worn daily. Individuals who perspire profusely need to change socks during the day.

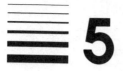

Orthotics

Orthoses are devices worn on the body for therapeutic purposes. They are sometimes designated as braces, or, if intended for temporary use, splints. They are usually made by orthotists, college graduates who are certified by the American Board for Certification in Prosthetics and Orthotics. Some physical therapists and physical therapist assistants construct temporary orthoses or apply prefabricated ones. The most frequently prescribed orthoses will be described, with indication of their relative advantages and drawbacks.

FUNCTIONS

Orthoses apply forces that support weakened segments by resisting gravity, assist joint motion, or counteract deforming forces provided by gravity or the action of antagonistic muscles.

Lower-Limb Orthoses

The patient with paralysis of one or both lower limbs may require orthoses to prevent the weak foot from dragging during the swing phase of gait or to resist inadvertent knee flexion. Paralysis may result from peripheral neuropathy, such as a severance of the sciatic nerve, or central neuropathy, including poliomyelitis, spinal cord injury, and cerebral trauma or vascular accident. Other indications for orthoses include muscular dystrophy, multiple sclerosis, and spina bifida. Those with extensive paralysis may benefit from orthoses that stabilize the hips, as well as the knees and ankles, thereby permitting standing and perhaps ambulation. An individual who presents with deformity of the foot, ankle, or knee joints may be provided with an orthosis that introduces stabilizing or corrective forces. Joint pain resulting from trauma or arthritis may be reduced by an orthosis that protects the part from unwanted stress. Patients with fractures may have an orthosis to limit injurious forces to the fracture site.

Trunk Orthoses

Orthoses may be prescribed to support a trunk that is paralyzed by poliomyelitis or spinal cord injury. Some patients with low back pain find relief from an orthosis that reduces motion and stress on trunk muscles and intervertebral disks. Similarly, individuals with traumatic or arthritic neck pain may benefit from an orthosis that limits motion or retains body heat to aid healing. Children with scoliosis or kyphosis may wear orthoses to limit the extent of deformity.

74

FOOT ORTHOSES

A shoe prescribed to apply specific forces to the foot may be considered as a foot orthosis. A basic shoe may be modified by the addition of external or internal components to enhance its capacity to reduce pain by transferring weight-bearing stresses to pressure-tolerant areas and by protecting painful areas from contact with the shoe. Comfort and mobility can be improved by realigning a flexible segment or providing additional contact area for feet with rigid deformity. Shoes also can be altered to equalize leg length when discrepancy exists. They also serve as the foundation of more extensive orthoses. Each portion of the shoe can contribute to its therapeutic effectiveness.

Shoe Parts

Upper

The upper covers the dorsum of the foot. The anterior portion usually contains lace stays with eyelets for laces. The Blucher pattern has a separation between the anterior margins of the lace stay that provides a wide inlet, making the shoe easy to don and adjust. These considerations are especially pertinent for individuals with edema or spastic or flaccid paralysis.

Low quarter Blucher shoe. (From Edelstein, JE: Orthotic assessment and management. In O'Sullivan, SB and Schmitz, TJ (eds): Physical Rehabilitation: Assessment and Treatment, ed 2. FA Davis, Philadelphia, 1988, p 591, with permission.)

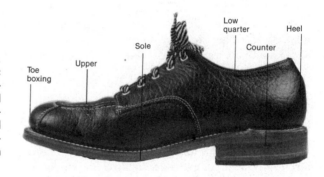

The posterior portion of the upper may terminate below or above the malleoli. A low shoe is less expensive, faster to don, and does not restrict ankle or foot motion. A high shoe is required to cover the foot with fixed equinus, as well as to support an unstable foot. If the patient is wearing a plastic orthosis molded about the ankle, then a high shoe is unnecessary.

Sole

A rubber sole, which absorbs shock and provides good traction, is suitable for a shoe to be worn with a plastic or metal insert. If the shoe is to be used with a riveted attachment for an ankle-foot or more extensive orthosis, then the sole should have leather outer and inner constituents. Between the two soles is a metal plate that receives the rivets. A leather sole is easier to augment with external modifications.

Heel

The heel usually is rigid with a rubber base. Ordinarily, a broad, low heel is preferable for most clinical purposes. A high heel shifts weight to the forefoot and may disturb ankle, knee, and hip control. A heel lift may be required for individuals with a short leg, calcaneal pain, or fixed equinus.

Reinforcements

The counter, made of firm leather, reinforces the upper in the vicinity of the anatomic heel. The patient with pes valgus should have a shoe with a long medial counter, which will resist the tendency of the foot to sag medially.

Most shoes with an inner and outer sole have a shank, which reinforces the sole under the metatarsals. If the shoe is to have a riveted orthotic attachment, then a steel shank is required so that the rivets can fasten securely.

Toe boxing reinforces the anterior portion of the upper. The individual with hammertoes or similar deformities should have a shoe with a high toe box to avoid abrading the digits.

Last

The last is the solid form, or its computerized replica, over which the shoe is manufactured. Although the last itself remains in the factory, the shape that the last imparts to the shoe determines the shoe's comfort. Shoes having the same numerical designation of length will fit differently if they were constructed over different lasts. Consequently, the clinician should judge the fit of the shoe on each foot by direct inspection, rather than by relying on the size. Patients with deformed feet require shoes made over special lasts. For example, the individual with rigid pes varus needs an inflare lasted shoe.

Special Shoes

A great variety of shoes are manufactured. The person who will be wearing a shoe insert may need an extra-depth shoe, in which the upper is spacious enough for the insert. The individual who has difficulty tying laces may appreciate pressure closures, either in a cinch or a flap design. If the toes are markedly deformed, then a shoe with an upper treated with plastic may accommodate the foot; this type of upper can be warmed with a heat gun, then shaped to conform to the contour of the foot. For the patient with healing foot ulcers, a shoe having a polyethylene foam upper and a resilient sole shields the foot, permitting the wearer to remain somewhat active.

Shoe Modifications

The therapeutic effectiveness of the shoe can be enhanced by bars, wedges, and other components that are attached externally or internally to the shoe, or by an insert placed inside the shoe. Occasionally the same disorder can be managed with either an internal or an external modification. An internal modification applies force directly on the foot and, because it is attached to the shoe, it will not displaced. It occupies room in the shoe; consequently, if the shoe fits snugly, the addition of an internal modification may crowd the foot. Another disadvantage of an internal modification is that it cannot be used with other shoes. A similar biomechanical effect is achieved with an insert that also contacts the foot and is hidden from public view; it can be used in any shoe having the same last. An insert, however, may slip inside the shoe and may be used in unsuitable shoes, unless the individual is instructed carefully. As with the internal modification, the insert uses space inside the shoe. An external modification known as an overlay does not disturb the fit of the shoe; however, it is conspicuous, it may erode as the user walks, and its force is attenuated by the intervening sole.

Internal Modifications and Inserts

Internal foot orthoses are commonly used for pes valgus and metatarsalgia. An insert may also be used to reduce the pain of a heel spur.

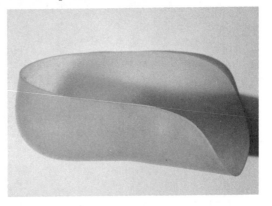

University of California Biomechanics Laboratory (UCBL) insert.

Pes Valgus

If the foot is flexible, it can be held in better alignment with a longitudinal arch support such as the University of California Biomechanics Laboratory (UCBL) insert. This semirigid plastic orthosis is molded over a plaster model of the foot taken with the foot in maximum correction. The UCBL insert applies medially directed force on the heel and laterally and superiorly directed force on the midfoot. The side walls of the insert encompass the heel, thereby applying stabilizing forces to it. A less expensive orthosis is the scaphoid pad, which applies force in a lateral direction against the sustentaculum tali and the navicular tuberosity. The resilient or semirigid pad may be glued inside the shoe or molded into an insert.

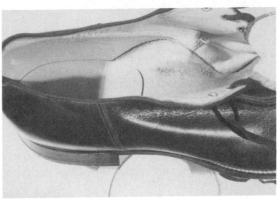

Leather scaphoid pad glued inside the shoe.

Fixed pes valgus may be accommodated with a rubber scaphoid pad, which increases the support area to lessen pressure and absorb shock.

Metatarsalgia

A metatarsal pad is a domed component that transfers weight-bearing pressure from the painful metatarsophalangeal joints to the less sensitive metatarsal shafts. The pad may be an internal modification affixed to the inner sole or can be incorporated in an insert.

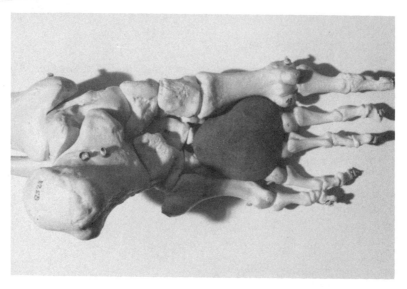

Rubber metatarsal pad. Whether used as an internal modification or as part of an insert, the pad should be oriented as shown on the skeleton.

Heel Spur

A resilient rubber or plastic pad wedged to slope anteriorly can benefit the patient with a heel spur. The pad reduces load on the painful heel. Heel spur pads also have an excavation under the spur to minimize pressure there.

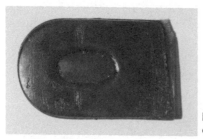

Plastic heel spur pad inferior aspect. Note the depression for spur.

External Modifications

Components on the outside of the shoe can also alleviate some of the discomfort of pes valgus and metatarsalgia, as well as compensate for leg length inequality.

Pes Valgus

A medial heel wedge shifts rearfoot load laterally. The wedge may be incorporated in a Thomas heel, the anterior border of which extends forward on the medial side to supplement the wedge. Occasionally the shoe may include a sole wedge to improve foot alignment.

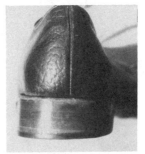

Medial heel wedge.

Metatarsalgia

In place of the metatarsal pad, or in addition to it, the shoe may have a leather metatarsal bar fixed to the sole immediately posterior to the metatarsophalangeal joints. The bar shifts load from the joints to the metatarsal shafts.

Short Leg

The patient with a leg length difference usually walks better with a shoe lift equal to the discrepancy, minus 1 cm. Part of the lift, as much as 0.8 cm, can be placed inside the shoe. The remainder is added to the sole and heel often with lightweight balsa wood, cork, or plastic.

ANKLE-FOOT ORTHOSES

Components of ankle-foot orthoses (AFOs) are a distal attachment, ankle control, foot control, uprights, and band. See figure on page 80.

Distal Attachments

The foundation for an AFO is either an insert worn inside the shoe or a metal fixture riveted to the shoe.

Shoe Insert

An insert or footplate is an excellent distal orthotic attachment. Modifications such as a longitudinal arch support or metatarsal pad can be incorporated in the insert. The insert facilitates donning the orthosis, which can be separated from the shoe. In addition, the patient can wear the AFO in any shoe made on the same last as the one for which the orthosis was originally made. Athletic shoes, for example, are often suitable with an insert attachment. The shoe, although separate, is an integral part of the AFO: consequently, the shoe upper should cover most of the dorsum of the foot.

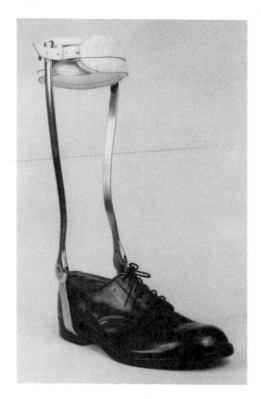

Metal and leather ankle-foot orthosis with stirrup attachment. (From Edelstein, JE: Orthotic assessment and management. In O'Sullivan, SB and Schmitz, TJ (eds): Physical Rehabilitation: Assessment and Treatment, ed 2. FA Davis, Philadelphia, 1988, p 595, with permission.)

Disadvantages of the insert attachment are its reduction of shoe volume, necessitating selecting a sufficiently roomy shoe, and the greater initial expense of the custom-made attachment. The patient who cannot be relied on to wear the orthosis with a suitable shoe should not have an insert attachment.

Riveted Attachments

Steel components can be riveted to the shoe, providing there is a steel shoe shank to accept the rivets.

Stirrups

Stirrups are the most common riveted attachment. Steel is bent into a "U" shape. With a stirrup, the orthotic ankle axis is in line with the anatomic joint. The combination of steel stirrup and steel shank makes the AFO heavier than one with a plastic insert. Stirrups are less expensive components; however, the cost savings will be lost when the wearer obtains replacement shoes, for the stirrup must be transferred from the old to the new shoes.

Solid Stirrup. This attachment consists of one piece of steel, the center portion of which is riveted to the shoe shank. The solid stirrup provides maximum stability of the orthosis on the shoe; however, donning is complicated because the patient cannot detach the shoe from the rest of the orthosis. See figure on page 81.

Split Stirrup. Constituents of the split stirrup are a box caliper, a receptacle that is riveted to the shoe, and medial and lateral arms that fit into the center piece. The

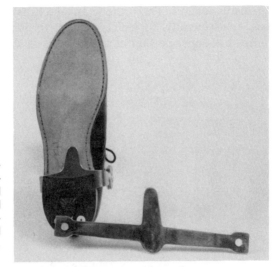

Steel solid stirrup. Note the placement on the shoe sole. (From Edelstein, JE: Orthotic assessment and
management. In O'Sullivan, SB and
Schmitz, TJ (eds): Physical Rehabilitation: Assessment and Treatment, ed
2. FA Davis, Philadelphia, 1988,
p 592, with permission.)

split stirrup enables the patient to detach the shoe from the proximal portion of the
orthosis, simplifying donning, and offering the possibility of interchanging shoes if
the other shoes are equipped with a box caliper. The drawbacks of the split stirrup are
added bulk and weight and the risk that the medial or lateral arm might slip out of
the caliper inadvertently.

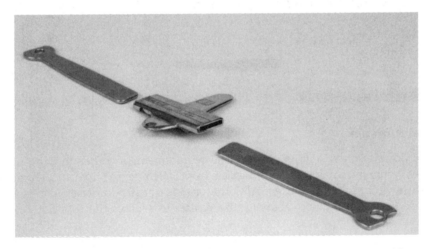

Steel split stirrup. (From Edelstein, JE: Orthotic assessment and management. In O'Sullivan, SB and Schmitz, TJ (eds): Physical Rehabilitation: Assessment and Treatment, ed 2.
FA Davis, Philadelphia, 1988, p 593, with permission.)

Caliper

Also a riveted attachment, the caliper consists of a metal tube on the sole into
which fit tonglike uprights. The caliper facilitates donning the orthosis, because the
shoe can be detached easily; as with the split stirrup, however, there is the chance
that the caliper might dislodge unexpectedly. The caliper presents a serious drawback

for many patients. The orthotic ankle axis is considerably lower than the anatomic axis. Consequently, for AFOs permitting dorsiflexion or plantarflexion, the caliper causes the upper portion of the orthosis to slide on the wearer's leg.

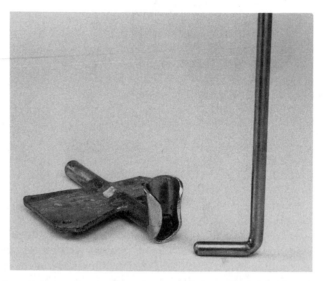

Steel caliper. (From Edelstein, JE: Orthotic assessment and management. In O'Sullivan, SB and Schmitz, TJ (eds): Physical Rehabilitation: Assessment and Treatment, ed 2. FA Davis, Philadelphia, 1988, p 593, with permission.)

Ankle Controls

The AFO is usually prescribed to assist or limit ankle plantarflexion or dorsiflexion.

Motion Assistance

Assisting dorsiflexion is a frequent orthotic requirement, in order to prevent the patient with paralyzed dorsiflexor muscles from catching the toe and stumbling during the swing phase of gait. An AFO that assists dorsiflexion also permits slight plantarflexion in early stance, allowing the wearer to achieve the foot-flat position easily.

Posterior Leaf Spring

The simplest dorsiflexion assistance is provided by the posterior leaf spring AFO. This is a plastic insert appliance with a semirigid posterior upright that yields slightly at heel contact and recoils when the brace is unloaded in swing phase. See figure on page 83.

Dorsiflexion Spring Assist

The medial and lateral arms of the stirrup can include a coil spring that is compressed in early stance and recoils in swing phase. To eliminate motion assistance, the clinician can adjust the springiness of the dorsiflexion spring assist or remove the spring. The component is bulky.

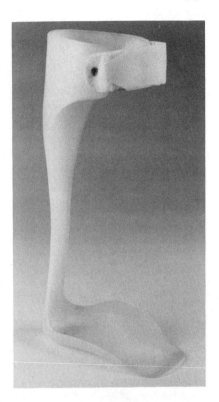

Plastic posterior leaf spring ankle-foot orthosis. (From Edelstein, JE: Orthotic assessment and management. In O'Sullivan, SB and Schmitz, TJ (eds): Physical Rehabilitation: Assessment and Treatment, ed 2. FA Davis, Philadelphia, 1988, p 594, with permission.)

Motion Limitation

Rather than assisting dorsiflexion, one may choose to restrict plantarflexion. Joint designs are also available that limit dorsiflexion or plantarflexion or both. See figure on page 84.

Posterior Stop

A posterior stop may be part of the side pieces of a stirrup or may be in a pair of metal joints attached to an insert. The stop limits plantarflexion in both swing phase (to prevent foot drag) and stance phase (when plantarflexion ordinarily occurs). The patient fitted with a posterior stop achieves the foot-flat position in early stance by flexing the knee or shifting weight forward. See figure on page 85.

Anterior Stop

An anterior stop in a metal joint restricts dorsiflexion, which can aid the individual with paralyzed plantarflexors during late stance.

Anterior and Posterior Limitation

Both plantarflexion and dorsiflexion may be prevented by a plastic solid ankle AFO with its borders in front of the malleoli. If a partial range of motion is desired, the plastic orthosis can be hinged and fitted with limited motion joints. The solid ankle orthosis also restricts mediolateral motion. Limited motion joints can also be used with a steel stirrup. Another way of controlling sagittal plane motion is with the use of the bichannel adjustable ankle lock. Its anterior and posterior springs may be replaced by metal pins, the length of which determines the amount of motion permitted by the orthosis.

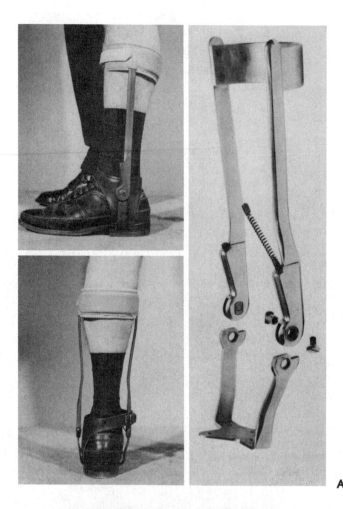

A

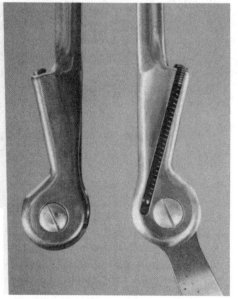

B

Steel dorsiflexion spring assist. A, Note the position of the spring in the channel. B, Component is incorporated in ankle-foot orthosis. (From Fishman, S, et al: Lower-limb orthoses. In American Academy of Orthopaedic Surgeons: Atlas of Orthotics, ed. 2. CV Mosby, St Louis, 1985, pp 200, 203, with permission.)

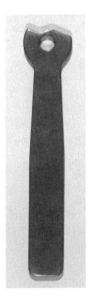

Steel stirrup with posterior stop at its proximal end. Stop is to the left.

Foot Controls

Solid Ankle

A plastic, solid ankle AFO provides maximum control of all motions of the ankle and the rearfoot and midfoot. This design conforms to the contour of the foot and leg, is lightweight, and cannot loosen to become noisy. As is the case with all insert orthoses, the solid ankle AFO requires a spacious shoe.

Valgus and Varus Correction Straps

Valgus or varus control with the orthosis having metal uprights requires the use of a leather strap. For valgus control, the triangular part of the strap is attached to the medial side of the shoe, near the sole. The upper portion of the triangle should cover the medial malleolus. The strap portion is then buckled around the lateral upright to

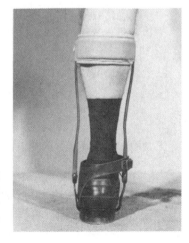

Valgus correction strap incorporated in metal and leather ankle-foot orthosis. (From Fishman, S, et al: Lower-limb orthoses. In American Academy of Orthopaedic Surgeons: Atlas of Orthotics, ed 2. CV Mosby, St Louis, 1985, p 200, with permission.)

apply a laterally directed force on the foot. A varus control strap is the reverse design. Straps are more adjustable than the solid ankle AFO but depend on the compliance of the wearer to buckle them correctly. Straps also take more time to don and are more conspicuous.

Uprights

The AFO has either one or two uprights extending from the shoe insert or the stirrup to the band. The uprights determine the leverage for the orthosis; consequently, higher uprights minimize proximal pressure better than shorter ones.

Plastic Uprights

The plastic AFO may have a single posterior upright or a calf shell. These uprights are form-fitting and lightweight. Well-finished plastic uprights will not injure insensitive skin. Because they are not readily adjustable, they may be unsuitable for patients with edema.

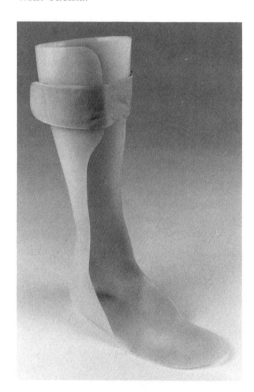

Plastic ankle-foot orthosis with a solid ankle and a calf shell. (From Edelstein, JE: Orthotic assessment and management. In O'Sullivan, SB and Schmitz, TJ (eds): Physical Rehabilitation: Assessment and Treatment, ed 2. FA Davis, Philadelphia, 1988, p 594, with permission.)

Posterior Upright

The posterior leaf spring AFO has a polyethylene upright extending from the shoe insert to the upper leg. The semirigid plastic post assists dorsiflexion in swing phase and permits slight plantarflexion in early stance phase. The posterior upright does not offer mediolateral foot control, although a specially contoured insert can contribute to foot stability.

Calf Shell

The insert orthosis may feature a polypropylene or polyethylene shell covering the posterior leg. The shell terminates immediately in front of the malleoli, thereby restricting all ankle and rearfoot and midfoot motion.

Metal Uprights

Steel or aluminum alloy uprights can be used with a stirrup or caliper attachment, or joined to an insert. Metal uprights may be embedded in a plastic calf shell or left exposed. The latter configuration is required by the individual who has volume fluctuation of the leg. Exposed uprights are conspicuous and somewhat bulky.

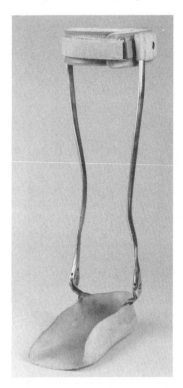

Ankle-foot orthosis with plastic insert, aluminum alloy uprights, and leather upholstered calf band. (From Edelstein, JE: Orthotic assessment and management. In O'Sullivan, SB and Schmitz, TJ (eds): Physical Rehabilitation: Assessment and Treatment, ed 2. FA Davis, Philadelphia, 1988, p 593, with permission.)

Band

The upper portion of the AFO may be a calf band, anterior band, or patellar tendon–bearing brim.

Calf Band

Most AFOs have a calf band that terminates immediately below the level of the fibular head to avoid impinging the peroneal nerve. Orthoses with a plastic upright have the band either as a continuation of the posterior upright or as the proximal border of the calf shell. The plastic band provides a large contact area to minimize pressure.

Orthoses with exposed metal uprights have a metal calf band upholstered in leather. Its position and biomechanical effect are similar to plastic bands. An AFO with a calf band is easier to don than those having other types of bands. Calf bands apply anteriorly directed force in the vicinity of the knee, tending to cause the knee to flex.

Anterior Band

An anterior band, usually plastic, terminates just distal to the tibial tubercle. Used in association with a solid ankle AFO, the anterior band applies a posteriorly directed force near the knee, assisting knee extension.

Patellar Tendon–Bearing Brim

Occasionally, a patient with a painful or very unstable ankle may benefit from a patellar tendon–bearing brim. It resembles the proximal portion of a below-knee prosthetic socket, although the orthotic contours are not as markedly defined. Used with a limited motion ankle, the brim bears some weight, thus reducing the stress on the distal part of the limb.

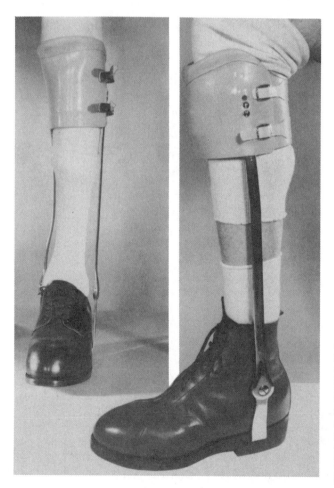

Ankle-foot orthosis with stirrup, steel uprights, and plastic patellar-tendon-bearing brim. (From Fishman, S, et al: Lower-limb orthoses. In American Academy of Orthopaedic Surgeons: Atlas of Orthotics, ed. 2. CV Mosby, St Louis, 1985, p 208, with permission.)

KNEE-ANKLE-FOOT ORTHOSES

More extensive bracing supports individuals with paralysis or deformity of the knee and ankle. A knee-ankle-foot orthosis (KAFO) may be prescribed to control the knee in the sagittal or frontal planes, or both planes. KAFOs have higher uprights with hinges, which restrict transverse and frontal plane motion. The infrastructure of the KAFO is similar to that of either a plastic/metal or a leather/metal AFO, and the suprastructure usually consists of one or two thigh bands joining the medial and lateral thigh uprights.

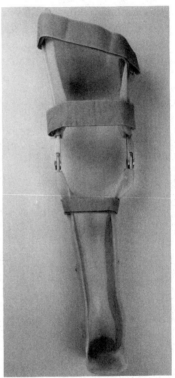

Plastic and metal knee-ankle-foot orthosis. (From Edelstein, JE: Orthotic assessment and management. In O'Sullivan, SB and Schmitz, TJ (eds): Physical Rehabilitation: Assessment and Treatment, ed 2. FA Davis, Philadelphia, 1988, p 597, with permission.)

Sagittal Knee Control

Various joints are manufactured to control knee flexion. Most joints include a lock that blocks all knee motion. The lock ensures stability during stance phase but interferes with swing phase and sitting, when knee flexion is desired. The joints are usually augmented by an anterior pad or band that applies posteriorly directed force to resist knee flexion.

Offset Knee Joint

This unlocked hinge has its axis of rotation more posterior than the axis of the anatomic knee. When the wearer stands, the line of gravity falls anterior to the mechanical hinge, preventing knee flexion. The offset joint does not impede swing phase or sitting. It is ineffective in the presence of knee flexion contracture and when the user stands on a downward-sloping surface.

Knee Locks

Most knee locks are designed for patients full passive knee extension. Special locks are required for those with flexion contracture.

Locks for Fully Mobile Knees

Drop Ring Lock. This is the most common knee lock because it is simple and inexpensive. A ring of metal slips over the proximal and distal uprights at the knee joint to prevent motion. The uprights must be fully extended for the lock to engage. Locks on the medial and lateral uprights provide maximum security. Managing the locks is inconvenient unless the locks have a spring-loaded retention button that permits the person to unlock one upright, then attend to the other one without having the first lock drop again. The buttons also allow the therapist to give the patient a trial period of walking with the knee joints unlocked.

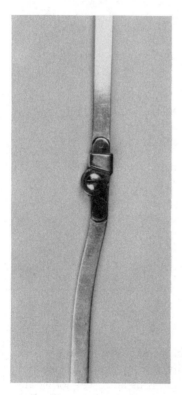

Aluminum alloy upright with drop ring lock. (From Edelstein, JE: Orthotic assessment and management. In O'Sullivan, SB and Schmitz, TJ (eds): Physical Rehabilitation: Assessment and Treatment, ed 2. FA Davis, Philadelphia, 1988, p 596, with permission.)

Pawl Lock with Bail Release. More complex than the drop ring lock, the pawl lock has a spring-loaded pin that fits into a notched disk. The bail, a thin bar of metal passing posteriorly between the medial and lateral pawl locks, permits the patient to unlock both locks by pulling the bail upward. When the knee is fully extended, the springs in the pawl locks recoil to engage the locks. Simultaneous locking and unlocking is convenient for the wearer and ensures maximum orthotic stability, but the bail is bulky and may be jostled into the unlocked position inadvertently.

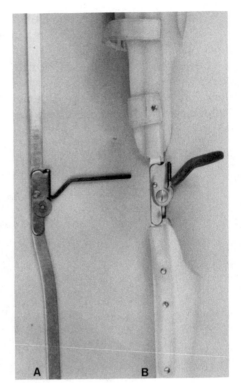

A, Pawl lock with bail release; bail has not yet been bent to curve behind the wearer's knee. B, Component is incorporated in metal and plastic knee-ankle-foot orthosis. (From Edelstein, JE: Orthotic assessment and management. In O'Sullivan, SB and Schmitz, TJ (eds): Physical Rehabilitation: Assessment and Treatment, ed 2. FA Davis, Philadelphia, 1988, p 597, with permission.)

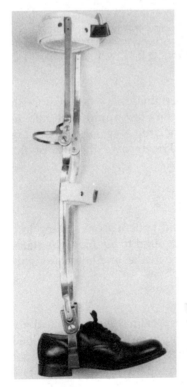

Knee-ankle-foot orthosis with a pawl lock with bail release, plastic prepatellar band, and steel bichannel adjustable ankle lock. (From Edelstein, JE: Orthotic assessment and management. In O'Sullivan, SB and Schmitz, TJ (eds): Physical Rehabilitation: Assessment and Treatment, ed 2. FA Davis, Philadelphia, 1988, p 598, with permission.)

Locks for Knees Having Flexion Contracture

Several locks are manufactured to accommodate flexion contracture, yet provide knee stability.

Serrated Lock. The distal upright of this lock has a serrated disk, which can be set to any angle to match the degree of contracture. The upper portion of the serrated lock has a drop ring lock. Although the component is streamlined, its angular adjustment is not congruent with the anatomic knee.

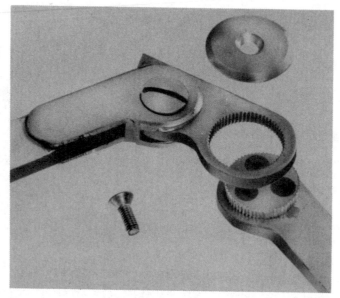

Serrated knee lock. Note the location of the knee hinge and the serrated disk. (From Fishman, S, et al: Lower-limb orthoses. In American Academy of Orthopaedic Surgeons: Atlas of Orthotics, ed. 2. CV Mosby, St Louis, 1985, p 213, with permission.)

Fan Lock. The lower end of the proximal upright terminates in a fan shape with five holes. The clinician screws the distal upright into the most appropriate hole to conform with the contracture. The fan lock includes a drop ring lock. It is more conspicuous than the serrated lock, but its axis lies directly over the axis of the patient's knee.

Anterior Bands and Pad

A knee lock is rarely sufficient to prevent the paralyzed patient from sinking into knee flexion. Consequently, an anterior component is required to augment the stabilizing effect of the lock. The band or pad is attached to the medial and lateral uprights of the KAFO.

Prepatellar Band

A fabric strap or semirigid plastic band over the proximal leg is particularly effective in complementing knee locks. The plastic band must be carefully molded over the tibial tubercle to avoid pressure concentration. The band or strap does not interfere with sitting and is relatively fast to don. If not properly fitted, it can irritate the sensitive skin that lacks much subcutaneous padding.

Suprapatellar Band

The strap or band may lie over the distal thigh. Its biomechanical effect is similar to the prepatellar alternative. It is easier to fit because it is cushioned by the fleshy thigh.

Knee Pad

The traditional leather knee pad, also known as a knee cap, has four straps that are buckled on the proximal and distal portions of the medial and lateral uprights. The straps permit substantial adjustment. Disadvantages of the knee pad are the greater time required for donning, and the need to loosen the straps when the user sits. Otherwise, the pad is apt to restrict knee flexion. When the wearer resumes the standing position, the straps must be retightened.

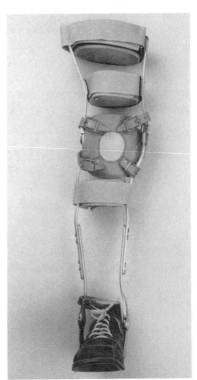

Leather knee pad buckled onto metal and leather knee-ankle-foot orthosis. Note the proximal and distal thigh bands. (From Edelstein, JE: Orthotic assessment and management. In O'Sullivan, SB and Schmitz, TJ (eds): Physical Rehabilitation: Assessment and Treatment, ed 2. FA Davis, Philadelphia, 1988, p 597, with permission.)

Frontal Knee Control

The patient with marked genu valgum or varum requires laterally or medially directed force, respectively, to control the deformity.

Plastic Calf Band Extension

An effective way of controlling frontal plane knee deformity is by extending the proximal margin of the plastic calf band. For genu valgum, the medial margin of the band terminates above the knee. The semirigid plastic provides firm laterally directed force and does not require that the patient fasten any buckles. The plastic extension must be carefully fitted and is not readily adjusted.

Puller Pad

The basic leather knee pad can be modified by the addition of a fifth strap and additional leather. For genu valgum, the extra strap and leather are on the medial side. The patient buckles the fifth strap on the lateral upright. The strap passes over the popliteal fossa, which may be irritated when the person sits.

Thigh Bands

The KAFO terminates with a plastic or upholstered leather thigh band joining the proximal metal uprights. The band determines the leverage that the KAFO exerts but must be lower than the perineum on the medial side and distal to the greater trochanter laterally. A distal thigh band adds to the stability of the KAFO and may be used in conjunction with the calf band to provide anteriorly directed force to control genu recurvatum.

A polypropylene thigh shell serves the same purpose as the proximal and distal thigh bands. The plastic is impervious to urine and applies pressure over a much larger area than do metal bands. Some individuals complain that the plastic shell retains too much body heat—especially in warm climates.

HIP-KNEE-ANKLE-FOOT AND TRUNK-HIP-KNEE-ANKLE-FOOT ORTHOSES

A hip-knee-ankle-foot orthosis (HKAFO) controls hip motion, in addition to motion of the distal joints. It consists of a pelvic band and hip joints added to a pair of KAFOs. The HKAFO is cumbersome to don, and wearers complain that sitting is uncomfortable even with a well-fitted orthosis. Use of the toilet is complicated by the hip joints, which ordinarily do not permit abduction. Although a pelvic band and a single hip joint can be attached to a KAFO, the orthosis will not control rotary motion of the hip very effectively. See figure on top of page 95.

Pelvic Band

An upholstered metal band may be made to anchor the HKAFO. The band is located between the greater trochanter and the iliac crest on each side. It provides rigidity to the orthosis, as well as being the attachment for the hip joints.

Hip Joints

The typical orthotic hip joint is a metal hinge with a drop ring lock. It restricts motion in all planes. The locked HKAFO limits the user to the drag-to, swing-to, and swing-through gait patterns. Without the drop ring lock, the joint would still control frontal and transverse motion. A two-position hip lock stabilizes the wearer in extension for standing and in 90-degree flexion for sitting. A few individuals wear HKAFOs with abduction hip joints that permit abduction and flexion but block adduction and rotation. See figure at bottom of page 95.

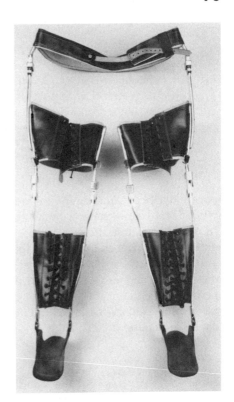

Metal and leather bilateral hip-knee-ankle-foot orthosis. The laced calf and thigh cuffs are time-consuming to don. (From Edelstein, JE: Orthotic assessment and management. In O'Sullivan, SB and Schmitz, TJ (eds): Physical Rehabilitation: Assessment and Treatment, ed 2. FA Davis, Philadelphia, 1988, p 598, with permission.)

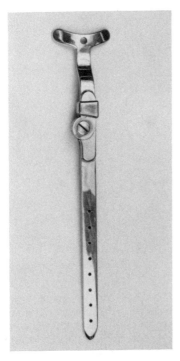

Steel hip joint with drop ring lock. (From Edelstein, JE: Orthotic assessment and management. In O'Sullivan, SB and Schmitz, TJ (eds): Physical Rehabilitation: Assessment and Treatment, ed 2. FA Davis, Philadelphia, 1988, p 598, with permission.)

Trunk Control

Addition of a trunk orthosis converts the HKAFO to a trunk-hip-knee-ankle-foot orthosis (THKAFO). Although this appliance provides maximum stability and is prescribed for patients with paraplegia, it is very difficult to don and is so heavy and cumbersome that few individuals wear it after being discharged from a rehabilitation program. Alternative orthoses provide standing stability, with or without provision for walking.

Standing Frames

Several types of standing frames are manufactured, primarily for children with spina bifida. The frames have a broad base, posterior nonarticulated uprights extending from the base to midtorso, anterior thigh and chest bands, and a posterior thoraco-lumbar band. The child wears ordinary shoes without any stirrups or calipers. Shoes are fastened to the base of the standing frame by straps or springs. The frame is inexpensive and can be adjusted easily to accommodate to the child's growth. It permits the child to stand without crutch support, freeing the hands for play activities. Unlike custom-made THKAFOs, the frame must be worn on the outside of the clothing, making it conspicuous.

Parapodia

An articulated version of the standing frame, the parapodium is also prefabricated with the same stabilizing points, provision for securing the shoes to the base, and the need to be worn over clothing. Parapodia, however, permit the wearer to flex the hip and knee joints to allow sitting, as well as leaning forward to pick objects from the floor.

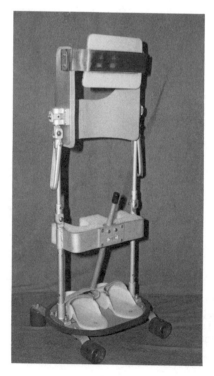

Parapodium. (From Edelstein, JE: Orthotic assessment and management. In O'Sullivan, SB and Schmitz, TJ (eds): Physical Rehabilitation: Assessment and Treatment, ed 2. FA Davis, Philadelphia, 1988, p 600, with permission.)

Some agile children are able to ambulate while wearing parapodia. Without crutches they shift weight to one side and rotate the trunk to advance the opposite side. Movement proceeds in a series of alternate rocking maneuvers. For faster travel, patients use crutches to perform the swing-to or similar gaits.

Reciprocating Gait Orthosis

A custom-made reciprocating gait orthosis (RGO) is an option for children and adults with paraplegia. The RGO consists of a pair of KAFOs attached to a special trunk orthosis that has a pair of metal cables connecting the hip joints. Reciprocal gait, whether two- or four-point, requires use of parallel bars or crutches. When the patient shifts weight to the right limb and transfers substantial load to the hands, the cables advance the left limb. Shifting to the left side advances the right leg. The patient releases the cables and knee locks for sitting. Some RGOs have offset knee joints, eliminating the need to manipulate knee locks. The orthoses have solid ankles to prevent any ankle or foot motion.

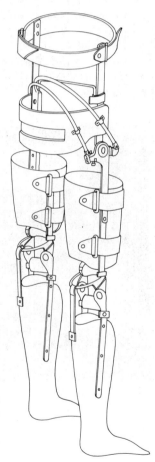

Reciprocating gait orthosis. Note the plastic solid ankles, pawl locks with bail releases, and plastic thigh cuffs. (From Edelstein, JE: Orthotic assessment and management. In O'Sullivan, SB and Schmitz, TJ (eds): Physical Rehabilitation: Assessment and Treatment, ed 2. FA Davis, Philadelphia, 1988, p 599, with permission.)

ParaWalker

Another type of THKAFO designed for individuals with paraplegia is the Para-Walker. Unlike the RGO, it does not have cables. Instead, the hip joints are particularly sturdy so they can withstand the laterally directed force applied as the patient shifts weight from one side to the other. The ParaWalker also permits reciprocal gait.

OTHER LOWER-LIMB ORTHOSES

Although most lower-limb orthoses are prescribed for patients with weakness, other specialized orthoses are sometimes required. Individuals with ankle sprains may benefit from prefabricated splints that afford mediolateral protection. A great many designs of knee orthoses are on the market. They are intended to stabilize the joint, particularly in the presence of sprain of the anterior cruciate ligament. Infants with congenital dislocation of the hips are often fitted with a Pavlik harness that permits the baby to move the hips, knees, and ankles in all directions, except for hip abduction, to retain the femoral head in the acetabulum. Children with Legg-Calvé-Perthes disease usually have an orthosis that maintains the desired position of the femoral head in the hip socket. The most common of these orthoses, the Scottish Rite, consists of a pair of thigh cuffs joined to a pelvic band. The orthosis has stout hip joints set in wide abduction for proper femoral positioning. The hip joints are not locked. Patients with tibial and femoral shaft fractures may be provided with fracture braces, in place of heavy plaster casts. The braces stabilize the fracture site without encumbering the adjacent joint, thereby speeding rehabilitation. Special orthoses are available to apply steady tensile stress to the ankle or knee, which prevents flexion contracture.

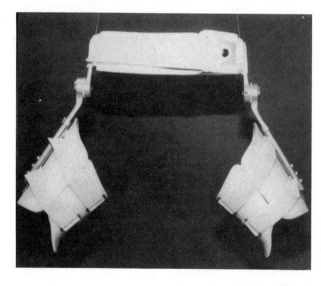

Scottish Rite Legg-Calvé-Perthes hip orthosis. (Courtesy of Durr-Fillauer Medical, Inc., Chattanooga, TN.)

TRUNK ORTHOSES

Orthoses are prescribed for the trunk either to be worn in conjunction with lower-limb bracing or as separate entities. Corsets and rigid orthoses benefit some patients by limiting painful motion, reducing muscular demand, stabilizing weak or sprained structures, or by introducing forces that oppose those tending to cause deformity.

Prolonged use of trunk orthoses is associated with lessened flexibility, muscular atrophy, and psychologic dependence. Consequently, the patient should be reevaluated periodically after receiving an orthosis.

Most orthoses are described by the region covered and the motions controlled. They may be custom-made or prefabricated.

Corsets

Corsets are orthoses that encircle the torso with sturdy fabric. Although the corset often has vertical reinforcements, it does not have horizontal rigid components. The most common corset covers the lumbosacral area. Occasionally, sacroiliac or thoracolumbosacral corsets are prescribed. Corsets relieve low back pain by reminding the wearer to limit irritating motion and by increasing intra-abdominal pressure, thereby decreasing stress on the back extensor muscles. Subjects who wear these orthoses also demonstrate reduced muscular activity.

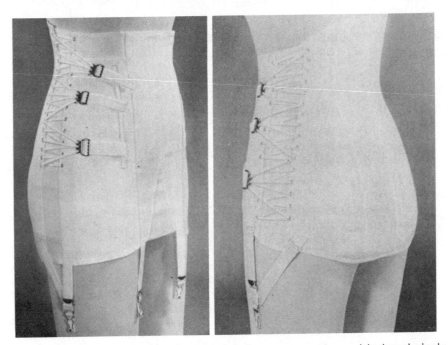

Women's model of a canvas lumbosacral corset. (This corset is provided exclusively by Camp International© 1991 BISSELL Healthcare Corporation.)

Lumbosacral Orthoses

Most rigid orthoses for the lumbosacral region of the trunk include thoracic and pelvic bands made of rigid plastic or metal. The bands are joined by two or more plastic or metal uprights. A fabric abdominal front or a full corset completes the orthosis. Bands, uprights, and abdominal front may be replaced by a plastic jacket encasing the lower trunk.

The thoracic band should lie horizontally on the torso, somewhat below the scapulae to avoid interfering with arm motion. The pelvic band is located between the iliac crests and the greater trochanters. It should not interfere with sitting. Both bands should conform to the contour of the trunk. The abdominal front extends from a point just below the xiphoid process to a point just above the pubic symphysis. The lower margin should be tailored to permit comfortable sitting.

Rigid orthoses impose more motion restriction than do corsets, and are equally effective in increasing intra-abdominal pressure.

Lumbosacral Flexion-Extension Control Orthosis

In addition to the thoracic and pelvic bands and abdominal front, this orthosis includes a pair of posterior uprights located on either side of the vertebral spines. The orthosis limits flexion by a three-point pressure system composed of posteriorly directed force applied by the top and bottom of the abdominal front, and anteriorly directed force from the midpoint of the posterior uprights. Extension control is achieved by anteriorly directed force from the pelvic and thoracic bands, together with posteriorly directed force from the midpoint of the abdominal front.

Lumbosacral Flexion-Extension-Lateral Control Orthosis (Knight Spinal)

This orthosis resembles the preceding one, with the addition of a pair of lateral uprights. Lateral flexion to the right is restricted by pressure from the top and bottom of the right lateral upright and the midsection of the left lateral upright.

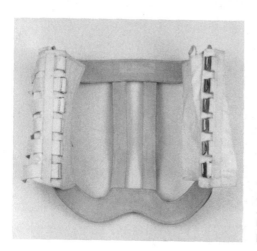

Lumbosacral flexion-extension-lateral control orthosis with leather-upholstered frame and canvas abdominal front. (From Edelstein, JE: Orthotic assessment and management. In O'Sullivan, SB and Schmitz, TJ (eds): Physical Rehabilitation: Assessment and Treatment, ed 2. FA Davis, Philadelphia, 1988, p 601, with permission.)

Lumbosacral Extension-Lateral Control Orthosis (Williams Brace)

Some patients with low back pain benefit from restriction of lumbar hyperextension but do not require flexion control. This orthosis has no posterior uprights that would hamper trunk flexion. Instead, there are oblique lateral uprights to increase the stability of the orthosis. The thoracic band pivots on the lateral uprights to permit unrestrained trunk flexion.

Lumbosacral Flexion-Extension-Lateral-Rotary Control Orthosis

A plastic jacket conforming to the contour of the lower trunk restricts all motions and compresses the abdomen.

Thoracolumbosacral Orthoses

Thoracolumbosacral Flexion-Extension Control Orthosis (Taylor Brace)

This orthosis includes the same pelvic band and abdominal front as used in lumbosacral devices. The posterior uprights are longer, terminating at midscapular level. An interscapular bar between the uprights provides structural stability. Axillary straps pass from each side of the interscapular bar to the front of the shoulder, then back again to the posterior uprights.

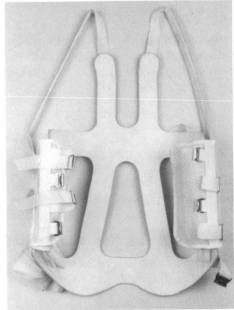

Thoracolumbosacral flexion-extension-lateral control with plastic frame and canvas abdominal front. (From Edelstein, JE: Orthotic assessment and management. In O'Sullivan, SB and Schmitz, TJ (eds): Physical Rehabilitation: Assessment and Treatment, ed 2. FA Davis, Philadelphia, 1988, p 601, with permission.)

Flexion is restricted by a three-point force system composed of posteriorly directed force from the axillary straps and the bottom of the abdominal front, and anteriorly directed force from the midpoint of the posterior uprights. Extension control is furnished by anteriorly directed force from the superior ends of the posterior uprights and the pelvic band, and posteriorly directed force from the midpoint of the abdominal front.

Thoracolumbosacral Flexion-Extension-Lateral Control Orthosis (Knight-Taylor Brace)

This orthosis is a combination of the preceding orthosis and the lumbosacral flexion-extension-lateral control orthosis. The thoracic band takes the place of the interscapular bar.

Thoracolumbosacral Flexion Control Orthosis

Two versions of this orthosis are manufactured. Both types limit flexion with sternal and suprapubic plates imposing posteriorly directed force and a thoracolumbar pad pushing anteriorly. In one version the plates are arranged on a oval frame, and in the other the plates are on the upper and lower ends of a plastic cross, with the posterior pad on the horizontal piece of the cross.

Thoracolumbosacral Flexion-Extension-Lateral-Rotary Control Orthosis

A custom-made or prefabricated plastic jacket limits motion in all directions and increases intra-abdominal pressure.

CERVICAL ORTHOSES

Unlike the preceding orthoses, which are named for the region covered and the motions controlled, cervical orthoses are categorized according to design—namely, collars, post orthoses, and cephalothoracic orthoses. Although the orthoses differ in relative degree of motion control, their generic names do not specify the motions that are limited.

Collars

A collar encircles the neck with flexible or rigid material. It does not limit motion very much but does remind the wearer to avoid abrupt movement. Collars also retain body heat, which can help sprained tissues to heal.

Soft Collar

Usually made of foam rubber or plastic, the soft collar is least restrictive. The resilient material is comfortable to wear and retains body heat very well.

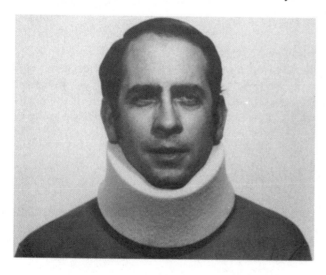

Soft foam rubber collar. (This collar is provided exclusively by Camp International © 1991 BISSELL Healthcare Corporation.)

Firm Collar

Semirigid plastic may constitute a firm collar that reminds the wearer to limit motion in all directions. Prefabricated firm collars usually are adjustable to permit the clinician to fit the patient in the most comfortable attitude of the neck.

Philadelphia Collar

This prefabricated orthosis is made of polyethylene foam that terminates at the lower margin of the chin anteriorly and the occiput posteriorly. The anterior and posterior midlines of the collar are reinforced with a rigid plastic strut. The Philadelphia collar is more restrictively than the soft or firm collar.

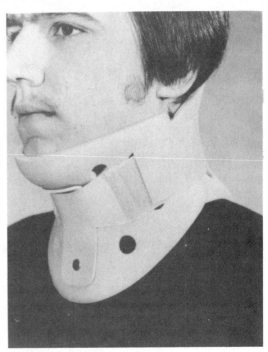

Philadelphia collar. (The Philadelphia collar is provided exclusively by Camp International © 1991 BISSELL Healthcare Corporation.)

Post Orthoses

When greater motion restriction is required, a prefabricated post orthosis is often prescribed. Reinforced pads on the occiput, chin, and chest are connected by adjustable uprights. These orthoses are cooler than collars.

Two-Post Orthosis

This design has an anterior and a posterior post to limit neck flexion and extension.

Four-Post Orthosis

In this model, the anterior and posterior pads are connected by a pair of posts in front and in back. The four-post orthosis is more effective than the two-post one in limiting lateral flexion and rotation of the neck.

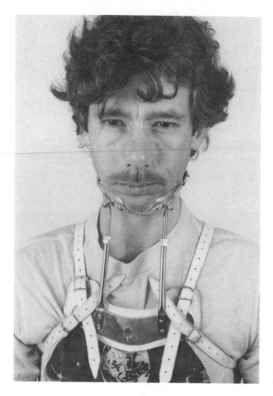

Four post orthosis. Note the two threaded metal anterior posts, leather straps, and leather-upholstered sternal and mandibular supports. (From Edelstein, JE: Orthotic assessment and management. In O'Sullivan, SB and Schmitz, TJ (eds): Physical Rehabilitation: Assessment and Treatment, ed 2. FA Davis, Philadelphia, 1988, p 601, with permission.)

Sterno-Occipito-Mandibular Immobilizer (SOMI)

A special design of a three-post orthosis, the SOMI can be applied to the supine patient without turning the individual. It limits flexion moderately well but offers little extension, lateral flexion, or rotational control.

Cephalothoracic Orthoses

Although post orthoses and the Philadelphia collar encompass parts of the head and thorax, the designation of cephalothoracic is usually reserved for orthoses that contact the superior part of the head and extend to the midchest. Cephalothoracic orthoses restrict motion substantially more than do collars and post orthoses but are more cumbersome.

Halo-Vest Orthosis

A halo is a metal ring stabilized by four pins, which the surgeon secures to holes drilled into the outer portion of the skull. Four posts extend from the halo to a fixture on a vest usually lined with sheepskin which is least apt to ulcerate the insensitive skin of a patient with quadriplegia. The halo vest provides the maximum restriction of motion, vital to prevent dislocation of a cervical fracture. Patients with spinal cord injury may also be fitted with a halo to facilitate early mobilization. The halo is an invasive orthosis. Some patients incur pin site infections with its use.

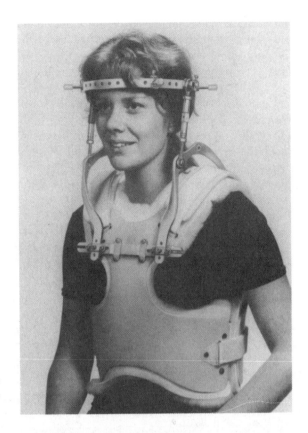

Halo-vest orthosis. (Courtesy Durr-Fillauer Medical, Inc., Chattanooga, TN.)

Minerva Orthosis

Named for the Roman goddess of wisdom who traditionally wore a helmet, the Minerva orthosis is a prefabricated or custom-made orthosis that has a band around the upper skull that leads to a broad section along the back of the neck terminating in a band around the upper torso. The Minerva orthosis compares favorably with the halo-vest orthosis in terms of motion control. It is noninvasive, but some patients object to its warmth.

SCOLIOSIS AND KYPHOSIS CONTROL ORTHOSES

The two most frequently prescribed orthoses for children with scoliosis and kyphosis are the Milwaukee and Boston orthoses. They apply a series of forces designed to prevent the trunk deformity from increasing as the child grows. Active reduction of spinal curvature is encouraged when the wearer moves away from the pads in the orthosis.

Milwaukee Orthosis

This custom-made appliance consists of a snugly fitting plastic or leather pelvic girdle to which are attached an anterior and two posterior uprights that terminate in a rigid ring encircling the upper chest. Corrective pads are strapped to the uprights and girdle.

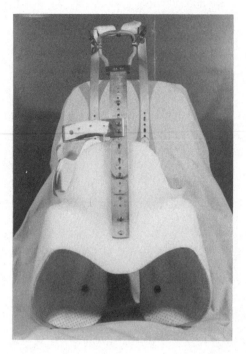

Anterior view of the plastic and metal Milwaukee orthosis.

Boston Orthosis

The basis of the Boston orthosis is a prefabricated plastic module encasing the pelvis and lower thorax. The orthotist fits various pads to counteract the direction of deformity. The Boston orthosis does not extend as high as the Milwaukee one and thus is not as conspicuous. Both are most effective for moderate thoracic, thoracolumbar, and lumbar curves.

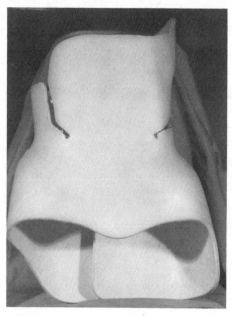

Plastic Boston orthosis.

ORTHOTIC MANAGEMENT

Orthoses should be evaluated on delivery to confirm that they fit and function properly and are well constructed. Particular attention should be directed at the condition of the underlying skin. Orthoses designed to limit motion should be checked to determine the effectiveness of control.

The patient should be instructed in the proper application of the orthosis. Lower-limb orthoses should be fastened snugly enough to provide the desired control force, without undue soft tissue compression. Lumbosacral and thoracolumbosacral appliances are best fastened from the bottom upward to support the abdomen most effectively. Cervical orthoses should be donned so that the neck is in the desired position.

Chapter 8 describes techniques used by individuals who wear a unilateral AFO or KAFO as they balance, walk, and climb stairs and curbs. Chapter 9 outlines the training program for patients wearing bilateral KAFOs, as well as HKAFOs and THKAFOs.

Regular follow-up visits are especially important to ascertain when maximum benefit has been derived from the orthosis and whether changes in design or adjustment are required. Many wearers of lumbosacral corsets and rigid orthoses, as well as those having scoliosis and kyphosis control orthoses, benefit from an individualized exercise program devised to counteract the tendency of the orthosis to limit flexibility and motor power.

CARE OF ORTHOSES

Orthoses deserve proper maintenance to provide the user with best service. The patient should have written instructions outlining basic care procedures.

Shoes and Hose

Shoes should be kept in good repair, with the sole and heel replaced as soon as moderate wear is evident. This is important whether the shoes are attached directly to the proximal portion of the orthosis or are used with an insert. Attention should be paid to maintaining the wedges, bars, and elevations. The patient who tends to strike on the toe may need metal toe plates to preserve the sole. Shoes that are outgrown or distorted interfere with function. Rivets in the stirrup or caliper may loosen, jeopardizing the wearer's stability; these need to be replaced by the orthotist promptly.

Hose or socks should be clean, without holes or repairs, to protect the feet, particularly for patients with insensitive skin. Those with plastic calf or thigh shells should wear long nylon or cotton hose to protect the underlying skin; cotton hose is more absorbent of perspiration.

Lower-Limb Orthotic Uprights

Routine inspection is especially important in children's orthoses. Their uprights are designed to accommodate for growth. In plastic/metal orthoses, uprights are screwed to the plastic calf and thigh shell. To lengthen the orthosis, the orthotist removes the old screws, drills new holes farther up the calf shell and down on the thigh shell, then reattaches the uprights. Screws are more apt to work loose in leather/metal orthoses that have overlapping uprights, reducing the stability of the appliance.

Joints and Locks

If joints do not move smoothly or if locks do not engage easily, they should be cleaned thoroughly. Sand, liquids, and similar substances can damage orthotic joints. Occasional lubrication may be required, although one should not use much oil as it will stain the wearer's clothing.

Bands, Trunk Orthotic Uprights, and Straps

Plastic components should be kept clean with a damp cloth, then dried thoroughly. Pressure closures lose effectiveness if they are infiltrated with too much lint; they need to be replaced if they cannot provide secure fit.

Leather upholstery absorbs perspiration, which causes it to become malodorous and eventually crack. Preventative care includes wearing clean undergarments, as well as periodically cleaning the leather with mild saddle soap. Brittle leather should be replaced to protect the patient's skin from contact with the underlying metal components. Leather straps that show signs of stretching or cracking also need immediate replacement.

Fabric Components

The corset or abdominal front of a trunk orthosis is usually designed to be detached from the rest of the orthosis so it can be washed. A clean undershirt should be worn to absorb perspiration.

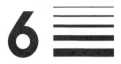

Wheelchairs, Assistive Devices, and Home Modifications*

Although the activities described in this chapter are designed for patients with one-sided involvement, bilateral lower limb and trunk weakness, or bilateral above-knee amputation, and weakness of all four limbs and trunk, they may be modified to suit any patient diagnosis.

The patient's wheelchair should be designed for comfort and ease of manipulation. Wheelchairs differ in design and construction based on the needs of individuals and the unique aspects of their disabilities. For example, a wheelchair for a bilateral above-knee amputee has a longer frame on which the rear wheels are set back to prevent the chair from tipping. Another example would be a chair with one-arm drive, which is propelled by wheeling with the right or left hand alone. Refer to Chapter 12 to compare wheelchair types.

WHEELCHAIRS

Frames

Wheelchair frames are either rigid or folding. The type of frame effects the maneuverability of the chair. A rigid frame is one solid piece, is lighter than a folding frame, and is used more for sports and other rugged activities (see figure at bottom of page 110). A folding frame is heavier and requires more effort to maneuver but is more convenient for storage in the home and for placing into areas such as automobiles. See figure at top of page 110.

Tires

The selection of tires depends on the use of the chair. Tires made with solid, hard polyurethane and having a smooth tread are designed for the indoor user, allowing for maximum ease of maneuverability on smooth surfaces. If used outdoors these tires offer no shock absorption and no traction.

Pneumatic (inflatable) tires provide for shock absorption and a smooth cushiony ride, particularly outdoors on uneven or rough terrain. These tires require more effort to maneuver and add slightly to the overall width of the chair. The tread depth and

*Information on wheelchair parts was obtained from a video, "New Moves, Program 4: Wheelchair Comfort and Performance, 1989," developed at Sacred Heart General Hospital, Oregon Rehabilitation Center, Eugene, OR.

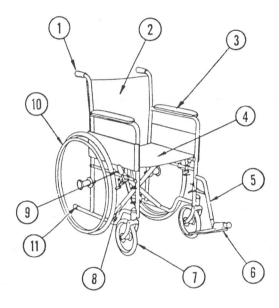

STANDARD CHAIR

1. Handgrips/Push Handles
2. Back Upholstery
3. Armrests
4. Seat Upholstery
5. Front Rigging
6. Footplate
7. Casters
8. Crossbraces (Serial No.)
9. Wheel Locks
10. Wheel and Handrim
11. Tipping Lever

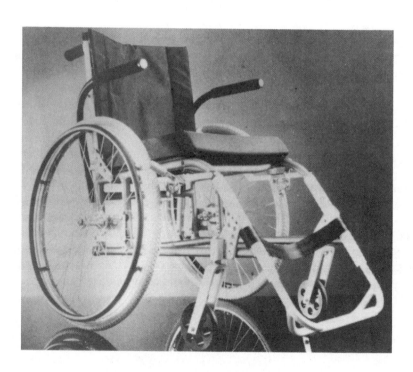

tire pressure determine the amount of traction. Greater tread depth and lower tire pressure provide more traction but requires more effort to propel the chair. The increase in tire tread depth has a disadvantage as well. Dirt tends to adhere and can then be tracked into buildings and homes. Some users compromise by having a pneumatic tire with a minimum tire tread depth.

Wheels

Two types of wheels are available: solid magnesium (mag) and spoke. Solid mag wheels never loose their shape and never need adjustments. Spoke wheels are lighter and therefore provide for easier maneuverability. The disadvantage of spoked wheels is the durability of the spokes: they are more easily broken and must frequently be checked for tightness. Broken or loose spokes will cause the wheel to lose its shape.

Wheel sizes may vary depending on the size and weight of the user. A smaller wheel size requires more strokes than a larger wheel size to propel the chair the same distance. An advantage to a small wheel is that there is less height to the wheelchair during transfers.

Quick-release wheels, found on the rigid frame chairs, are convenient when transporting the chair. The wheel is removed by pushing on a button, which releases the lock, allowing the wheel to slide off the axle of the chair. When ready for use the wheel is placed on the axle and locks into place.

Push Rims (Handrims)

The type of push rim depends on the extent of the user's grip. There are basically three types: (1) standard metal rims, (2) friction rims, and (3) rims with projections. Standard metal rims are used when grip is not a problem. Friction rims are standard rims with friction tape or surgical tubing added to provide additional traction on the rim surface for users who have a limited grip. Projection rims are used by people with limited reach and grip. The projection knobs are placed at intervals to suit the needs of the user. The greater the number of knobs the greater the convenience: it is more likely that a knob will be in position when needed. Projection knobs may be either at an oblique angle or vertical. The new user will have the knobs placed at an oblique angle, which provides a greater surface area for propulsion. Later, as the user gains skill and coordination, the knobs should be changed to a vertical position. The vertical knobs lessen the overall width of the chair and allow for greater maneuverability. See figure at top of page 112.

One-Arm Drive

As the name implies, the one-arm drive wheelchair is propelled and steered by the use of one upper limb. This type of wheelchair is designed for those who have no functional use of the lower limbs and one upper limb. This chair allows control of both large wheels from one side of the wheelchair. The chair has two rims on the propelling side, one rim activating each wheel. Using the two rims simultaneously, the individual can move the chair in a straight line. The outside handrim is smaller than the other. The smaller handrim provides control of the opposite wheel. Propul-

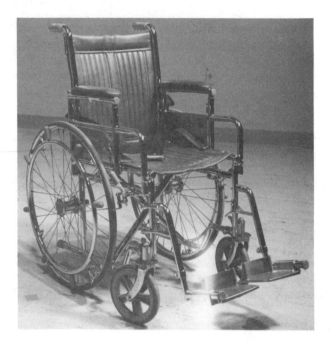

sion using the outer rim turns the wheelchair toward that side and propulsion of the inside or standard rim turns it in the opposite direction.

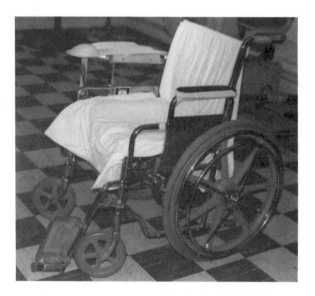

Footrests

Footrests, either fixed or swing-away removable, support the lower limbs. Swing-away footrests are more convenient but increase the length of the chair, which affects turning maneuverability. Footrests tend to lack durability and require frequent repair. Heel loops or leg straps can be added to the footplate. Either or both of these accessories add length to the wheelchair, however.

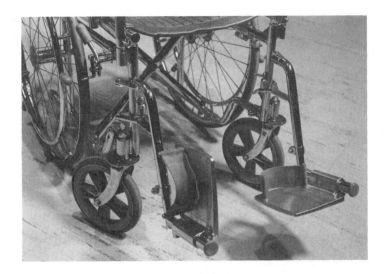

Spacers

Spacing between the push rim and the tire is adjustable to suit the user's hand size. The tubing and screws are longer for a greater distance between the rim and the tire.

Casters

Casters are pneumatic, semipneumatic, or solid. Solid casters allow for better front-end maneuverability on smooth surfaces. The semipneumatic type is better on uneven terrain. Pneumatic casters provide for greater shock absorption; however, the increased drag during propulsion adds considerable effort to wheelchair propulsion. Casters may also have locks. The advantage of locks on the casters is to keep the chair from pivoting during transfer activities; their primary disadvantage is that they may inadvertently lock unexpectedly.

Tilt Bars

Tilt bars, which project from the back of frame, usually 2 to 3 inches above the floor, are used by the individual who is pushing the wheelchair. By placing the foot on the tilt bar and pushing down with the foot, the person can tilt the wheelchair back, allowing the casters to rise off the surface, thus enabling them to clear objects such as a curb or a rug.

Chair Backs

High wheelchair backs provide trunk support and are ideal for a high-level quadriplegic. However, a disadvantage of the high back is that it gives the person in the chair a feeling of being pushed forward. Also, it may interfere with the power stroke and does make the chair somewhat more cumbersome to stow.

Low chair backs provide a greater freedom for movement and are preferred by individuals with low-level spinal cord lesions and by those who participate in sporting activities.

Armrests

Removable armrests are convenient, provide support, and make transferring easier when removed. However, the removable armrest does restrict movement during the power stroke. Armrests can also be fixed or adjustable in height and may be desk-length or full-length. Wraparound armrests provide the desired arm support without substantially increasing the width of the wheelchair. It is also possible to order a wheelchair without armrests. Chairs without armrests are equipped with sideguards to protect the user's clothing.

Cushions

Important for the health and comfort of the wheelchair user, cushions are used to achieve the most comfortable and supportive position possible. A few of the companies that manufacture cushions are listed here.

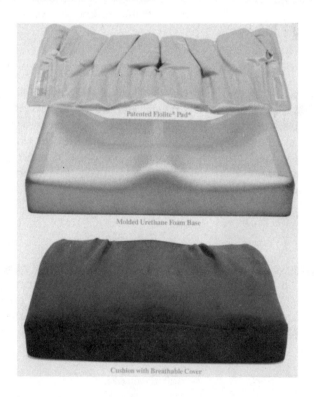

1. *Jay Medical:* Jay offers various cushions and backs made of foam and Flolite with a variety of accessories to achieve optimal positioning.
2. *Otto Back:* This manufacturer offers contoured cushions, headrests, and other

accessories. The Otto Back contour U molded seat and back is custom-molded to the person's body.

3. *Roho Company:* Roho offers cushions with individual inflatable air cells, which are available in high and low profiles and can be customized to variable cell height for posture control and pressure relief.

Wheel Locks

Wheel locks prevent the chair from rolling and can assist in slowing and stopping the momentum of the chair. They are mounted either in a high or low position. The high-mount locks, with or without extensions, are usually designed for individuals with limited upper limb use and with poor trunk support. These locks are easily accessible but can get in the way when propelling the chair. The low-mount locks require a greater degree of trunk flexion to reach the lock handles but do permit a greater freedom of movement during propulsion.

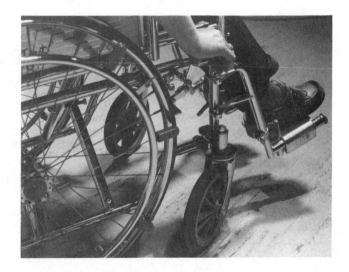

Hill Holders

Hill holders prevent the chair from rolling backward between strokes, which can be a necessity on inclines—particularly for individuals with upper limb weakness. On occasion hill holder may engage unexpectedly. As users gain strength and experience, the hill holders are generally discarded.

Antitip Bars

Antitip bars keep the chair from tipping too far backward. They are used primarily by new users and by those with a high-level spinal cord injury. The bars do have a tendency to catch when the chair is tilted back to ascend or descent curbs, causing a loss of balance.

WHEELCHAIR DIMENSIONS

Proper fit of the wheelchair includes consideration of the patient's size, disability, and needs. Chairs have adjustable features that can adapt as specific needs change.

Balance of the chair is key to safety and performance. Axles can be adjusted: the farther forward the axle is mounted the less weight is applied to the casters. This position allows for ease to turn, propel, and perform "wheelies." When the axle is positioned farther back, the chair's center of gravity shifts forward, placing more weight on the caster and thereby allowing for more stability.

Feature	Objective or Purpose
Casters	To provide steering capability
Wheels	To aid in propulsion, hand or power (higher wheels have an advantage in propulsion because they have a greater surface area covering a greater distance with less effort; their disadvantage is that their height causes difficulty in performing transfers)
Footrests/legrests	To support weight of lower extremities and provide elevation of the limb(s) if necessary
Arms	To provide lateral stability, security, and comfort
Back	To provide trunk stability, support, and comfort
Seat	For support; weight should be distributed over the maximum area, consistent with user's disability; seat height should allow for foot clearance 3 inches above the ground; thighs should be horizontal or angled downward slightly to help distribute pressure. Low seats fit under tables more easily but expose more wheelrim making it more difficult to perform transfers.
Seat angle	To provide greater stability and balance: if the seat is angled backward more of the trunk is supported and the weight is off the casters
Brakes	Safety device, required on all wheelchairs
Overall weight	Should be as light as possible (to extend the user's degree of independence and to reduce secondary disabilities of both user and attendant)
Overall width	Minimum overall width, 26 inches
Wheel camber	This is the angle of the wheelrim to the chair (increasing the angle will increase the width of the chair, but will also increase chair's stability and make turning easier)

WHEELCHAIR MAINTENANCE

The wheelchair should be cleaned regularly. Mild, soapy water and wax should be used on the painted surfaces. A lightweight oil may be used for all moveable parts, except bearings. Nuts and bolts, which tend to loosen over time, must be tightened. Tire pressure should be checked; normally the pressure is between 50 and 70 pounds. Low pressure in the tires will damage rims and make the chair more difficult to propel. As spokes keep the wheel round, they should be tightened periodically and replaced immediately if broken. The wheel and caster bearings should be checked for freedom of spin and smoothness.

Pneumatic tires should be checked weekly for proper inflation; solid tires for cracks and worn areas. The spokes should all be tight and the wheel should run "true" — in a straight line.

Monthly, the metal parts should be sprayed and wiped clean, followed by an application of car wax. The upholstery should be cleaned and the screws checked for tightness. Telescoping tubes (armrests) should be waxed to aid in sliding.

Once every 6 months, the wheelchair should have a complete overhaul, particularly if it is used outdoors.

HOW TO CONSTRUCT A BATHTUB CHAIR*

Materials

Wooden, straight-back chair
Two 1- by 2-inch boards, 25 inches long
Eight 2-inch, number 8 galvanized nails
Waterproof paint (enamel or spar varnish)

Measurements

Height of inside of bathtub
Width of inside of bathtub

Modification of Chair

Cut the legs of the chair so the seat height equals the height of the bathtub when the chair is in the bathtub. Cut both of the 1- by 2-inch boards to equal the width of the bathtub minus 1 inch. These boards will prevent the chair from turning.

Completion of Chair

Nail the 1- by 2-inch boards at the front and back of the chair, 2 inches below the top of the seat. After sanding the chair, paint it completely with waterproof paint.

METHODS OF STANDING A PATIENT AT HOME

Using a Sturdy Board or Prone Standing Table

Materials

Large, sturdy board, approximately 3 by 6 feet
Posterior splints with anterior knee cages and two additional straps each
Three or four restraints

Procedure

Place restraints on bed, one each at upper trunk, hip, and knee levels.
Place board on restraints on bed.
Apply posterior splints to patient.
Place patient with splints on top of board in bed.
Tie restraints around the patient.
Slide the board to the foot end of the bed and tilt it to the standing position.

Note. Eliminating the posterior splints may be possible if there is some lower
limb function.

---

*Adapted from Rancho Los Amigos Hospital, Department of Physical Therapy, Downey, CA.

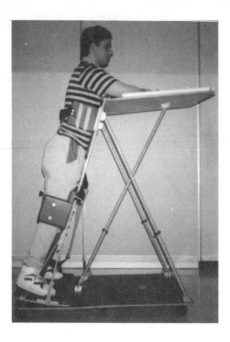

Using a Wall

Materials

Wall with studs, approximately 16 inches apart
Six to eight ½-inch diameter screw eyes with 1⅛-inch shanks
Three to four strips of webbing of various lengths (20 inches and longer)
Four copper rivets for each strip of webbing
Six to eight harness snaps
A drill with ³⁄₁₆-inch bit
Pliers
Hammer

Procedure

Knock on wall or use a stud finder to find studs.
Place eye screws at the levels of hip, knee, and upper chest, as patient would be
   standing against wall.
Put the screws into the studs.
Make straps to fit across chest, hips, and knees.
Rivet two harness snaps on each end of the straps.
Apply posterior splints to patient.
Stand the patient against the wall and strap in place.

Note. If there is some lower limb function, use same procedure but eliminate the
   posterior splints.

Using a "Hinder Binder"

Materials

Posterior splints with anterior knee cages and two additional straps each
Pelvic sling with harness snap at each end
Sturdy table or counter with two screw eyes about 16 inches apart

Procedure

Apply posterior splints to patient while he or she sits in the wheelchair.
Place wheelchair facing screw eyes.
Scoot patient forward in wheelchair until feet are on ground.
Place wheelchair as close to table or counter as possible with patient's lower
   limbs extended in front and feet on floor.
Lock wheelchair.
Pull patient to standing and strap pelvis with sling fastened to screw eyes.

Note. Padded board may be needed in front of chest if patient does not have
   trunk control or cannot hold trunk with upper limbs.

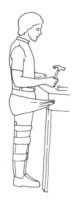

Using a Hand-Propelled Wheel Stretcher

Strap patient in supine position onto stretcher with feet at large wheel end of
   stretcher.
Lock brakes.
Tilt small wheel end of stretcher up until patient is standing.

AMBULATORY AIDS—CRUTCHES, CANES, AND WALKERS

Axillary Crutches, Used with Good to Normal Upper Limb Muscle Strength

Construction: Metal or wood, adjustable or nonadjustable
Types: Standard or Lumex ortho

Advantages: Lateral stability, inexpensive if made of wood, fits stairs
Disadvantages: Cumbersome, tendency to exert axillary pressure, especially on
   stairs

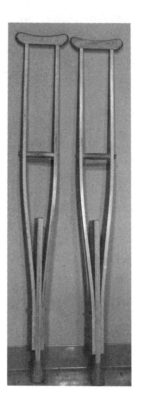

Upper Arm Crutches, Used with Weak Elbow Extensors

Types: Triceps, Everett, California, Warm Springs
Advantages: Aids weak elbow extensors, fits stairs
Disadvantages: Somewhat cumbersome; cuffs difficult to remove

Forearm Crutches (Canes), Used with Good to Normal Upper Limb Strength

Types: German, Lofstrand, Canadian, Lumex ortho
Advantages: Handgrip, in addition to cuff, gives more support than standard
   cane; may release grip without dropping crutch; less cumbersome and more
   easily used than aforementioned two types; fits stairs
Disadvantages: Cuff difficult to remove; requires better control than aforementioned two types; more expensive than wooden axillary

Note. Both the upper arm crutch and the forearm crutch should be ordered with
   plastic-covered cuff. Metal cuffs cut patient's arm.

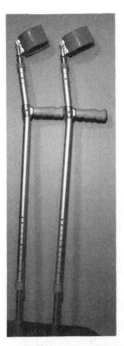

Platform Crutch, Providing a Platform for Forearm Weight-Bearing

Advantages

Patients with below-elbow amputations

Patients who cannot bear weight on wrists or hands (often used with arthritic patients and patients who have severe wrist or finger deformities from increased muscle tone or contractures)

Patients who cannot extend the elbow passively

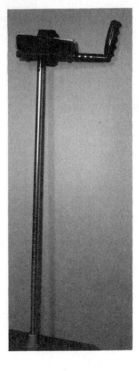

Platform Rolling Walker, Providing Unilateral or Bilateral Forearm Weight-Bearing

Advantages

Larger base of support for patients with poor balance and coordination
Patient who cannot bear weight on wrists or hands owing to pain, increased muscle tone, or instability
Patients with elbow flexion contractures

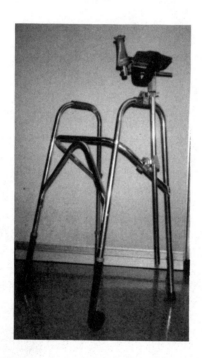

Standard Cane

Types

Crook handle
Metal or wooden
Adjustable or nonadjustable

Advantages

Wooden cane is inexpensive
Fits stairs

Disadvantages

Point of support in front of hand
Small base of support, no arm support

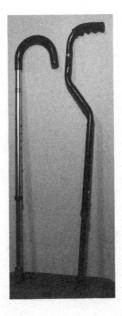

Lumex Ortho Cane

Molded handgrip
Adjustable

Advantages

Point of support directly below hand
Fits stairs

Disadvantage

Small base of support, no arm support

Quadriped Cane

Bases available in several sizes
Adjustable

Advantage

Wide base of support

Disadvantages

Point of support not centered
Large size does not fit stairs
Difficult to carry up stairs while using handrail

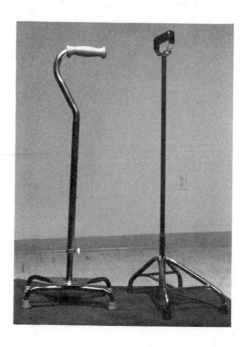

Walkane

Wide base for support
Greater stability than quadriped cane

Disadvantages

Cumbersome
Large size does not fit stairs
Difficult to carry up stairs while using handrail

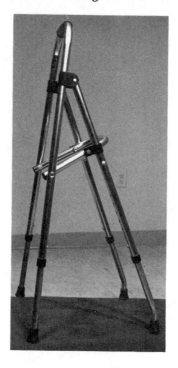

Crutch and Cane Accessories

Axillary Pad

Helps hold crutch in place

Disadvantage

May encourage patient to lean on axillary piece

Handgrip covers

For axillary crutches, upper arm, and forearm crutches; often necessary to reduce pressure on palms

Crutch Tips

Use large suction tips: Saf-T-Grips
Maintain contact with ground at any angle of crutch
Absorb shock with floor or pavement
1.5-inch size good for crutches
Must be replaced often

Arm Cuffs

Rubber-covered most comfortable
Side opening types will not accidentally pop off from forearm pressure
Front opening types may pop off accidentally if not kept tight, but are easier to remove when necessary

Pick-Up Walker

Types

Adjustable or nonadjustable
Folding or nonfolding
Reciprocal
Stair-climbing

Advantage

Provides stability with bilateral lower limb weakness

Disadvantages

Requires use of both hands
Does not fit through all passages
Questionable stair-climbing ability

Walker with Casters

Comes with seat attached
Can be ordered with brakes

Advantages

Provides stability for bilateral lower and upper limb involvement and poor
balance

Disadvantages

Cumbersome, cannot fit through all passages
Unable to be used on stairs
Caster locks do not stabilize walker well enough

Reciprocal walker

The left side of the walker and the right lower limb move forward together

Advantages

Allows for a two-point gait
Provides for greater stability than a cane
Permits fast gait

Disadvantages

Cumbersome and cannot be used on stairs

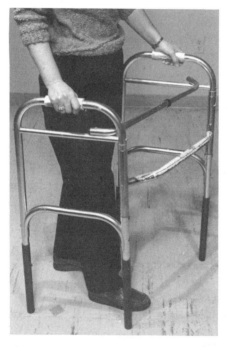

Shopping Cart with Attached Poles

Advantages

Encourages upright posture
Easily fabricated
Easily used

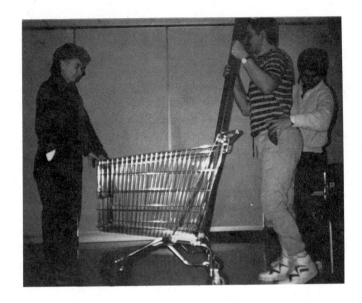

Rolling Bedside Table

Advantages

Adjustable in height for more or less weight-bearing on upper limbs
Weight-bearing on forearms—aids in decreasing upper limb flexor tone

Note. One or two tables may be used, depending on stability.

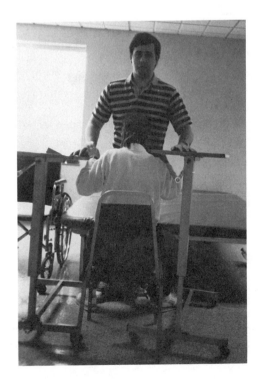

HOME IMPROVEMENTS FOR THE
HANDICAPPED INDIVIDUAL

Removal of architectural barriers in the home or apartment will permit greater independence and provide a safer environment. Modifications, alterations, or remodeling of the home may be done without detracting from the home. The expense may vary depending on the complexity of the modifications. It may be as simple as removing a throw rug or as involved as constructing a ramp to substitute for stairs at the entrance to the house from outside. A one-story home is ideal; this eliminates the need to negotiate stairs. Home modifications are of greater concern when the handicapped individual is using a wheelchair than when external devices such as a cane or crutches are used.

Identified here are some suggestions for improving the physical environment of the home to allow for the greatest amount of safety and independence. These suggestions were developed by the Commonwealth of Massachusetts Architectural Barrier Board, reprinted in 1984. The specifications are based on average wheelchair dimensions and characteristics; the sample used is a collapsible model of tubular metal construction with cloth or plastic upholstery.

Wheelchair Dimensions

Length: 48 inches
Open width: 28 inches
Folded width: 13½ inches
Height of seat from floor: 19 inches
Height of armrest to floor: 29 inches
Height of lap from floor: 27 inches
Eye level: 43 to 51 inches

Wheelchair Use Characteristics

Space for wheelchair to turn 360 degrees: 60 inches
Vertical reach: 60 inches above floor
Horizontal reach (tables, desks): 30 inches
Diagonal reach (wall-mounted phones, towel dispenser, shelves): 48 inches

Width of Path for Crutch User

If user is 5½ feet tall: 31 inches
If user is 6 feet tall: 32½ inches
If user is 6 feet 6 inches: 34 inches

Ramps

A ramp leading into the home should be constructed of weather-resistant materials such as 2- by 8-inch pressure-treated wood planks. The slope of the ramp should not exceed 1 inch for 12 inches in length. The ramp width should be not less than 48 inches, measured at the railings. Handrails should be set on both sides of the ramp and should extend 12 inches beyond the ramp if possible. The surface of the ramp should be covered with a nonslip material. At the top of the ramp there should be a 48-inch platform, unobstructed by doors, to allow for manipulation of a wheelchair.

Doors

An average wheelchair width of 28 inches will require a minimum door width of 36 inches with a clearance opening of 34 inches. The threshold should not exceed ½ inch in height. Door handles should be placed 36 to 42 inches above the floor. Individuals with limited grip may prefer levers or latches rather than knobs. Doors should be operable with one hand.

Stairs

If stairs are unavoidable within the home, they should be constructed without the projection of tread lips. An advanced wheelchair user may be able to negotiate stairs but not as a routine daily activity. Individuals who can ambulate may find that stairs are not a barrier if constructed properly. Handrails should be set on both sides of stairs at a height of 34 inches above the step and should extend 12 inches beyond the steps. The handgrip portion of the rail should be not less than 1¼ inches and not more than 2 inches in diameter; 1½ inches is ideal. A nonslip material should be applied to each step.

Floors

Floors should have a nonslip surface. If carpeting is used, it should be a high-density, low-pile type. It should be stretched tautly and securely anchored at all open edges.

Bathroom

Ideally, there should be a 60-inch clearance around the toilet to allow for the manipulation of the wheelchair. These dimensions may not be reasonable in many homes. Therefore, the doorway into the room should be 36 inches, with enough clearance to propel the wheelchair up to the side of the toilet. The door should open outward. Two grab bars may be installed to add to the safety features of the room. One bar is placed on the wall behind the toilet, the other along the side wall. The toilet seat should be set at 15 to 17 inches above the floor. The grab bars should have an outside diameter of 1¼ inches, should have a 1½-inch clearance between the bar and the wall, and should be set 30 inches above and parallel to the floor. The bars should be nonrusting and acid-etched or roughened. If the tank of the toilet prevents location of the rear grab bar, a bar may be installed 3 inches above the tank. Grab bars should end at least 6 inches from the corner of the wall. They should be capable of supporting 250 pounds of weight for 5 minutes.

The toilet paper dispenser should be placed at least 24 inches from the floor.

The sink should be set at a height of 27 inches to the bottom of the rim or counter and should extend at least 22 inches from the wall. The pedestal type, without legs, will allow the individual's knees to clear the sink. The open knee space should be approximately 30 inches. Ideally grip strength will determine if the faucets can be knobs or lever handles.

The bottom of a mirror or medicine cabinet in the bathroom should be 38 inches above the floor. If the mirror must be placed higher than 38 inches, it can be tilted at the top.

All towel racks should be placed no higher than 42 inches above the floor.

A shower stall is more appropriate than a bathtub for most wheelchair users. The stall should be 36 inches by 60 inches minimum, with a 36-inch door opening. The floor should be pitched to drain within the stall at the corner farthest from the entrance. The floor should have a nonslip surface. The easiest type of control to operate a shower is a single lever with a pressure balance mixing valve. All controls should be located on the center wall adjacent to a hinged shower seat. The shower head should be attached to a metal hose with a wall mounting adjustable from 42 inches to 72 inches above the floor.

A hinged, padded seat should be installed in the shower stall. Its dimensions should be at least 16 inches deep, at least 24 inches long, and set at a height of 18 inches to the top of the seat. The seat should fold upward and be securely attached to the side wall. Two grab bars should also be installed in the shower. One should be 32 inches long and the other 48 inches long. They should be placed horizontally 36 inches above the floor or should be a continuous L shape. Soap dishes should *not* be used as grab bars.

If a bathtub is installed it should not be less than 16 inches nor more than 20 inches from the floor. A built-in seat 18 inches deep should be available. The bottom of the tub and the tub seat should have a nonslip surface. A tub enclosure should not have tracks mounted on the rim of the tub.

Kitchen

Floor space should be sufficient to allow turning mobility for the wheelchair user. Countertops should be from 30 to 40 inches high, measured from the floor to countertop. The depth of the counter should be at least 15 inches and have clear space underneath for feet and knees. Space under sinks and counters should be 30 inches wide. Access space under the counter should be continuous, at a height of 27 inches to the underside of the counter.

The bottom of wall cabinets should be set at 42 to 56 inches from the floor. The hardware should be operable with a closed fist for those with minimal upper limb strength.

Sink depth should not exceed 6 inches. Traps and drains should be located as close to the rear wall as possible. Plumbing pipes should be recessed, insulated, or padded.

Cooking units should have the controls placed at the front with an open space underneath. The controls should be no higher than 54 inches above the floor. Ovens should be 30 inches above the floor. The doors to ovens should be either bottom- or side-hinged.

If refrigerator and freezer units are combined, the bottom of the door to the higher unit should be no more than 44 inches from the floor.

Bedroom

Floor space should be sufficient so that a wheelchair user can reach the windows and closet poles. There should be 60 inches of space allowed on one side of the bed. Closet shelves and poles should be 42 to 72 inches. Electrical outlets should be located at least 18 inches above the floor.

Modifications may be incorporated into the plans during construction or remodeling of a home or apartment or alterations may occur in an existing structure. Refer to Chapter 12 for a home evaluation form developed by the Greenery Rehabilitation and Skilled Nursing Center, Boston, MA.

7

Body Mechanics and Guarding Techniques

The activities included in this chapter are designed for patients with one-sided involvement, bilateral lower limb and trunk weakness, and weakness of the four limbs and trunk. Some alternate methods for the activities are described. These may be modified and varied to meet individual patient requirements. Assistive devices to aid the patient in becoming functionally independent are identified throughout this chapter and in Chapter 6.

To aid the patient in performing bed or mat activities, the bed should be sturdy and have a firm mattress with a tight-fitting bottom sheet. The mattress should be topped with an egg crate foam. Although this may make the bed hotter during summer, it provides a greater opportunity for ease of rolling and redistributing pressure. Individuals who are unable to change bed position should use a soft-sider (water bed). This type of mattress has longitudinal tubes filled with water, allowing an even distribution of the body weight and decreasing the possibility of developing bed sores. Any assistive equipment should be firmly attached to a stable part of the bed frame. Brakes or rubber tips are necessary to prevent the bed from slipping or sliding on the floor while the patient is moving.

GENERAL PRINCIPLES OF GUARDING AND ASSISTING THE PATIENT

Each daily activity skill should be analyzed for elements of danger before it is taught to the patient. The therapist should consider all the guarding techniques for an activity and decide on the most efficient. Also, preventive measures should be heeded when apparatus and equipment are used. Before beginning the activity, the therapist should always check the patient's appliances and the functional training equipment. Successful guarding methods should be the concern of the therapist as well as the patient because guarding, in the final analysis, is simply a matter of handling and controlling weights.

The application of proper body mechanics is an essential aspect of any functional activity to protect oneself and to guard a patient effectively. Most often, when guarding a patient, the therapist assumes a position of trunk flexion, slight anterior tilt of the pelvis, hip and knee flexion, with the arms in front of the body. The position of trunk rotation combined with trunk flexion should be avoided because of the forces it places on the vertebral disks, the ligaments, and the erector spinae muscles. Prolonged physical stress may alter the vertebra and surrounding structures, resulting in chronic pain. Awareness of body position while lifting and guarding should reduce the potential for strain, fatigue, and injury.

The normal curves of the trunk—in particular, the lumbar lordosis—should be maintained during lifting and guarding techniques. This position maintains the normal alignment of the spine and decreases the stresses otherwise placed on the ligaments, muscles, and intervertebral disks.

Body Mechanics

1. Maintain a normal lordotic curve in the low back while flexing the hips, knees, and trunk. This can be achieved by tilting the pelvis anteriorly and then posteriorly slightly to ensure a coactivated trunk with both posterior and anterior musculature supporting the trunk and pelvis. With the low back and pelvis in a coactivated anterior pelvic tilt, flex the hip and knee joints.
2. Keep the object being lifted or guarded as close to your body and the vertical line of gravity as possible.
3. Rotate or turn your body from the hips and feet, not from the trunk.
4. Move slowly, avoid twisting or jerking.
5. Assume a wide stance, feet a shoulderwidth apart and in a side-to-side position, or the leading foot slightly ahead of the other, to allow for proper shifting of body weight with the patient.
6. Hip and knee flexion should not exceed 60 degrees, to maintain maximum efficiency of the knee and hip extensors.

The person guarding should stay as close to the patient as possible and remain near enough to anticipate and prevent falls.

Assisting the Patient

1. Assist the patient as much as necessary, but allow the patient to perform as independently as possible.
2. Allow enough room for the patient to perform the activity.
3. Watch the patient's performance at all times.
4. Be ready to prevent the patient from falling or to ease the patient to the floor without injury to the patient or self.

GUARDING THE PATIENT

Rolling

1. Position yourself so that the patient will roll toward you.
2. Be in a position to guide the hips and shoulders, if necessary. This will give assurance that the patient will not roll off the edge of the bed.

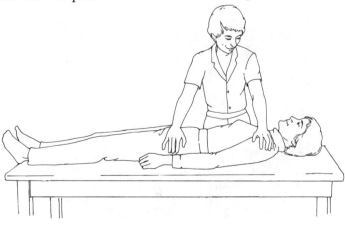

Short Sitting

1. Stand in front of the patient.
2. Place your hands near the patient's shoulders to be ready to prevent the patient from falling.

Note. Initial short sitting activities should be performed in the most stable positions and then progress to more challenging, less supportive positions (e.g., feet not in a weight-bearing position).

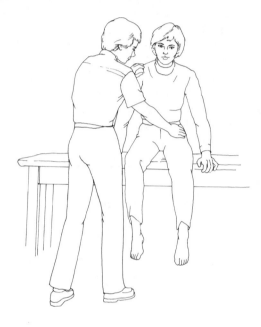

Long Sitting

1. Kneel behind patient on mat.
2. Stand beside patient in bed.
3. Place hands near patient's shoulders to be ready to prevent patient from falling.

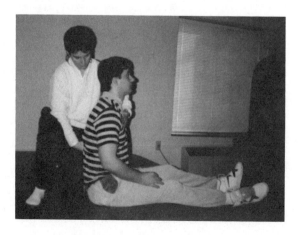

Guarding on One Knee

1. Keep the knee nearest the patient on the mat.
2. Use one hand to support the patient at the shoulder and the other hand to steady the hips.
3. Always stay close to the patient and never permit the patient to get away from you. Guarding at arm's length is not effective.

Guarding From a Crouched or Semicrouched Position

1. Position legs far enough apart to provide a broad base of support.
2. Place one hand on the patient's shoulder and the other on the guarding belt.
3. Use the thigh of the advanced leg as an effective lever in helping to force the patient's hips forward if "jacking" occurs.

GUARDING DURING WHEELCHAIR TRANSFERS

When guarding the patient during wheelchair transfers, the therapist should stand with flexed knees and pelvis in a slight anterior tilt with the shoulders in line or slightly in front of the hips. The therapist should stand with a broad base of support, close to the patient, without obstructing their movement or vision.

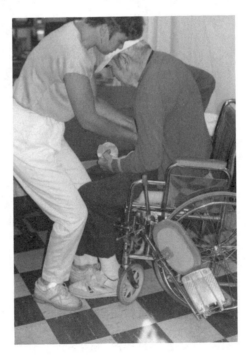

When assisting the patient during a transfer, the therapist should ask the patient, or assist the patient, to scoot forward in the wheelchair. When the patient is forward in the chair, with the feet flat on the floor and the leading foot slightly in front the therapist helps facilitate an upright sitting posture with a coactivated trunk in a slight anterior pelvic tilt. The therapist, with key points of control at the shoulders or pelvis, should assist the patient in shifting the body weight forward over the lower limbs. When giving assistance the therapist should always lift with the lower limbs, not the back, and guide the patient toward the transfer surface. Always allow the patient to perform the transfer actively, giving them only as much assist as they need and no more. The therapist must be in a position that does not block the patient's movement or vision. If the patient is unable to transfer in this fashion, then a sliding board or another therapist may be needed to assist the patient from behind.

Alternate Method

If the patient needs little or no assistance, guard from behind, using a safely belt.

Guarding Against a "Wheelie"

The therapist stands behind the wheelchair with the hands close to the push handles. When the forward motion of the wheelie is performed during a descent over a curb, one of the therapists hands should be close to the shoulder to prevent inadvertent trunk flexion.

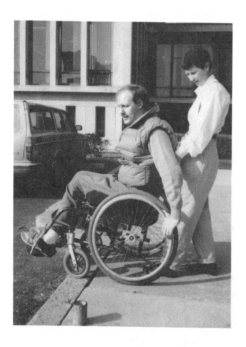 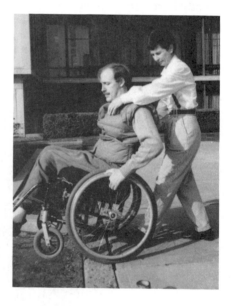

TECHNIQUES OF GUARDING AND ASSISTING

Crutch Balancing (Axillary and Forearm Crutches)

Forward and Backward Method

> *Patient:* Performing crutch balancing drills
> *Therapist:* Guarding in front or at the rear of the patient
> *Instructions to therapist*

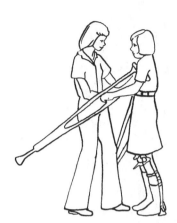 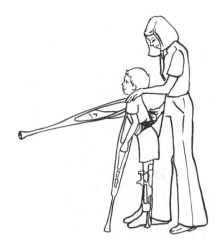

1. Stand either in front of or behind the patient, according to preference. Some who teach functional training believe that it is better to guard from behind a patient. Their contention is that the patient becomes too dependent on the therapist when the therapist stands in front. Those who prefer to guard a patient from the front assert that they can recognize fear and hesitation more easily by watching the patient's facial expressions. They believe, too, that when patients, as beginners, see a therapist in front, their attention is diverted from the dangers of the exercise or activity. The patient has only to think of the fundamentals for proper execution. Fear causes tension and distracts attention from the task to be performed. Regardless of which location is preferred, the stance and the principles involved are the same.
2. Use a broad base of support. Standing with one leg in advance of the other allows the therapist to rock the body weight forward and backward depending on the movements of the patient, keeping the center of gravity and the line of gravity within the base of support.
3. Stand as close as possible to the patient without impeding any motions.
4. Be ready to help at any time during the activity. Place one hand on the patient's shoulder and the other hand on the safety belt to control the patient's movements. When in front of the patient, the therapist is ready to pull the hips forward and push the shoulders back; when to the rear, the therapist is in a position to push the hips forward and pull the shoulders back to restore the patient's balance.

Ambulation Activities

Moving With the Patient's Feet

Patient: Performing four-point gait with braces and crutches
Therapist: Guarding behind the patient
Instructions to therapist

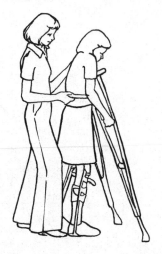
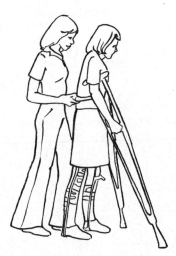

Stand with the feet in a walk-stand position, one foot advanced as in boxing position. Foot movements should be synchronized with the patient's foot movements; for example, when the patient advances the right crutch and left foot, the therapist advances with the left foot, keeping close to the patient at all times. Avoid reaching and never let the patient get too far away. Observance of this simple rule will reduce muscle tension and fatigue and generally conserves the therapist's energy during gait training.

Moving With the Gait Pattern

Patient: Performing a swing gait with braces and crutches—for example, the swing-through gait
Therapist: Guarding behind the patient
Instructions to therapist

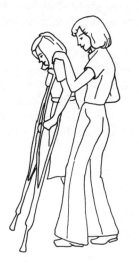
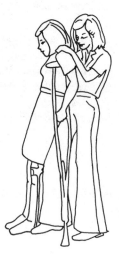
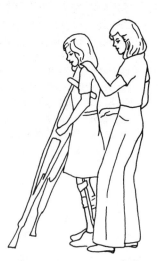

1. It is necessary to assist the beginner through the gait many times, gradually reducing physical assistance. At first, guarding is a matter of lifting with all

safety rules heeded. Lift with the lower limb muscles, not with the upper limbs or back. The patient should not try the swing-through gait until after preliminary training.

2. Keep close to the patient, to anticipate and prevent falls. Avoid reaching, as a sudden mishap may strain your back while you attempt to break the fall or restore the patient's balance.

3. Stand behind the patient and slightly to one side, to assist or follow the patient without interfering with his or her movement.

4. As the patient travels, synchronize movements with the gait pattern, advancing the outside leg with the crutches and the inside leg with the patient's feet. The thigh of the inside leg can be an effective lever in forcing the patient's hips forward if "jacking" occurs.

5. Place one hand on the patient's shoulder and the other on the guarding belt, to be ready to push the patient's hips forward and pull the shoulders back. As the patient swings through, assist by lifting the patient at the hips and controlling the shoulders, giving the patient the feeling of arching the back.

Teaching Functional Activities — Basic Methods

Sitting Activities

Patient: Sitting down and getting up to erect position with braces and crutches —for example, from wheelchair to crutches and return
Therapist: Guarding in semicrouch stance
Instructions to therapist

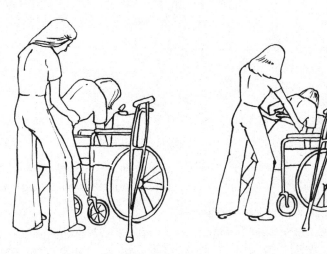

1. Protect the patient in the same way as for wheelchair transfers. Stand to the rear of the patient and slightly to one side to avoid interfering with motions of the patient. Assume and maintain a semicrouch position with a broad base of support, the feet in a walk-stand position. Be careful to keep the center of gravity within the base of support.

2. Use your feet to brace the patient's feet. The patient need never worry about his or her feet slipping when they are supported in this manner.

3. Place hands on each side of the patient's hips, grasping the guarding belt.

During rising, guide or lift the patient's hips around and upward until balance is established.

4. Steady the patient's hips as he or she reaches for the crutches and assumes the crutch stance. One hand may be placed at the patient's shoulder and the other hand on the hips in order to lift the patient's shoulders backward and to push the hips forward while the patient comes to the erect position. In such a stance, the thigh of the advanced leg can be an effective lever.

Stairs With Handrail

Patient: Performing stair climbing with handrail
Therapist: Guarding on the stairs at the side of the patient
Instructions to therapist

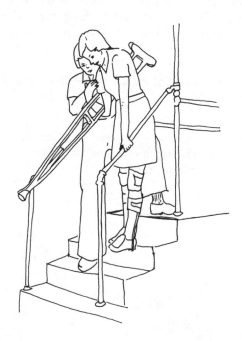

1. Stand at the side, in the front, or to the rear of the patient, depending on the method of stair climbing employed (e.g., backjack, forward leg swinging, or push-up method), and also according to preference. Regardless of location, the stance and the principles involved are essentially the same. Guarding at the side seems the most favorable location and is recommended for guarding a patient using stairs with a handrail. The other locations for guarding are proposed as variations or adaptations of the basic method with full realization of their limitations.

2. Place one hand on the patient's shoulder and the other hand on the safety belt, permitting assistance in either ascending or descending stairs. If the patient is ascending, the therapist can easily prevent the patient from losing balance backward by pushing the hips forward and the shoulders backward. Patients who have difficulty in raising the feet to the step above can often be

given confidence and assistance from the rear by being lifted at the hips and being supported at the shoulders with the other hand. In descending, if the patient falls forward, the therapist can restore the patient's balance in the same manner as for ascending. Until descending stairs is well learned, the therapist can control the rate of descent by holding back on the safety belt while supporting the patient under the shoulder. After each step the therapist's position should be readjusted on the stairs so that a broad base of support is maintained and so that the therapist can stay as close to the patient as possible. The therapist must never let the patient (weight or mass) disturb the relationships among the therapist's center of gravity, line of gravity, and base of support.

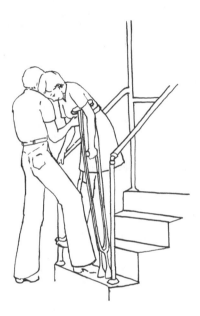

3. When descending, guard in front of the patient, keeping one hand on the safety belt and the other hand on the shoulder. In this case, the patient moves into the therapist's base of support, whereby adequate stability can be maintained. If the patient falls forward, the therapist can easily check the fall with the shoulders. However, if the patient completely loses balance, the load may force the therapist off balance backward, especially when at the top of the staircase; therefore, extreme care must be taken so that both therapist and patient are protected from falling. When the patient ascends the stairs, guarding in front of the patient is a poor position, because the patient then moves away from the therapist's base of support. There is a resultant shift of the therapist's center of gravity and a disturbance in the relationship of the line of gravity to the patient's base of support. Eventually, the therapist will be guarding at arm's length, which is almost never effective. Guarding in front of the patient with both hands on the hips or safety belt allows the therapist to assist a beginner in lifting the feet to the step above or lowering the feet to the step below, but the therapist is in a poor position to guard a patient who suddenly and completely loses balance.

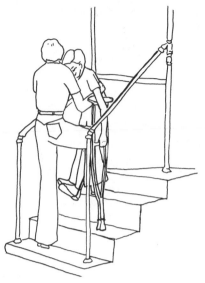

4. Guarding from the rear with one hand on the shoulder and the other hand on the safety belt permits a good position when ascending the stairs. The patient moves into the therapist's base of support and can be easily and quickly checked by the therapist when falling off balance backward. If the patient requires assistance to lift the feet to the step above, the therapist is in a poor position, as all the factors of stability are being violated. When descending the stairs, the patient moves still farther away from the therapist's base of support. If the patient falls forward he or she can get completely away from the grasp of the therapist.

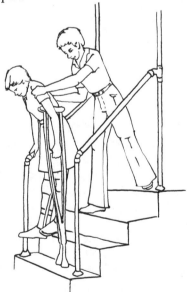

For Curbs

Patient: Performing curb activities— for example, ascending or descending curbs with braces and crutches

Therapist: Guarding at the side of the patient
Instructions to therapist

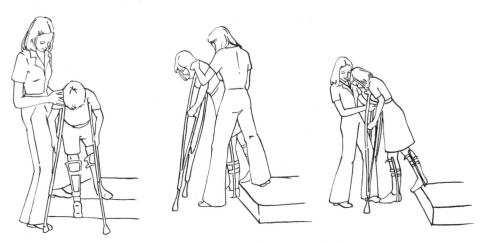

1. Guard the patient in the same way as for using stairs with a handrail.
2. Stand at the side, in the front, or to the rear of the patient. The position suggested as the basic method is from the side of the patient. Guarding in the front and to the rear is suggested as alternate methods. Guarding at the side is an excellent position from which to help the patient in either ascending or descending curbs. The therapists work within their base of support and can keep close to the patient so as to anticipate and prevent falls. Guarding in front of a patient is a good position for descending curbs but is a difficult position from which to maintain an adequate base of support when the patient ascends. Guarding a patient from behind is a good position if the patient is ascending, but it is a poor position for descending from a curb. A fall forward would place the patient completely out of reach.

For Stairs Without a Handrail

Patient: Performing stair climbing without a handrail
Therapist: Guarding on the stairs at the side of the patient
Instructions to the therapist

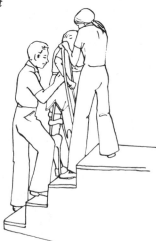

1. The patient should learn to use stairs with a handrail and climb curbs before attempting this activity. Guard the patient in the same way as suggested for using stairs with a handrail and for curb activities. Two therapists should help the beginner for the first few times. One should be in front and to one side of the patient, with one hand on the crutches and the other hand on the shoulders. One therapist should stabilize the crutches and push the shoulders back if the patient falls off balance forward or "jacks." The other therapist should be behind the patient and off to the side opposite that taken by the partner, with both hands on the safety belt. This therapist should help the patient lift the feet to the step above when ascending stairs or lower the feet to the step below when descending stairs, and should also prevent or correct jack-knifing. Both therapists should maintain a solid base of support, stay as close to the patient as possible, and observe the rules of safe lifting.

2. When one therapist works alone, the basic method is guarding at the side. The stance is the same as for using stairs with a handrail and for curbs, with this exception: The therapist's hand is placed under the patient's arm instead of on the shoulder. If this is not done, the therapist can easily interfere with raising and lowering movements of the patient and the stability of the crutch, which is an essential part of the patient's base of support.

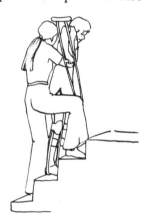

3. If the therapist guards in front of the patient, the stance illustrated on the left should be used. The stance and method illustrated on the right may be disastrous when using stairs without a handrail because the patient is completely out of the therapist's base of support, causing the therapist to guard at arm's length. The result is strain on the back and arms.

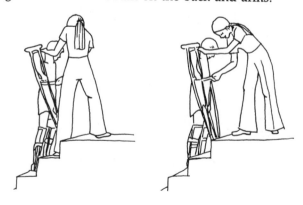

Using a Bedside Table

Patient: Being supported on a rolling bedside table (the table should be high enough to support weight on the forearms)
Therapist: Guards from behind to avoid impeding forward ambulation. Initially, guarding may occur in front of as well as behind the patient.

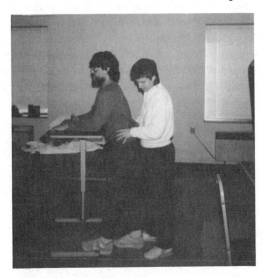

Using a Shopping Cart With Poles

Patient: Ambulates with hands on the poles approximately shoulder height.
Therapists: One therapist stabilizes the cart while the other guards the patient from behind. As the patient's balance and stability improve, it may no longer be necessary for one therapist to stabilize the shopping cart.

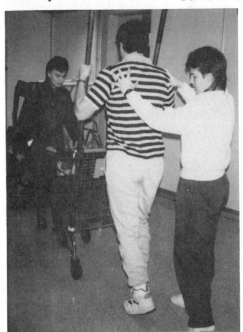

Getting Down To and Up From Floor

Patient: Getting down to and up from the floor with braces and crutches
Therapist: Assisting patient in getting up from the floor
Instructions to therapist

1. Teaching the patient to get down to or up from the floor is very much a matter of handling weights. Weights are always lifted with the large leg muscles, not with arms or back. The principles that govern stooping, lifting, and carrying apply. The therapist stoops in preparation to assist the patient to jack-knife up onto feet, controls the patient at the hips, and helps the patient to lift the hips to a level higher than the shoulders and to get the weight onto the feet.

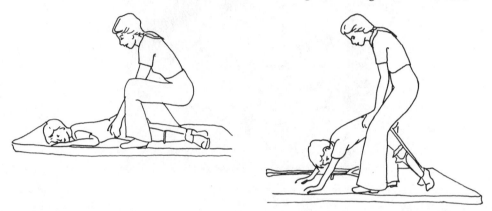

2. Assist the patient in extending the trunk to assume the erect position and in placing the crutches under the arms to assume the proper crutch stance. If the patient uses forearm crutches, the therapist assists by using both hands to stabilize the hips to help the patient get the feel of the proper trunk and arm action. Stand with one leg placed between the patient's braced legs. In this way, the therapist can be effective in the event the patient requires total assistance.

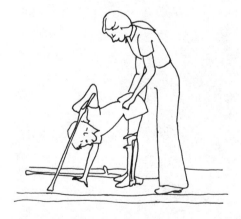

3. If the patient uses full-length underarm crutches, assist by placing one hand on the crutches and the other on the safety belt. The crutches are stabilized with the therapist's hand, thereby making it easier for the patient to climb up

the crutches to the erect position. The therapist's other hand on the patient's hips can help the patient feel how to roll the pelvis forward and under the trunk.

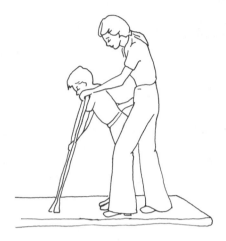

Multiperson Assist

The number of therapists who assist and guard the patient will be determined by the ability of the patient and the availability of therapists.

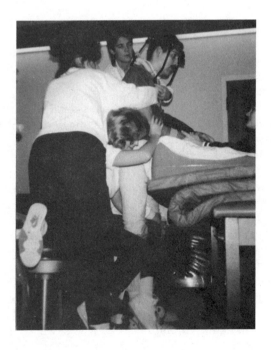

8

Functional Activities for One-Sided Involvement

Individuals with one-sided involvement usually have suffered a cerebral vascular accident, traumatic head injury, peripheral injury resulting from a neuropathy, or any degenerating disease that is unilateral. Functional training activities should begin with the least difficult and less demanding activities such as lying and sitting and mat activities. As the patient becomes stronger and develops new motor patterns it is usually possible to progress to wheelchair and upright activities. Independence in one activity does not have to be completely achieved before moving on to the next higher level of performance as long as guarding and assistance are provided for the safety of the patient.

BED ACTIVITIES

I. Moving in Bed
   A. Toward head of bed—supine
      1. Flex nonaffected hip and knee with foot flat on bed.
      2. Push against bed, extending nonaffected foot, forearm, and hand.
   B. Toward foot of bed—supine
      1. Flex nonaffected hip and knee, keeping foot flat on bed.
      2. Pull against bed with nonaffected foot, pulling trunk toward foot.
      3. Extend arm against bed at same time, digging elbow into bed.
   C. Toward foot of bed—lying on side
      1. Roll to nonaffected side.
      2. Abduct nonaffected arm until weight is on forearm.
      3. Push forearm against bed, forcing trunk toward feet, hips flexing.
      4. Lift foot off the bed and extend hip and knee joints.
      5. Replace foot on bed and repeat procedure.
   D. Toward head of bed—lying on side
      1. Roll to nonaffected side.
      2. Abduct nonaffected arm until weight is on forearm.
      3. Flex nonaffected hip and knee.
      4. Adduct nonaffected arm, push foot against the bed and extend and abduct nonaffected leg. The affected limb can be assisted with the nonaffected (or less affected) limb.
   E. Toward side of bed—supine, no equipment
      1. Flex nonaffected hip and knee, keeping foot flat on bed.
      2. Extend nonaffected arm until weight rests on forearm.
      3. Push against nonaffected foot and forearm, lifting body.
      4. Swing body to side.

F. Toward side of bed—supine, using trapeze bar
Same as E except nonaffected arm pulls on trapeze.

II. Rolling from Supine to Side or Prone Position
Scoot to opposite side of bed before rolling.

A. No equipment, turning to affected side
1. Flex nonaffected hip and knee, keeping foot flat on mattress.
2. Position affected arm at side, slightly anterior to trunk.
3. Grasp edge of mattress with nonaffected hand.
4. Push against mattress with nonaffected foot and pull with nonaffected arm until lying on side or prone.
5. Roll to opposite side if affected shoulder is painful.

B. No equipment, turning to nonaffected side
1. Place affected arm across chest or abdomen.
2. Flex nonaffected hip and knee, keeping foot flat on mattress near affected knee.
3. Grasp edge of mattress with nonaffected hand.
4. Push against mattress with nonaffected foot and pull with nonaffected arm until lying on side.
5. If affected leg begins to lag behind, hook the nonaffected foot under the affected knee and pull it forward.
6. Before becoming prone, place the affected arm on bed at least one foot from trunk.
7. Continue rolling prone.

C. Using the arm of the chair or side rail of the bed turning to nonaffected side
1. Move to the far side of the bed (to the side of the affected limbs).
2. Place affected arm across chest or abdomen.
3. Grasp rail or arm of chair with nonaffected hand.
4. Pull strongly with nonaffected arm until lying on side or prone.
5. If affected leg begins to lag behind, hook the nonaffected foot under the affected knee and pull it forward.

III. Coming to Sitting Position

A. From side-lying position
1. Lie on nonaffected side.
2. Abduct and extend nonaffected arm until weight is on forearm.
3. Hook nonaffected foot around affected ankle.
4. Flex nonaffected hip and knee, carrying affected hip and knee along into flexion.
5. Extend nonaffected elbow until weight is on hand.
6. Walk nonaffected hand toward hips, coming to sitting position.
7. At same time, use nonaffected leg to carry both legs off the edge of the bed. (See figures at the top of page 150.)

B. Alternate method
1. Lie on nonaffected side.
2. Hook nonaffected foot around affected ankle.
3. Flex nonaffected hip and knee, carrying affected leg over the edge of the bed.
4. Abduct and extend nonaffected arm until weight is on forearm.
5. Extend nonaffected elbow until weight is on hand.
6. Walk nonaffected hand toward hips, coming to sitting position.

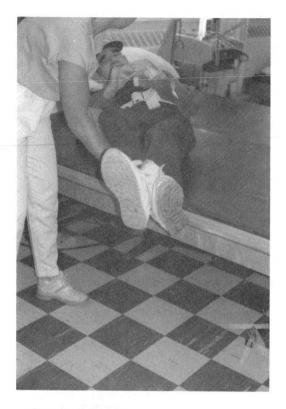

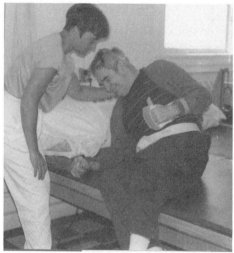

IV. Lying Down
   A. Reverse procedure IIIA or IIIB
V. Balancing Activities
   A. Sitting with hips and knees flexed, feet on foot.
      1. Assume a coactivated trunk position in an anterior pelvic tilt.
      2. Weight shifting side to side with appropriate elongation of the trunk on the weight-bearing side; incorporate reaching activities.
      3. Incorporate affected limb in a weight-bearing position.

      a. At patient's side

      b. In front on supportive table

      c. In front on slow-moving surface on a table

    4. Regain balance when challenged from all directions, continue to facilitate coactivated trunk.

  B. Creep position (hands and knees)

    1. Shift weight to side, forward, backward.

    2. Regain balance when pushed quickly to left, right, front, and back.

VI. Self-Assistive Range of Motion (ROM)

  A. Supine (assume right-sided weakness—no function of the right side; if patient has some function, it should be used)

    Activities should be performed slowly, as quick movements may increase spasticity.

    1. Shoulder flexion

      a. Grasp right wrist and hand with left hand (usually will have to raise head and left shoulder.)

      b. Raise right arm with elbow straight until it is overhead.

      c. Flex right elbow, continuing to move arm overhead until it is lying on the bed close to head.

    2. Elbow flexion and extension

      a. Grasp right wrist and hand with left hand.

      b. Flex elbow bringing hand toward shoulder and keeping arm on bed.

      c. Extend elbow until forearm and hand rest on bed.

    3. Hip and knee flexion

      a. Flex left hip and knee and slip left foot under right knee.

      b. Slide left foot down until it is under right ankle.

      c. Flex left hip and knee to chest, bringing right leg along.

      d. Using left hand, pull right knee to chest.

      e. Reverse procedure for extension.

  B. Sitting (assume right-sided weakness)

    1. Shoulder flexion and extension

      a. Same as supine except keep elbow extended—more difficult if patient has limited ROM or spasticity.

    2. Shoulder abduction or flexion

      a. Cradle upper limbs with the right resting on the left.

      b. Maintaining a cradle position, move upper limbs toward the right and toward the left.

      c. Maintaining a cradle position lift upper limbs above the head.

      d. Use overhead pulley with wrist cuff on right.

    3. Elbow flexion and extension

      a. Same as supine

      b. Difficult to get full extension of elbow.

    4. Wrist flexion and extension

      a. Rest right forearm on arm of chair, hand over edge.

      b. Supinate forearm.

      c. Place left thumb in right palm, fingers on dorsum of right hand, leaving fingers free.

      d. Alternately flex and extend wrist.

    5. Finger flexion and extension

      a. Rest forearm, supinated, in lap with wrist neutral.

    b. Using thumb of left hand on dorsum of distal phalanges, flex interphalangeal (IP) joints.

    c. With IP joints flexed, use fingers of left hand to flex metacarpophalangeal (MP) joints.

    d. Using thumb of left hand on volar surface of distal phalanges, extend fingers.

    e. Individual finger flexion and extension as needed.

  6. Thumb

    a. Rest forearm, supinated, in lap with wrist neutral.

    b. Using left hand, grasp right thumb.

    c. Abduct, oppose, and flex thumb.

    d. Extend and repose thumb.

VII. Dressing Activities (assume right-sided weakness)

  A. Putting on a pullover shirt

    1. Begin sitting with shirt in lap, backside up, neck away from patient (label is facing down).

    2. With left hand gather up the back of the shirt to expose the right armhole.

    3. Using left hand, lift right hand and place it through the armhole and sleeve.

    4. Place left arm through left armhole and sleeve up to the elbow.

    5. Using left hand, push right sleeve above right elbow.

    6. Gather back of shirt from collar to hemline.

    7. Continue holding shirt and work shirt up both arms toward the shoulders.

    8. Duck head and pull shirt over it.

    9. Pull shirt down in back and front.

  B. Putting on a cardigan garment

    1. Begin sitting with shirt in lap, inside up, and collar away from body.

    2. Using left arm, place right hand in right armhole (the armhole is diagonally opposite arm).

    3. Pull sleeve over hand, grasp collar, and pull sleeve up onto the right shoulder.

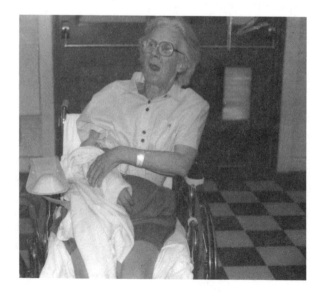

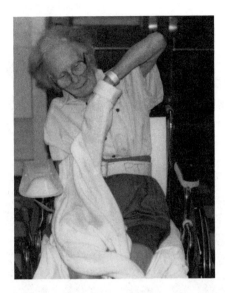

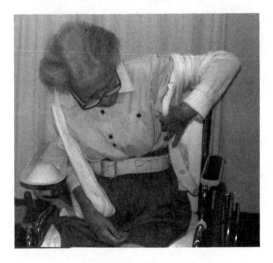

4. Toss the rest of the garment behind body.
5. Reach left hand back and place it in armhole.
6. Work sleeve up arm and straighten shirt.
7. Button shirt (easier to start from bottom).
C. Putting on trousers
1. Begin sitting on side of bed.
2. Using left hand, cross right leg over left.
3. Check to see that trousers are opened completely.
4. Grasp trousers at bottom of front opening and toss down toward right foot.
5. Pull right trouser leg up and over right foot.
6. Place right foot on floor and put left leg in other trouser leg.
7. Pull trousers up over knees.
8. Lie down, bend left hip and knee, push against bed, and raise buttocks.
9. Pull pants over hips; fasten. If patient can stand, omit step 8 and pull trousers on while standing; sit to fasten trousers.

D. Putting on socks
   1. Cross legs and pull on with left hand.

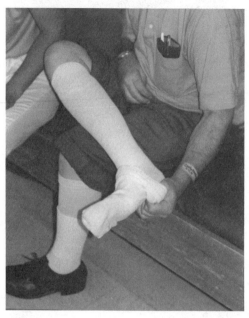

E. Putting on shoes or orthosis
   1. Sew tongue to top of shoe at one side to prevent it from doubling over.
   2. If brace is attached to shoe, be sure that the leg is in front of brace when putting shoe on.
   3. Begin sitting on side of bed with right leg crossed over left.
   4. Slip shoe on foot as far as possible.
   5. Place a shoehorn in heel of shoe and place foot on floor.
   6. Push down on knee making sure shoehorn stays in place.
   7. Fasten shoes (buckles, Velcro, or one-handed tie).

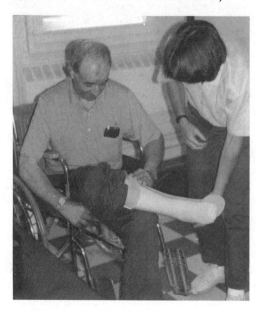

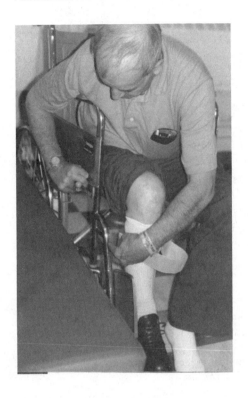
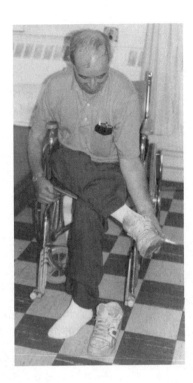

F. Tying a shoe one-handed
    1. Knot one end of the shoe string and lace the shoe, leaving the knotted end at the lowest eyelet.

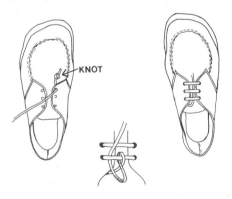

    2. In the top eyelet feed the end of the shoe string from outside to inside. Throw the end over the top of the laces.
    3. Make a loop, in the free end of the shoestring and pull it, loop within a loop, as shown in center position of illustration.
    4. Pull the lace tight, being careful not to pull the free end all the way through.
    5. To untie, pull the free end.
G. Alternative method of lacing one-handed (shoe is laced before putting shoe on)

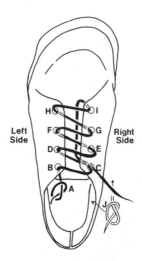

1. Tie knot A in one end of an extra long shoelace.
2. Begin lacing from underside of eyelet B on left side.
3. Cross to opposite eyelet C and continue to lace shoe to eyelet I (last eyelet on right side).
4. Bring lace under layers of cross threads toward eyelet C.
5. Thread lace through eyelet C underside up.
6. Make knot J at end of lace (like knot A). This prevents accidental unlacing. Leave all strands loose.

Putting on shoe: After lacing shoe completely, place foot inside of shoe.
1. Tighten lace. Start at eyelet B and pull up all cross strands at each eyelet on left side of shoe only.
2. Pull tightly on knot J and tuck knot and excess lace into right side of shoe (or if preferred, into left side of shoe).

Taking off shoe: Once shoe is laced properly, it need not be unlaced. To take off shoe, simply release tension of shoelace as follows:
1. Release excess lace and knot J from right side of shoe.
2. Loosen shoe by pulling down on cross strand at eyelet I as far as it will go (lace will be stopped by knot J).
3. Loosen each following cross strand on right side, leaving a loop in each strand, until . . .
4. Shoe is opened sufficiently and can be taken off.
H. Alternatives to lacing (may be preferred because of ease)
   1. Use of elastic shoe laces and long-handled shoe horn.
   2. Use of Velcro strap and shoehorn.
I. Putting on a back-fastening bra
   1. Place bra around waist with back in front, fasten hooks.
   2. Turn bra around to proper position.
   3. With left hand place right hand inside right strap and pull strap up arm.
   4. Insert left hand in left strap; pull strap up arm to shoulder.
   5. Push right strap up arm to shoulder; adjust.
   Note: Some patients may prefer front-fastening bras that are easier to put on and take off.

MAT ACTIVITIES

Mat activities for patients with one-sided weakness are designed to meet the initial goal of preventing contractures as well as to assist the individual in preparing for activities of daily living.

Guarding techniques should be employed with all mat activities for the safety of the patient when balance and coordination are of concern. Refer to Chapter 7 for specific guarding techniques.

I. Supine Position
   A. Rolling to affected side
      1. *Position:* Supine with uninvolved hip and knee flexed on the mat and unaffected shoulder extended
      2. *Action:* Extend hip and knee and hyperextend the shoulder joint, rotate head to the side of the turn.
      3. *Functional carry-over:* Bed mobility, preliminary to come to sitting
     Caution: If affected shoulder is painful, be aware of its position or elect not to roll onto that side.

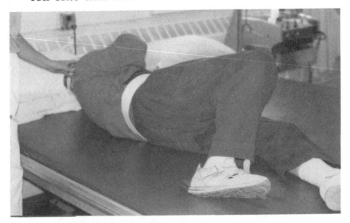

   B. Moving on the mat
      1. *Position:* Same as previously described
      2. *Action:* Extend the hip, knee, shoulder, and head, pushing on the mat moving toward the head, and reverse moving toward the feet.
      3. *Functional carry-over:* Moving in bed and using the bedpan

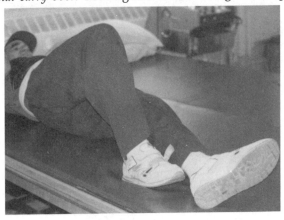

    C. Moving sideways on the mat
       1. *Position:* Supine with the noninvolved lower limb flexed and the foot flat on the mat
       2. *Action:* Extend and abduct the lower limb scooting toward the affected side; extend and adduct the lower limb scooting toward the nonaffected side. Upper limb and head will extend and direct the movement sideways.
       3. *Functional carry-over:* Moving in bed preliminary to rolling or coming to sitting
    D. Leg mover
       1. *Position:* Noninvolved foot placed under the involved ankle
       2. *Action:* Abduct or adduct the noninvolved lower limb carrying the involved limb
       3. *Functional carry-over:* Moving in bed and preliminary to come to sitting
    E. Pelvic tilter—anterior and posterior
       1. *Position:* Supine with lower limbs extended
       2. *Action:* Flatten and arch the low back
       3. *Functional carry-over:* Erect sitting and standing
    F. Bridger
       1. *Position:* Supine with the lower limbs flexed and the feet flat on the mat
       2. *Action:* Raise the buttock off the mat by extending hip and knee joints.
       3. *Functional carry-over:* Moving in bed, off and on bedpan, preliminary to come to standing

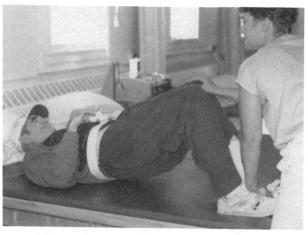

 II. Prone position
    A. Weight shifting
       1. *Position:* Prone on elbows and forearms
       2. *Action:* Shift weight from elbow to elbow, lift, and reach with free arm.
       3. *Functional carry-over:* Develop stability in shoulders and scapula and balance for dressing, transfer, and ambulation activities
III. Sitting Position
    A. Sit-ups
       1. *Position:* Supine, lower and upper limb extended
       2. *Action:* Adduct the lower limb with the uninvolved limb, abduct and extend the nonaffected upper limb until weight is on forearm, extend the elbow until weight is on the hand.
       3. *Functional carry-over:* Assume sitting for transfers

B. Lying down: Reverse the aforementioned procedure.
C. Weight shifting
   1. *Position:* Sitting with the lower limbs flexed over the edge of the mat (short sitting)
   2. *Action:* Shift weight forward, backward, and side to side.
   3. *Functional carry-over:* Sitting balance and wheelchair transfers

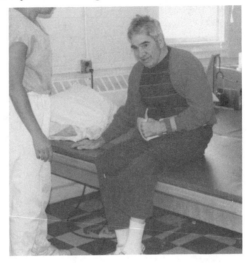

D. Scoot forward and backward
   1. *Position:* Sitting with lower limbs flexed over the edge of the mat (short sitting)
   2. *Action:* Unweight pelvis on unaffected side and hike hip backward, pulling the lower limb; attempt with the involved side. Reverse action to move forward.
   3. *Functional carry-over:* Sitting balance and wheelchair transfers.

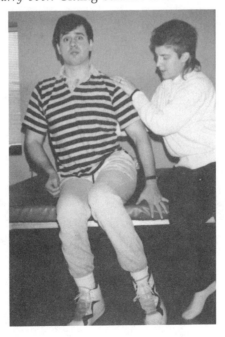

E. Scoot to right or left
   1. *Position:* Short sitting with the upper limb at the side and hand in a weight-bearing position
   2. *Action:* Abduct the nonaffected hip, then adduct it while weight-bearing to move the affected limb. The upper limb may be used to help unweight the pelvis by performing a partial sitting push-up.
   3. *Functional carry-over:* Positioning oneself for sitting transfers
F. Pelvic tilter—anterior or posterior
   1. *Position:* Short sitting
   2. *Action:* Flatten and arch the low back.
   3. *Functional carry-over:* Erect sitting and standing

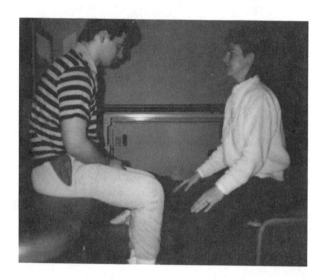

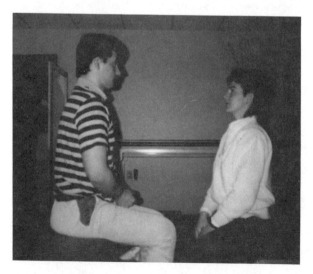

G. Pelvic rotator
   1. *Position:* Short sitting
   2. *Action:* Move pelvis in the horizontal plane toward the right and left; the trunk should naturally follow.
   3. *Functional carry-over:* Upright activities

H. Trunk motions
   1. *Position:* Short sitting
   2. *Action:* Flex and extend; laterally flex to right and left; rotate to right and left.
   3. *Functional carry-over:* Sitting balance, manipulating wheelchair parts, dressing, and upright activities.

IV. Hand-Knee Position
  A. Assume the hand-knee position
    1. *Position:* Sitting with both lower limbs extended
    2. *Action:* Flex and rotate lower limbs toward the unaffected side to assume a side-sitting position; twist trunk and bear weight on all four limbs (may need to support the involved elbow).
    3. *Functional carry-over:* Getting up from the floor with brace and cane, standing transfers with brace and cane.
  B. Weight shifter
    1. *Position:* Hand-knee position with as much weight bearing as possible on the involved side.
    2. *Action:* Shift weight forward, backward, and side to side.
    3. *Functional carry-over:* Transfers, getting up from the floor, ambulation, and elevation activities.
  C. Pelvic tilter
    1. *Position:* Same as aforementioned position
    2. *Action:* Arch and lower the low back
    3. *Functional carry-over:* Getting up from the floor; standing from the wheelchair and ambulation activities

V. Kneeling
  A. Assume kneeling
    1. *Position:* Hands and knees
    2. *Action:* Hold onto edge of raised mat, stool or seat of chair, shift weight onto unaffected forearm, extend elbow, and straighten trunk to upright position.
    3. *Functional carry-over:* Getting up from the floor

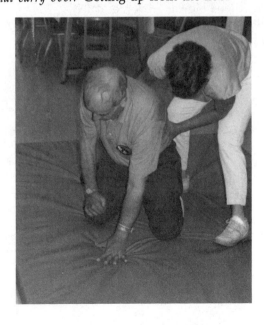

B. Weight shifter
   1. *Position:* Kneeling with support for balance and weight bearing on the upper limbs
   2. *Action:* Shift weight forward, backward, right and left.
   3. *Functional carry-over:* Ambulation activities (see figure at the bottom of page 161)
C. Pelvic tilter
   1. *Position:* Kneeling, using support for balance; encourage weight-bearing bilaterally
   2. *Action:* Anterior and posterior pelvic tilt
   3. *Functional carry-over:* Assuming the upright position and ambulatory activities
D. Pelvic rotator
   1. *Position:* Kneeling with support for balance
   2. *Action:* Rotate the pelvis in the horizontal plane toward the right and left.
   3. *Functional carry-over:* Transfer and ambulatory activities
E. Knee-standing
   1. *Position:* Kneeling using a bench or chair for balance, place uninvolved foot forward
   2. *Action:* Shift weight side to side, forward and backward.
   3. *Functional carry-over:* Getting up from the floor
VI. Standing
A. Come to standing
   1. *Position:* Knee-standing with uninvolved foot forward, using a bench, cane, or seat of a chair for balance
   2. *Action:* Extend uninvolved hip and knee and trunk to assume an upright position.
   3. *Functional carry-over:* Getting up from the floor, assuming standing from wheelchair, bed, toilet, and so forth
B. Standing to floor
   1. *Position:* Standing with weight shifted to uninvolved side
   2. *Action:* Flex both lower limbs and reach for the mat with the uninvolved upper limb. Slowly lower self onto mat.
   3. *Functional carry-over:* May be necessary in an emergency that the patient assume a position on the floor

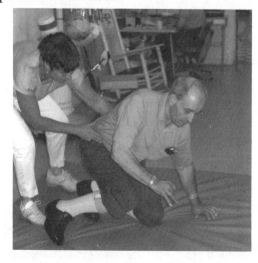

WHEELCHAIR ACTIVITIES

Wheelchair activities include balancing skills, propulsion, and transfer activities. Transfer activities refer to the patient moving from the wheelchair to another surface and vice versa.

Wheelchairs have been designed for both comfort and performance. There are many choices of frames with all features. The chairs are made of lightweight alloys, which adds to the maneuverability and convenience for the user. A standard wheelchair usually seen in most clinical facilities consists of a metal, collapsible frame with a vinyl seat and back and padded armrests. The front wheels or casters are small, and the back wheels large. Most standard wheelchairs are equipped with footrests and hand brakes. Individuals with one-sided weakness may find this type of wheelchair suitable for limited chair use. Young individuals who depend on their wheelchair for mobility for most functional activities often request the lightweight chairs. For all transfer activities be sure to reinforce an upright posture with the pelvis in a slight anterior pelvic tilt with coactivated abdominal and back extensors.

I. Balance Activities
   A. Shift weight forward in the wheelchair, maintain balance without arm support, regain upright sitting.
   B. Shift forward and touch floor (often patients collapse or fall down when doing this because they have not maintained a coactivate trunk using their abdominals and back extensors); regain upright sitting.
   C. Shift weight to right and left, alternating unweighting the opposite hip and thigh.
   D. Maintaining a weight shift to the right, scoot left hip forward. Scoot back to original position in the same manner, moving one hip at a time.
II. Manipulation of Wheelchair Parts
   A. Leaning toward involved side, lock and unlock brake with uninvolved hand.
   B. Leaning toward uninvolved side, lock and unlock brake with uninvolved hand.
   C. Assist placing foot on and off the foot pedal with uninvolved or less involved hand or foot.
   D. Leaning forward, raise and lower the foot pedal with uninvolved or less involved hand or foot.
   E. Remove and replace armrests.
III. Wheelchair Mobility
   A. Level surface
      1. Forward propulsion
         a. Place uninvolved hand on wheelchair rim and push forward (hand gives momentum).
         b. Simultaneously, pull with uninvolved foot in a heel-toe sequence (foot guides direction of wheelchair according to angle of pull of foot).

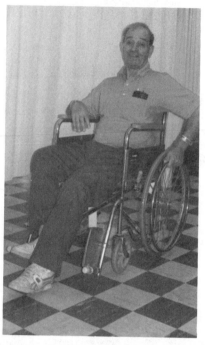

2. Backward propulsion—to ascend ramps
   a. Place uninvolved hand on wheelchair rim and pull backward.
   b. Simultaneously, push with uninvolved foot in a toe-heel sequence.
3. Turning to involved side
   a. Push forward on handrim.
   b. For a sharper turn, guide with foot also.
4. Turning to uninvolved side
   a. Pull backward on handrim.
   b. For a sharper turn, guide with foot also.
B. Inclines
   1. Ascending
      a. If strength and trunk balance are adequate, use same method for forward propulsion on level surface.
      b. *Alternate method:* Ascend backwards, pulling on handrim and pushing with foot.

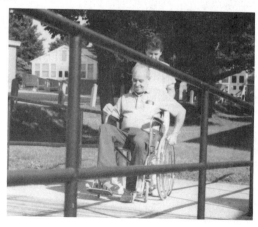

2. Descending
   a. Control speed with hand and direction with foot.
C. Open door
   1. Approach door toward the involved side.
   2. Use door handle to pull door open
   3. Push the wheelchair backward with the uninvolved foot until the door clears the footrest.
   4. Maneuver chair through the open door.
   5. Turn the wheelchair around and pull the door closed.

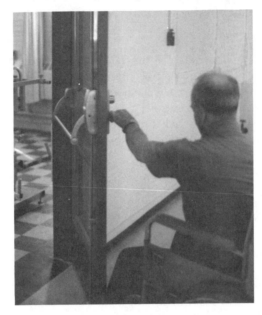

IV. Transfers

A transfer is the shifting of the patient from one surface to another or from one object to another by means of a specified pattern of movements that are safe and efficient. Head-injured persons may not be independent in transfers secondary to memory disorders or inability to sequence the task. Written cue cards attached to the wheelchair may allow the patient to be independent.

While doing independent transfers the patient moves without assistance. At first the patient may require considerable assistance; however, as cognitive ability, endurance, and strength improve, less assistance will be necessary.

The patient transfers in either a standing, sitting, or squatting position. (If patients have extensor tone in the lower limbs or trunk they may be unable to break to extensor pattern to sit back down after standing. In this case, a squatting or sitting transfer will be more effective.) When possible, a standing transfer is preferred.

For patients to transfer independently, they must be able to:

- Demonstrate adequate safety awareness
- Move in bed
- Maintain a coactive trunk in sitting
- Follow directions (simple verbal or written)

The patient should:

1. Rehearse transfers to both sides. Often patients can only transfer in and out of bed, on and off a toilet or in and out of a car because of the location of the surface they are transferring to; for example, because the toilet is too close to the wall to transfer to either side, they must get off toward the same side from which they got on.
2. Move toward the edge of the sitting surface (bed, chair, toilet) using appropriate scooting method and maintaining an erect posture before transferring.
3. Shift body weight forward maintaining a coactive trunk.
4. Make use of all possible function.

The therapist should:

1. Explain and demonstrate the procedure to the patient.
2. Stand where the patient can be protected from falling.
3. Place hands on patient's pelvis, shoulders, or upper thorax or a combination of these key points of control.
4. Allow patients to use what function they have.
5. Allow patients to see in the direction they are moving.

The surface on which the patient will transfer should be:

• Immoblized
• Firm, to give good support
• The same level height as the wheelchair

The wheelchair:

• Should be locked
• Foot pedal should be raised
• Should be positioned so that the less involved side of the patient is closest to the surface he or she is transferring on to

As mentioned earlier, this is not always possible; therefore, it is imperative that transfer training is performed to both sides.

I. Techniques
   A. To and from wheelchair and bed or mat
      1. Lock wheelchair brakes, remove feet from footrests.
      2. Place feet flat on floor, uninvolved foot slightly behind involved foot. (Alternate method: Place involved foot behind to avoid extensor thrust as in hemiplegia.)
      3. Lean trunk forward, pushing down on handrail or wheelchair armrest nearest bed.
      4. Come to a standing position.
      5. Maintain balance.
      6. Grasp middle of far arm of wheelchair.
      7. Pivot on feet.
      8. Lower body into chair slowly.
      9. Lower foot pedal, place involved foot on pedal.
     10. Reverse procedure for wheelchair to bed.
     11. Procedure for a high bed transfer would necessitate the use of a foot stool.

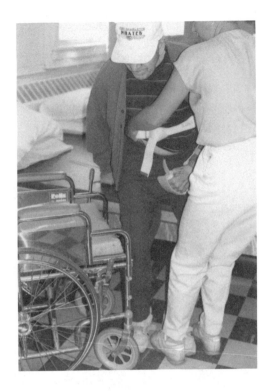

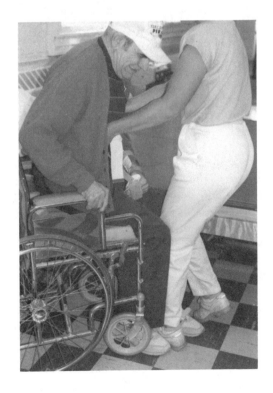

B. *Alternate method:* Assist to standing, stabilizing the patient's lower limbs from a sitting position.
   1. The therapist sits with feet crossed at the ankle joints, feet resting on the floor.
   2. Applying pressure with legs, the therapist pushes against the legs of the patient to support the lower limbs in extension.
   3. The therapist's upper limbs are used to control the pelvis and trunk.

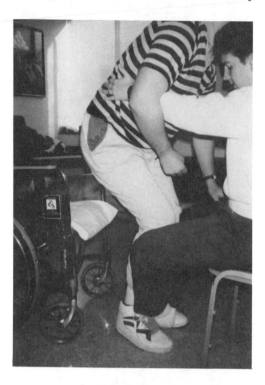

C. To and from wheelchair and toilet. In most cases a bathroom is so small that manipulation of wheelchair is difficult, and only one approach may be feasible. For the patient's safety and ease of transfer, a raised toilet seat and a handrail may be installed.
   1. Approach toilet with uninvolved side closest to the toilet seat.
   2. Lock wheelchair brakes, remove foot from footrest, and swing footrest away (clothing may be loosened at this time).
   3. Slide forward in chair; push down on armrest.
   4. Come to standing; pivot until standing in front of toilet.
   5. Lower clothing; sit down on toilet.
   6. From toilet to wheelchair, reverse the procedure.
D. To and from wheelchair and tub or shower. Getting in and out of the bathtub is one of the most hazardous transfers. This transfer should be made in a sitting position from a chair or stool onto a shower chair or stool placed in the shower or tub. Whenever possible the patient should transfer toward the involved side

when getting into the tub. The temperature of the water must be checked to avoid any danger of burning the patient. All clothing should be removed prior to transfer.

1. Position chair so that the involved side is closest to the tub.
2. Lock wheelchair brakes, remove foot from footrest, and swing footrest away.
3. Push down on chair seat, move toward edge of chair and onto the edge of tub.
4. Place involved leg in tub.
5. Push down, moving onto the chair in the tub.
6. Bring uninvolved leg into the tub.
7. From tub to chair, reverse procedure.

E. To and from wheelchair and floor
   1. Lock wheelchair brakes, remove foot from footrest and swing footrest away.
   2. Move to edge of chair, twist body toward involved side.
   3. Bend involved knee, placing involved foot behind uninvolved foot.
   4. Place hand on wheelchair seat, shift weight to uninvolved hand.
   5. Slowly lower body onto knees.
   6. Place uninvolved hand on floor, gently lower body to floor.
   7. Floor to wheelchair, reverse position.

F. To and from wheelchair and front seat of car
   1. Park car on level ground with emergency brakes on.
   2. Place wheelchair on passenger's side, facing the front of the car, and get the wheelchair as close to the front seat as possible.
   3. Lock wheelchair brakes, raise footrests and place feet flat on the ground; scoot hips forward.
   4. Come to standing by leaning forward at the waist and pushing with arm.
   5. Pivot so the back is turned toward the seat.
   6. Place uninvolved hand on any nonmovable part of the car (do not grasp the door or window).
   7. Sit down slowly on the front seat.
   8. Flex head to avoid hitting it on the top of the car.
   9. Lift legs into the car, use uninvolved leg to lift involved leg.
   10. Fasten seat belt.
   11. Reverse procedure to go from car to wheelchair.

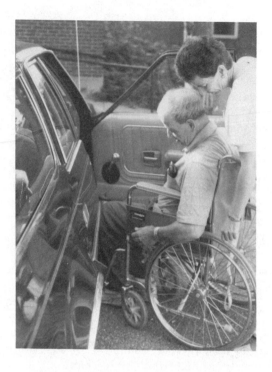

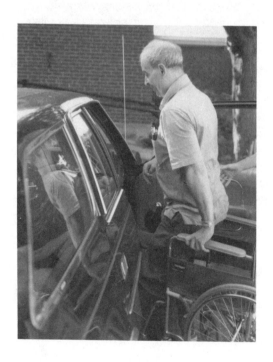

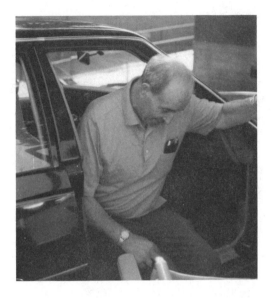

UPRIGHT ACTIVITIES

Measuring for a Cane

The patient stands erect, wearing shoes, and holds onto cane with uninvolved hand. A rubber suction tip, free of dust and lint, must cover the end of the cane. The cane is placed 6 to 8 inches from the toe and side of shoe. The top of the cane should be at the level of the greater trochanter. With the shoulder relaxed and level, the elbow should have 20 to 30 degrees of flexion.

Orthotic Management

Orthotic management should address the patient's current and anticipated functional status. Because an orthosis applies force it can assist the patient to stand with greater stability and to walk with fewer deviations, and it can counteract the tendency for development of specific deformities. Sometimes it may be necessary to compromise some of these treatment goals in the interest of reducing or eliminating bracing for the patient who complains about the appearance or cost of orthoses. Some individuals will accept a cane or other auxiliary aid rather than an orthosis.

Peroneal Neuropathy

The principal immediate problem experienced by the individual with a disorder of the common peroneal nerve is the tendency of the foot to drag during the swing phase of gait because of dorsiflexor paralysis. To reduce the risk of stumbling, the patient may resort to exaggerated hip flexion to raise the leg high enough to clear the floor. This gait pattern is unsightly and fatiguing. Also, some patients may experience slapping of the foot in early stance, which occurs because of the inability to strike the floor with the heel and control the downward motion of the foot. Chronic peroneal neuropathy is apt to result in pes equinus because the functioning triceps surae muscles is unresisted by the paralyzed dorsiflexors.

An orthosis can resist plantarflexion or assist dorsiflexion during the swing phase of gait. The same appliance will also prevent the foot from abrupt plantarflexion in the early stance phase. Wearing the orthosis on a regular basis will maintain the full length of the Achilles tendon in the presence of muscle imbalance, thus sparing the patient from pes equinus.

Orthotic Options for Peroneal Neuropathy

Posterior Leaf Spring Ankle-Foot Orthosis
This is the simplest orthosis for peroneal neuropathy. The insert portion will recoil when the leg is unloaded in swing phase, bringing the ankle to the neutral position, thereby preventing the foot from dragging. In the stance phase, as the wearer applies weight to the braced limb, the insert portion yields slightly, moving plantarward, to allow the foot to achieve the foot-flat position in a controlled manner.

Stirrup with Dorsiflexion Assist
This is an alternate orthosis with the stirrup terminating proximally with dorsi-flexion spring assists on the medial and lateral ends of the stirrup. The stirrup may be either solid or split and may be attached to the shoe with rivets and/or embedded in an insert. The orthosis achieves the same effect in swing and stance phase as does the posterior leaf spring orthosis. The spring assists, while bulky, are adjustable, so that the clinician can select the amount of springiness.

Posterior Stop
A third option involves posterior stops as part of the stirrup. The biomechanical effect in swing phase is identical to that of posterior leaf spring or dorsiflexion spring assists. In the stance phase, however, the posterior stop prevents any plantarflexion. Consequently, the individual reaches the midstance portion of gait by flexing the knee slightly. If the patient has normal neuromuscular and ligamentous control of the knee, there will be minimal risk of collapse. This orthosis may be indicated in the presence of mediolateral instability or deformity, particularly if the peroneal lesion is incomplete. Any tendency toward pes varus or valgus can be countered preferably by the use of an insert of the UCBL design, or the installation of a varus or valgus correction strap if the stirrups are riveted to the shoe.

Cerebral Vascular Accident

Patients with a stroke tend to drag the foot during swing phase because of persistence of the extensor synergy initiated during weight-bearing in stance phase of gait. The problem of advancing the lower limb is complicated by the inability to swing the upper limbs freely or rotate the trunk symmetrically. Perceptual disorder may cause the patient to lean toward the less involved side. The patient may discover that flexing the hip causes the distal joints to flex in reflex fashion, thus avoiding the chance of catching the toe on any object on the floor. Stance phase may begin with floor contact with the lateral border of the forefoot. Contact with the floor may trigger the extensor synergy, which causes excessive stability. The knee may be hyperextended either involuntarily in response to the synergy or voluntarily as the patient attempts to guarantee stability. Repeated hyperextension produces pain in the knee joint as ligaments are stretched. The patient who presents with flaccidity may fear that the knee joint will give way during stance. Forcible backward thrusting thus offers a semblance of protection against falling. Some patients then proceed very rapidly into a collapsed position of the foot as the medial border lowers quickly. Unless neurologic recovery occurs rapidly, the patient is likely to develop contracture of the Achilles tendon.

Safety during gait is the primary goal. The foot should be kept from dragging in swing phase, and in early stance the patient should be able to strike on the heel without excessive inversion. Protection of the knee is important to avoid pain, eventual ligamentous laxity, and arthritic changes, and for the patient with flaccidity, preventive flexion. One should also be concerned about development of pes equinus as the hypertonic triceps surae muscles overpower the dorsiflexors.

Orthotic Options for Cerebral Vascular Accident

Posterior Leaf Spring Ankle-Foot Orthosis

This orthosis is designed for patients with flaccidity or mild to moderate spasticity. It is simple to don and keeps the foot from dragging in swing phase, yet offers little resistance to reaching the foot-flat position in stance phase without jeopardizing the knee. Orthotic wear, in conjunction with regular exercise, should prevent Achilles contracture. If inversion is a conspicuous feature of early stance, then the basic posterior leaf spring orthosis will control foot placement. The shoe may need a lateral sole flare to resist overloading the lateral border. A more versatile approach is to alter the insert of the posterior leaf spring orthosis. The insert would include sidewalls to stabilize the subtalar joint in optimum position.

Stirrup with Posterior Stops

This orthosis is very sturdy and effective during swing phase of gait. During early stance phase, the patient may guard the knee against the flexion moment of force introduced by the calf band by thrusting the knee posteriorly. After several weeks of such force, the patient may cause the posterior stops to erode so much that the orthosis no longer provides a 90-degree stop. A control strap may be required. If varus persists during most of early stance, then the varus control strap should be used. If the foot reverses rapidly to eversion, then a valgus control strap will provide some stability.

Dorsiflexion Spring Assist

When spasticity is moderate or severe, the assist should be modified by replacing the coil spring with metal pins. The modification converts the joint to one that controls the ankle by limiting its motion. As spasticity reduces, the pins can be discarded in favor of springs.

Solid Ankle-Foot Orthosis

This orthosis is used in the presence of severe mediolateral instability or deformity. It offers maximum frontal and sagittal plane control.

Knee-Ankle-Foot Orthosis

Useful during early rehabilitation for patients with knee joint instability. Typically, a drop-ring lock is used. It is somewhat easier for the patient to manipulate if the lock is placed on the medial upright. The lock should be fitted with a spring-loaded retention button so that as the patient regains ambulatory skill, the therapist can place the locking ring in the unlocked position. It is also useful to prevent knee joint flexion contracture, which may develop if the patient spends extended periods sitting in a wheelchair. While the knee-ankle-foot orthosis is appropriate for institutional use, it is rarely satisfactory for continued use at home. It is cumbersome to don, especially by the patient who must manipulate with one hand. The severely involved patient may become confused about the need to unlock the knee when sitting.

I. Balancing Exercise*
   A. Kneeling
     1. Assume kneeling position from hand-knee position.
     2. Balance with one or no mat crutches.
     3. Shift weight from side to side.
     4. Maintain balance when pushed by therapist.
     5. Walk on knees; therapist may use resistance.
   B. Standing
     1. Assume standing from kneeling position by pushing with uninvolved leg and arm.
     2. Keep uninvolved foot forward, involved foot behind.
     3. Lean forward.
   C. Balance with aid of one parallel bar
     1. Shift weight from side to side.
     2. Lift uninvolved leg momentarily.
     3. Perform shallow knee bends using both legs and one leg at a time.
II. Walking on Level Surfaces
   A. From sitting to standing
     1. Lock both brakes and raise foot pedals.
     2. Place both feet firmly on floor with uninvolved foot slightly behind involved foot.
     3. Grasp armrests with uninvolved hand and slide forward in wheelchair.
     4. Shift weight to foot, lean forward, and extend elbow and knees.
     5. Balance in standing position and grasp parallel bars or assistive device.
     6. Reverse procedure to sit.

---

*Refer to Chapter 5 for more details on orthoses.

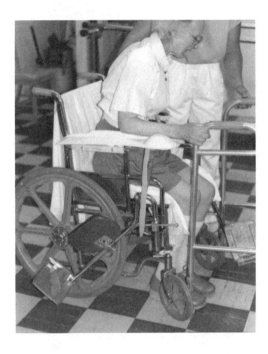

B. Parallel bars
   1. *Forward:* Three-point gait
      a. Advance uninvolved arm.
      b. Advance involved leg.
      c. Advance uninvolved leg.
      d. Key points
         (1) Steps of equal distance, step through pattern.
         (2) Equal weight distribution on both feet.

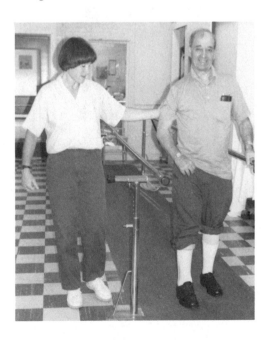

2. *Forward:* Two-point gait
   a. Uninvolved arm and involved leg advance simultaneously.
   b. Advance uninvolved leg.
   c. Key points
      (1) Steps of equal distance, step through pattern.
      (2) Equal weight distribution
3. *Backward:* Same technique as for forward.
4. *Sideward:* Facing one parallel bar, move in direction of involved side.
   a. Advance uninvolved arm toward involved side.
   b. Advance involved leg.
   c. Advance uninvolved leg.
   d. Key points
      (1) Steps of equal distance.
      (2) Equal weight distribution on both feet.

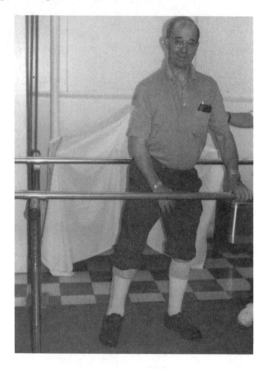

5. *Sideward:* Facing one parallel bar, move in the direction of uninvolved side.
   a. Advance uninvolved arm away from body.
   b. Advance uninvolved leg.
   c. Advance involved leg.
   d. Key points
      (1) Steps of equal distribution distance.
      (2) Equal weight distribution.
6. Turning toward affected side
   a. Cross uninvolved leg in front of involved leg.
   b. Grasp parallel bar on opposite side.
   c. Move involved leg.

7. From standing to sitting
   a. Back up toward wheelchair until wheelchair seat is touching legs.
   b. Grasp armrest with uninvolved hand.
   c. Bend head and trunk forward.
   d. Slowly lower body into wheelchair.
C. Cane
   1. Balance with a cane.
   2. Walk in parallel bars using cane.
   3. Follow same methods as described for parallel bars; forward, backward, sideward, and turning.
   4. Walk on level surface outside parallel bars using method described in parallel bars: forward, backward, sideward, and turning.
D. Hemiwalker, walker with casters, or standard walker
   1. Perform balance activities using walker.
   2. Ambulate on level surfaces by picking up or sliding walker forward.

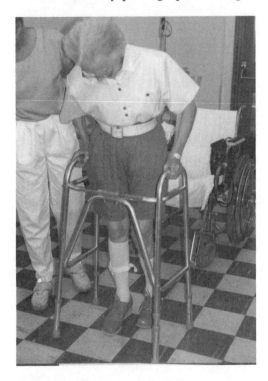

3. Standing and sitting with a walker from a wheelchair.
   a. Same procedure as for parallel bars.
E. Open, walk through, and close door
   1. Approach door.
   2. Grasp door handle with uninvolved hand, continue to hold cane.
   3. Step sideward while opening door.
   4. Turn and face door, close it.
F. Using platform rolling walker
   1. The platform may be adjusted to suit the need of the patient's involved upper limb.
   2. Perform the same activities as one would with a walker.

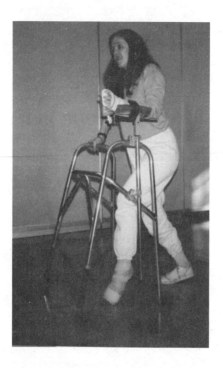

G. Ambulate with quad cane.
   1. This provides more stability than a cane.
   2. Perform the same activities as one would with a cane.

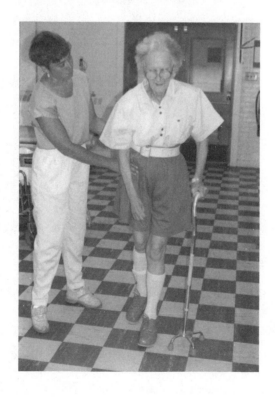

III. Transfers
  A. To and from bed
    1. Move toward the edge of bed.
    2. Sit up and place both feet on floor, uninvolved foot slightly back.
    3. Place uninvolved hand on bed, cane in easy reach.
    4. Lean forward, extend elbow and knees, shifting weight to both feet.
    5. Balance in standing position and grasp cane.
    6. Reverse procedure to sit.
  B. To and from toilet
    1. Approach front of toilet
    2. Turn, back facing toilet seat.
    3. Lower clothing.
    4. Grasp grab bar or back of toilet.
    5. Flex head and trunk forward, lowering self slowly onto toilet seat.
    6. Reverse procedure to stand.
  C. To and from bathtub
    1. Sit in chair, which is placed next to tub.
    2. Remove clothing.
    3. Proceed as described using sitting transfers.
  D. From standing to floor
    1. Move uninvolved foot forward.
    2. Shift weight to uninvolved side.
    3. Bend forward reaching floor, flexing hips and knees.
    4. Lower body gently to the floor, supporting most of weight on uninvolved side.
  E. Come to standing
    1. Assume kneel-standing position.
    2. Place uninvolved foot flat on floor.
    3. Lean forward, push to standing position.
    4. Lift cane while coming to standing position.
  F. To and from automobile
    1. Approach car door.
    2. Open door with uninvolved hand while holding cane.
    3. Turn backward and lean against front seat.
    4. Place cane in car.
    5. Grasp seat of car, back of seat, or dashboard.
    6. Flex hips, tuck chin, sit down slowly.
    7. Place feet in car.
    8. Reverse procedure to get out of car.
IV. Elevation Activities (When Using Handrail, Carry Cane)
  Always ascend leading with uninvolved foot and descend leading with involved foot.
  A. Ascending stairs with handrail
    1. Lead with uninvolved foot.
    2. Place uninvolved hand closer to hips of involved limb.
    3. Raise involved leg to same step.

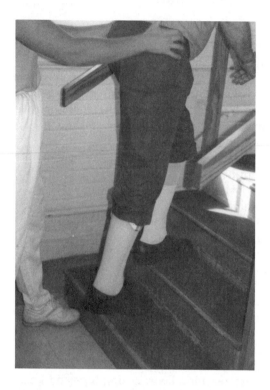

B. Descending stairs with handrail
   1. Lead with involved foot.
   2. Place hand near hips of involved limb.
   3. Step with uninvolved foot, bringing it to the involved foot on the same step.

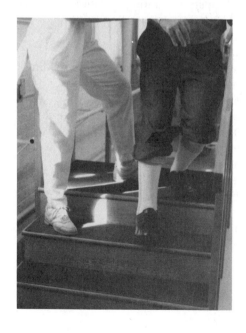

C. Ascending curbs using cane
   1. Stand with both feet near edge of curb.
   2. Place uninvolved foot on curb.
   3. Cane remains with involved foot below curb.
   4. Shift weight to uninvolved leg, simultaneously extending uninvolved leg.
   5. Raise cane and involved foot up onto curb.
D. Descending curbs using cane
   1. Shift weight to uninvolved foot on street.
   2. Place cane and involved foot on street.
   3. Shift weight to involved leg and cane.
   4. Bring uninvolved foot down to street.
E. Stairs without handrail, using cane
   1. Both feet placed at edge of stairs.
   2. Ascend, lead with uninvolved foot.
   3. Place cane with involved foot.
   4. Bring involved foot and cane up to step with uninvolved foot.
   5. Proceed until top of stairs has been reached.
   6. Reverse procedure to descend.

≡9
Functional Activities for Bilateral Lower Limb and Trunk Involvement

Paraplegia may result from a sudden onset of a spinal cord lesion such as a motor vehicle accident or a fall or it may be the result of an insidious onset such as multiple sclerosis or infection of the spinal cord. The degree of functional independence will vary according to the level of the lesion and function of the residual musculature.

The individual with a thoracic lesion has paralysis of the hips, knees, and feet. Depending on the level of lesion, trunk stability and respiratory capacity may also be compromised. The motor loss is compounded by tactile and proprioceptive anesthesia, so that the patient is aware of neither floor contact nor movement excursion. Further complicating rehabilitation is the risk of hip flexion contractures developing from prolonged sitting; contractures cause a disturbance of alignment when the individual tries to stand. Hip adductor spasticity may also cause problems by narrowing the standing and walking base. Bowel and bladder incontinence influence the selection of materials from which orthoses are made; urologic care may occupy considerable time that would otherwise be devoted to standing and walking. Although paraplegia spares the upper limbs, patients differ with regard to muscular development in the shoulder girdle and elbows. Wheelchair activities are limited only by the motivation and interests of the patient. The patient requires assistive devices for standing, as well as some means to advance the limbs during swing phase of gait.

LYING AND SITTING ACTIVITIES

I. Rolling from Supine to Side or Prone Position
   A. Strong upper limbs
      Grasp the edge of mattress with one hand and pull body over.
   B. Good upper limbs
      1. Grasp the edge of mattress with one hand.
      2. Pull with that hand and abduct opposite shoulder until weight is on forearm. Extend elbow to assume desired position.
      3. Lower limbs should follow.
      4. If moving to prone position, continue pulling on edge of mattress with hand until prone.
   C. Alternate method
      1. Come to sitting position.
      2. Cross one leg over the other.

      3. Reach one arm in front of trunk on bed, the other arm in back of trunk on bed lower self to prone position.

II. Coming to Sitting from Supine

  A. Strong upper limbs and at least 90 degrees of hamstring range

     1. Prop on elbows; shift weight to forearms.

     2. Extend elbows until weight is on hands.

     3. Walk hands forward until long sitting.

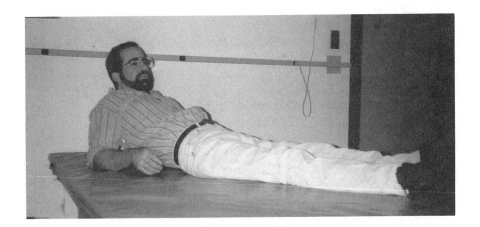

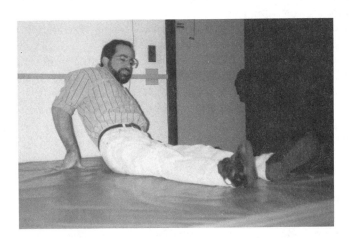

  B. Strong upper limbs and less than 90 degrees of hamstring range

     1. Come to side position, flexing hips slightly.

     2. Push up on both arms, by extending elbows.

     3. Walk hands toward hips.

     4. When able to reach back of thighs, use top arm to pull legs over edge of bed; other arm is supporting trunk.

     5. Continue walking hands toward hips until sitting.

   C. Alternatives
     1. Pull up with a long rope attached to foot of bed.
     2. Pull up on trapeze bar.
III. Moving in Bed
   A. Toward head of bed—sitting; must have 90 degrees of hamstring range
     1. Come to long sitting position.
     2. Place extended arms at sides and posterior to hips.
     3. Push arms against bed, elevating buttocks.
     4. Swing body weight through arms and set buttocks down behind hands.
   B. Toward foot of bed—sitting; must have 90 degrees of hamstring range
     1. Come to long sitting position.
     2. Place extended arms at sides and anterior to hips (hips should be flexed).
     3. Push arms against bed, elevating buttocks.
     4. Swing body weight through arms and set buttocks down in front of hands.
   C. Toward side of bed—sitting (to the right)
     1. Come to long sitting position.
     2. Place extended right arm in front of right hip and about a foot to the right side.
     3. Place extended left arm in front of left hip and close to left side of hip.
     4. Push against bed, elevating buttocks.
     5. Set buttocks down close to right hand.
     6. Keeping trunk flexed forward at hips, use hands to move and realign legs.
IV. Balancing Activities—Preliminary to Moving in Bed and Dressing
   Long sitting (unless hamstring range of motion [ROM] is less than 90 degrees). Need to do short sitting also.
   A. Shift trunk anteriorly, posteriorly, and laterally, facilitating trunk control with upper limbs in a weight-bearing position.
   B. Regain balance when pushed quickly to left, right, front, and back, using trunk musculature to facilitate trunk elongation and shortening appropriately.
   C. Protective falling—allow balance to be lost, catch weight on forearm, and resume sitting.
   D. Raise arms overhead; abduct.
   E. Throw and catch a ball.
   F. Can perform steps A through E also on a tilt board to further challenge sitting balance.
 V. Self-ROM*
   All patients with paraplegia are taught lower limb self-ROM. As soon as they learn, they are given the total responsibility for doing it themselves, and ROM aid by the hospital staff is discontinued. They are encouraged to range their legs daily before getting up in the morning and several times a day if they have a tendency to develop tightness easily. The motions should be performed in the sitting position. Patients should assume the position as described, count to 10

---

*Adapted from Rancho Los Amigos Hospital, Department of Physical Therapy, Downey, CA.

slowly, then slowly replace limb to resting position. This is to be repeated 10 times.

A. Hip and knee flexion

    1. Place the right hand under the right knee and pull the knee up toward the chest.

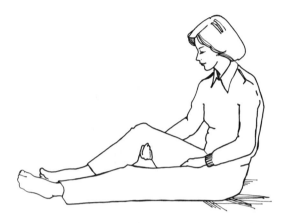

    2. Place your left hand on the shin and the right near the knee and pull it as close to your chest as possible

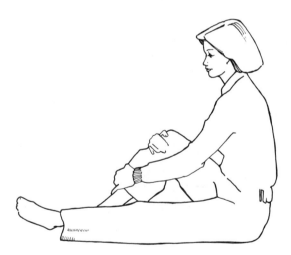

B. Hip lateral rotation and abduction

    Hold your right foot against the left leg with the left hand and gently push down on the knee with your right hand.

    Note: Do not force the leg down. The hip can dislocate or fracture easily in this position.

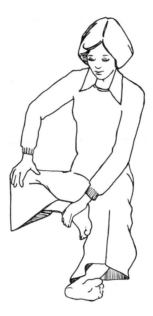

C. Ankle dorsiflexion

Begin with leg in position illustrated in step B. Balance on the right arm. Place the heel of the left hand under the forefoot (ball of the foot) and push it toward your knee.

Note: Toe flexion and extension may also be done in this position.

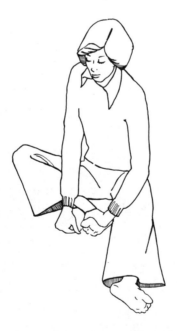

D. Dorsiflexion (this is the preferred method for patients with 120 degrees of hamstring length). However, the gastrocnemius muscle cannot be adequately stretched with the knee in flexion (step C). A towel can be used by hooking it around the forefoot and gently stretching the foot into dorsiflexion pulling on the towel. Sit with both knees straight. Lean forward helping balance with your right hand on the right leg. Place the left hand under the forefoot (ball of the foot) and pull toward your knee. If there is inadequate hamstring range, harmful stretching will be done to the back.

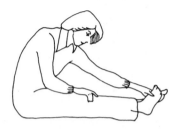

E. Hip medial rotation and adduction
  1. Balance on the left arm. Begin with your right hip and knee flexed and the foot flat on the mat. Place the right hand on the lateral border of your knee and gently push it across the other leg or as far as possible.

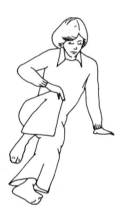

  2. Repeat previous steps for left leg.
F. Straight leg raising
  1. Lie on your back, grasp your right thigh or trousers with your right hand, and pull the leg toward your chest.
  2. Grasp the right ankle with your left hand.
  3. Place your right palm on the front of your knee.
  4. Pull the leg toward your chest with the left hand, keeping the knee straight by pushing on it with your right hand.
  Note: The right leg should not be pulled up beyond the point where the left leg leaves the surface. This will cause a stretch to the low back instead of the hamstring muscles.

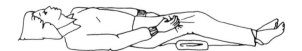

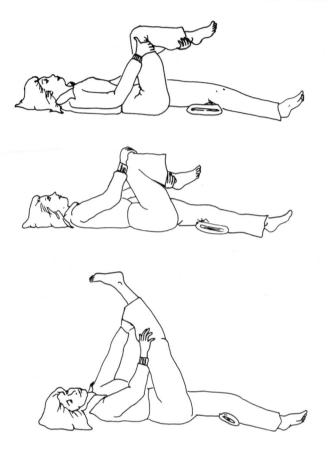

     5. Repeat step for left leg.

VI. Skin Inspection*

    A. Look at all parts of your body. Use a mirror for the hard-to-see parts, such as the tail bone, buttocks, the crease at the top of your leg where it joins the body at your buttocks, the groin (between legs), under breasts, under heels, shoulders, and elbows. If you are unable to use a mirror, get someone to help you, such as a nurse, attendant, or member of your family. Areas that have the greatest potential for skin breakdown are where sensation is decreased or lacking.

    Practical Suggestions

- Keep dry. Change clothing and/ or linen that has become wet from any cause: perspiration, spilled flood or liquids, urine, bath water, or rain.
- Keep your clothing and bed linen smooth and free of wrinkles. Make sure there are no food crumbs in your bed.
- Do not rub your skin across the bed.
- Changing your position relieves pressure.
- Because there is more pressure on bony prominences when sitting in a wheelchair, pressure must be relieved every 15 minutes. This can be done by shifting your weight from side to side and from back to front by "depressing and lifting," also called "push ups."

*Adapted from Rancho Los Amigos Hospital, Department of Physical Therapy, Downey, CA.

- Skin must be inspected in the morning before getting up and at night right after undressing for bed.
- Take skin inspection seriously, it may prevent irreparable damage.

VII. Dressing Activities

Upper limb dressing presents no problem for a patient with bilateral lower limb and trunk involvement. This activity is usually performed in the wheelchair after dressing the lower limbs.

A. Putting on trousers, long sitting in bed.
  1. Grasp waistband; toss trousers toward foot of bed.
  2. Put feet into legs of trousers; work trousers up over feet.
  3. While sitting, pull trousers over knees up to the hips.
  4. Lie down and roll from side to side, pulling pants into position.

B. Putting on skirt or dress, long sitting in bed.
  1. Put skirt or dress on over head.
  2. Lie down; pull skirt down over hips, rolling from side to side.

C. Putting on shoes and socks, long sitting in bed. Same positions as described for putting on trousers. (*Caution:* Avoid wrinkles in socks.)

MAT ACTIVITIES

The aim of a mat exercise program is for the patient to develop good physical condition and to improve his or her ability to learn and perform daily activity skills. These exercises should have functional carry-over to daily activities, not only in the development of strength, but also in the development of balance, coordination, and speed. Although most of the following activities are designed primarily for patients with bilateral lower limb weakness, a similar progression and a variation of these activities may be included in a treatment program for the patient with any disability, including patients with amputations, neuromuscular, musculoskeletal, and cardiopulmonary disorders. The activities should be selected to meet the individual needs of the patient.

Purposes of mat activities are to teach the following skills:

1. Changing position—prone to supine and supine to sitting
2. Sitting balance—moving trunk and/or arms
3. Movement in all directions while sitting
4. Handling of affected limbs
5. The patient's strengthening of muscles—push-ups, abdominal exercises, chin-ups, sitting push-ups, barbells, and dumbbells.
6. Stretching—active or passive
7. Coordination and skills—ball games, preparation for standing and walking in parallel bars, wheelchair transfers, and self-care activities
8. Deep breathing and chest mobility

Mat exercises may be appropriate for various diagnoses and may be taught to classes or an individual. Classes may include patients with similar or varied diagnoses.

When teaching mat activities to a group or an individual, remember to do the following:

1. Give an explanation of the activities

2. Demonstrate them
3. Participate by stabilizing and guarding
4. Correct errors in performance

Several methods of giving the exercises are:

1. Verbal counting (1 through 10)
2. Direction (up, down, in, and out)
3. Setting the rate (slower or faster)
4. Having patient give commands

Variations within the mat activities are helpful to maintain interest, such as a ball game in the middle or at the end of a class.

Advantages of mat classes are as follows:

1. Motivation of patient through socializing and competing with others
2. Reduction in boredom by changing the pace or routine
3. Opportunities to participate in group activities, such as ball games for balancing and coordination
4. Reduction in personnel required
5. Homogeneous classes may improve individuals attitude toward rehabilitation by participating with others having the some disability. Heterogenous classes are often the case depending on the situation. These individuals may vary in age, sex, and disability.

I. Supine Position
  A. Supine roller
    1. *Position:* Supine, arms raised to a vertical position, hands clasped together
    2. *Action:* Use pendulum chopping action of arms to initiate rolling.
    3. *Functional carry-over:* Develop coordination and strength necessary for changing bed position

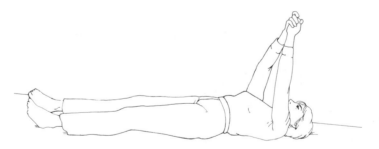

  B. Chest raiser
    1. *Position:* Supine, shoulders abducted to 90 degrees, elbows flexed, forearms perpendicular to mat
    2. *Action:* Upper back raised by hyperextending neck and shoulders and adducting scapula.
    3. *Functional carry-over:* Develop coordination and skill necessary for changing bed position
  C. Bridger (pelvic lifter)
    1. *Position:* Supine, hips and knees flexed, elbows close to trunk and forearms perpendicular to mat

2. *Action:* Hyperextend back, lifting hips off mat (making a bridge).
3. *Functional carry-over:* Transfer off and on bedpan, in and out of braces, and dressing activities

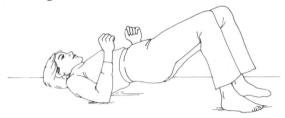

D. Pelvic tilt (anterior and posterior)
   1. *Position:* Supine, legs extended, arms at sides
   2. *Action:* Flatten and arch lower back.
   3. *Functional carry-over:* Assume erect position during ambulation
E. Hip hiker
   1. *Position:* Supine, legs extended, arms at sides
   2. *Action:* Approximate iliac crest to lower ribs.
   3. *Functional carry-over:* Ambulation and elevation activities.

II. Prone Position
   A. Prone push-up
      1. *Position:* Prone, hands in line with shoulders
      2. *Action:* Straighten elbows lifting trunk from mat.
      3. *Functional carry-over:* Getting up from floor with crutches and braces, standing from a wheelchair, and performing standing transfers with braces and crutches

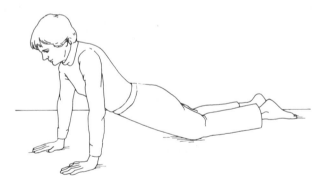

   B. Prone mover
      1. *Position:* Prone on elbows and forearms
      2. *Action:* Shift weight from elbow to elbow pulling body forward and pushing body backward.
      3. *Functional carry-over:* Develop coordination and strength for moving in prone position
III. Sitting Position
   A. Sit-ups
      1. *Position:* Supine, legs extended, arms at sides
      2. *Action:* Hyperextend shoulders and flex neck, flex elbows, raise head and shoulders off mat, assume forearm position, extend elbows, and come to sitting.

     3. *Functional carry-over:* Being able to assume sitting position for dressing and putting on braces

B. Leg mover
     1. *Position:* Sitting, legs extended
     2. *Action:* Abduct and adduct the opposite leg with hands.
     3. *Functional carry-over:* Wheelchair transfers, placing legs in braces

C. Sitting push-ups
     1. *Position:* Sitting, arms at sides opposite hips, palms flat on the mat or on blocks
     2. *Action:* Straighten elbows, depress shoulders, lift buttocks from mat.
     3. *Functional carry-over:* Off and on bed pan, in and out of braces, wheelchair transfers

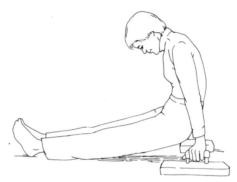

D. Sitting balance
     1. *Position:* Sitting, legs extended, progress to short sitting
     2. *Action:* Trunk shifting, arm raising, protective falling, shift body weight by using the arms and head, throwing and catching a ball, self-ROM
     3. *Functional carry-over:* Develop balance and coordination in sitting position

E. Trunk twister and hip raiser
     1. *Position:* Sitting, legs extended, arms at sides
     2. *Action:* Twist the trunk, place both hands to one side, straighten elbow, and raise hips from mat.
     3. *Functional carry-over:* Getting up from floor with braces and crutches, assume hand-knee position

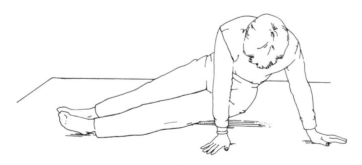

F. Toe toucher
     1. *Position:* Sitting, legs extended and slightly abducted, arms at side

      2. *Action:* Bend trunk forward and downward, touching both hands to one foot.

      3. *Functional carry-over:* Moving legs, transfers, and dressing

  G. Sitting hip-hiker

      1. *Position:* Sitting, legs extended, hands opposite hips

      2. *Action:* Hike hip on one side, moving hip backwards, shift weight to that side, repeat.

      3. *Functional carry-over:* Wheelchair transfers, changing bed position ambulation and elevation activities

  H. Sitting swing-through

      1. *Position:* Sitting, legs extended, arms at sides, opposite hips, or on blocks

      2. *Action:* Moving backwards, place hands 6 inches behind hips, lift buttocks from mat, and swing hips back through hands. Repeat moving forward and to the side.

      3. *Functional carry-over:* Wheelchair transfers, ambulation and elevation activities

IV. Hand-Knee Position

  A. Assume hand-knee position

      1. *Position:* Prone, hands in line with shoulders

      2. *Action:* Push on hands, straighten elbows, tuck chin, round back, align hips over knees.

      3. *Functional carry-over:* Getting up from the floor with braces and crutches, standing transfers with braces and crutches

  B. Assume hand-knee position (from sitting)

      1. *Position:* Sitting, legs extended and crossed (leg opposite direction of turn should be crossed over the other leg). Place both hands at hip opposite direction of turn.

      2. *Action:* Swing arms in direction of turn, place hands on mat next to hip, push up on hands and twist trunk, keeping head tucked and back rounded.

      3. *Functional carry-over:* Getting up from the floor with braces and crutches, standing transfers with braces and crutches

  C. Hip swayer

      1. *Position:* Balance on hands and knees

      2. *Action:* Sway hips from side to side, forward and backward.

      3. *Functional carry-over:* Wheelchair transfers with braces and crutches, ambulation and elevation activities

  D. Cat and camel (trunk flexion and extension)

      1. *Position:* Hands and knees, head up, low back in lordotic position

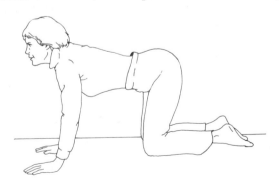

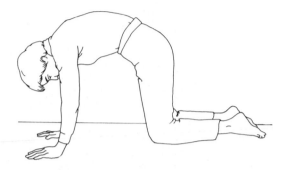

    2. *Action:* Lower head between arms, rounding back.

    3. *Functional carry-over:* Getting up from the floor, standing from wheelchair with braces, ambulation and elevation activities

  E. Forward and backward reacher

    1. *Position:* Hands and knees

    2. *Action:* Shift weight to legs and one arm, reach backward and touch buttocks, reach forward.

    3. *Functional carry-over:* Getting up from the floor with braces and crutches, standing from wheelchair, locking and unlocking braces

  F. Hip hiker

    1. *Position:* Hands and knees

    2. *Action:* Shift body weight to arms and one leg, hike opposite hip.

    3. *Functional carry-over:* Ambulation and elevation activities

V. Kneeling Position

  A. Assume kneeling

    1. *Position:* Hands and knees using mat crutches

    2. *Action:* Crutches placed on each side of body with top toward feet. Grasp handpiece of one crutch, palms forward; place crutch semivertical on the floor by pronating forearm (crutches cane style). Brace crutch against arm and shoulder, bring other crutch to same position, push up erect and roll pelvis forward, walk crutches back and place under arms.

    3. *Alternate action:* Crutches on same side of body, grasp both crutches by hand grips, palm forward, lift crutches to semivertical position by pronating forearms (crutches cane style). Brace crutches against shoulder, shift weight and place other hand on lower shaft of crutches, walk hand up crutches, tuck pelvis, establish balance, remove top crutch and place under axilla, reverse grip on other crutch and place under axilla.

    4. *Functional carry-over:* Getting up from floor with braces and crutches, standing from wheelchair with braces and crutches, ambulation and elevation activities

  B. Kneeling balance

    1. *Position:* Kneeling with crutches, bench, or chair

    2. *Action:* Weight shifting, forward and sideward, arm and crutch raising, forward, backward, sideward; hip swayer; crutch placer, forward, backward, and sideward.

    3. *Functional carry-over:* Develop balance and coordination for all upright activities

  C. Jack-knife and return

    1. *Position:* Kneeling with crutches, opposite hips

2. *Action:* Place crutch 8 to 10 inches behind hips, shift body weight to hands, allow hips to jack-knife, shoulders stabilized, pull trunk forward and upward extending hips, by pushing down on handgrips, bring hands forward to starting position.
3. *Functional carry-over:* Ambulation and elevation activities

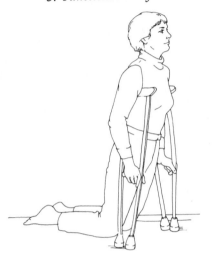

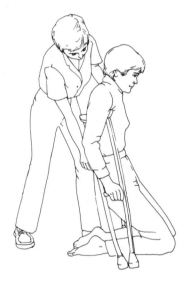

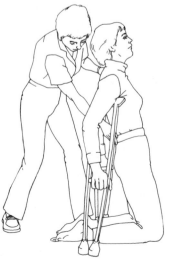

D. Dipper
　　1. *Position:* Kneeling with crutches or bench
　　2. *Action:* Hands forward of hips, shift body weight onto hands, flex elbows and hips until trunk is parallel to mat, straighten elbows and return to starting position.

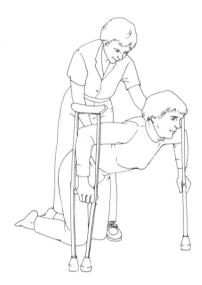

　　3. *Functional carry-over:* Wheelchair to standing, floor to standing
E. Hip hiker
　　1. *Position:* Kneeling with crutches or bench
　　2. *Action:* Shift weight to one side, raise hip on opposite side.
　　3. *Functional carry-over:* Ambulation and elevation activities
F. Return to floor
　　1. *Position:* Kneeling with crutches or bench
　　2. *Action:* Reverse of "Assume knee standing, V, A2."
　　3. *Functional carry-over:* Standing to wheelchair, standing to floor
G. Falling
　　1. *Position:* Kneeling with crutches
　　2. *Action:* Discard crutches by supinating forearms, extending elbows and abducting shoulders, catch fall on hands and quickly roll onto forearms, turning head to one side.
　　3. *Functional carryover:* Protective falling from an upright position using crutches

WHEELCHAIR MOBILITY

To begin learning manual wheelchair skills, it is necessary for patients to learn something about themselves, their wheelchair, and wheelchair skills and techniques. With this combination of knowledge, good judgment, desire, patience, and practice, patients will be able to develop the skills necessary to be an independent wheelchair user. They should be aware of their physical condition, limits of endurance, strength, and disability in order to understand their needs and limitations both for safety and attaining independent wheelchair performance.

Several factors may affect the level of safe wheelchair performance such as spasticity, pain, weight distribution, visual impairment, or decreased ROM. Each wheelchair technique is adapted to meet the individual needs. Wheelchair selection should consider the needs of the individual, including activity level, safety, and comfort.

Paraplegic individuals will be able to perform almost all wheelchair activities unless there are some unusual circumstances such as severe spasticity. Learning the techniques initially will require work, practice, and patience.

I. Preliminary Activities
1. Leaning forward in chair, balance trunk without use of arms if trunk control is present.
2. Leaning forward and reaching floor, then regaining sitting position. Patient may hook one arm behind wheelchair handle if necessary.
3. Shift weight from side to side.
4. Shoulder girdle depression (push-ups)

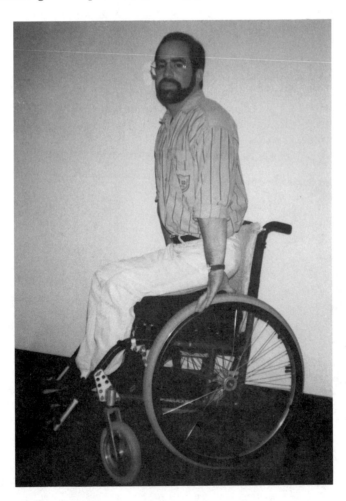

B. Manipulation of wheelchair parts

1. Remove feet from foot pedals.
2. Pull heel loop forward.
3. Raise foot pedal.
4. Swing away legrests.
5. Remove armrests, place on wheelchair handle.
6. Replace armrests.
7. Swing legrest into place, pull heel loops back.
8. Lower foot pedal.
9. Place feet on foot pedal.

II. Level Surface
  A. Forward propulsion
    1. Starting position—Grip the pushrim or handrim and the tire. Place thumb on the surface of the tire and hold the fingers around the handrim. The upper limbs are back with the elbows slightly flexed and the trunk erect.
    2. Action: The forward push is from a 10 o'clock to a 2 o'clock position, or at the limits of one's ROM.
      a. Lean forward with a forward head.
      b. Flex the elbows applying pressure down on the handrim past 12 o'clock.
      c. Snap the wrists as the elbows extend and the shoulders rotate medially and depress.
      d. As the power stroke is completed, the hands drop in a relaxed position.
      e. Reposition the hands on the handrims.
    3. Teaching tip: The wrist snap is important for controlled forward motion and momentum of the wheelchair. The action is like that of throwing a frisbee.

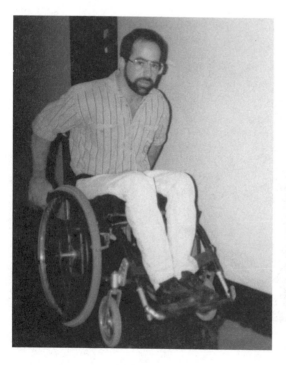
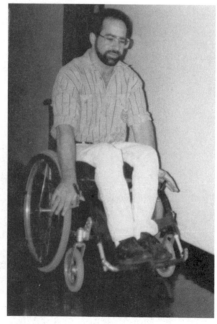

Note. Keep the upper limbs extended and relaxed as they swing back for the next stroke. Do not pull the upper limbs up and back, which seems to be a natural tendency for most wheelchair users. The first few strokes are power strokes until momentum is built up, then one can loosen the grip and catch the tire and develop strokes in a smooth rhythm. Once momentum is established it is possible to coast every few strokes to rest the upper limbs. Speed is controlled by applying even pressure on the tires and handrims. Uneven pressure would cause the wheelchair to turn.

B. Backward propulsion
   1. Starting position—Grip the handrims as stated earlier for forward propulsion.
   2. Motion—The thrust of the motion is from the 2 o'clock to the 10 o'clock position.
       Note. Caution: A forceful backward motion with a sudden stop can cause the wheelchair to tip over backward. A slight forward lean of the trunk will counteract this tendency.
C. Turning
   1. Starting position—Propelling forward.
   2. Action: Apply pressure (squeeze) on the rim and wheel to create a drag on the tire in the direction of the turn while applying forward motion on the opposite tire.

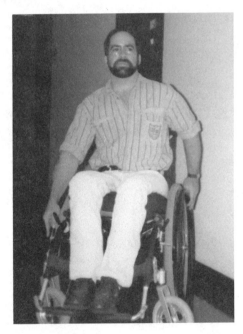

   3. Tip: The greater the pressure, the quicker the turn.
D. Cornering (using the wall)
   1. Starting position—Adequate momentum is necessary for a smooth turning of a corner.
   2. Action: Approach the corner.
       a. Reach out and contact the wall with the hand in the direction of the turn. The center of gravity will pivot the wheelchair around the corner.

      b. Also pivot by trailing the arm along the object or wall to guide the turn.

   3. Tip: Use the object and momentum to do the work.

E. Through door

   1. Staring position—Reduce forward momentum of chair.

   2. Action

      a. Approach the door, pulling or pushing the door open.

      b. Propel the chair forward with one hand while guiding the direction of the chair with the other hand on the door.

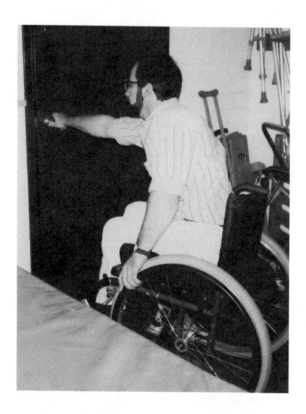

F. Lateral hopping—This is an advanced sill that is necessary in order to maneuver the wheelchair in small or tight places. It requires strength, grip, and the ability to shift weight.

   1. Starting position—Grip the handrims and tires firmly.

   2. Action

      a. With a quick, forceful motion pull up on the rims.

      b. At the same time lift and shift the weight, either to the left or right, sliding the wheelchair under you.

   3. Tip: The procedure should be performed in one fluid motion.

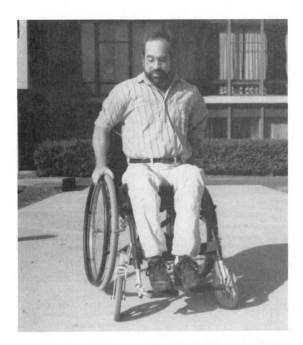

G. Falling from wheelchair (backward)—Wheelchair users should experience and practice this activity so they know what to expect and will be prepared to protect themselves from injury.
   1. Starting position—Tuck chin, place hands on top of knees. This position will protect both the upper limbs and the head from serious impact.
   2. Action
      a. Get out of the wheelchair
      b. Right it and use the techniques described in getting up from the floor and into the wheelchair.
H. Static "Wheelie"—Mastering wheelies will allow the wheelchair user independently and safely to maneuver curbs, curb cuts, ramps, and, in some cases, stairs. A static wheelie may be used to rest or for pressure relief by leaning the back of the chair against a wall or a corner of a room.
   1. Starting position
      a. Align wheelchair casters in a forward direction.
      b. Lean trunk slightly forward.
      c. Place hands slightly behind hips about the 2 o'clock position on the handrims.
   2. Action
      a. Extend trunk, hitting the back of the chair to give the chair momentum to raise the casters.
      b. At the same time pull forward on the tires by bending the elbows.
      c. Slightly flex the head to assist in raising the wheels to balance the chair in the wheelie position.
      d. Once up in the wheelie position, the head should be slightly forward.
      e. Once in the wheelie position, a change in the head position will alter the balance of the chair.

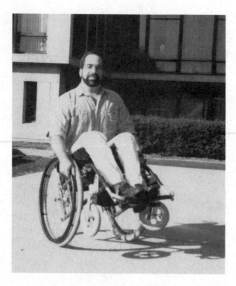

3. Teaching tip—Once in the wheelie position, the front of the chair is weightless. It is important to feel when the chair is balanced and the front end is weightless. Try to keep forward motion to a minimum to reduce the need for stopping the motion, which causes the front end of the chair to drop down. Keep hands at 12 o'clock to maintain position and to be ready to correct for changes in balance. If the chair falls backward, pull back on rims; if chair falls forward, push forward on rims.

4. *Caution:* Do not take hands off handrims; slide them forward or back. Once the hands are removed from the rims, the chair will fall forward or backward.

   I. Dynamic Wheelie—Dynamic wheelies are used to descend curbs and curb cuts, and, in some cases, to descend ramps and stairs.

1. Starting position—Static wheelie.

2. Action—Maintaining the chair in a wheelie position, propel the chair forward using a power stroke.

3. Teaching tip—The speed at which one descends is controlled by using friction applied with pressure from the palms of the hands.

III. Inclines (it requires more effort to ascend an incline than to propel on level terrain)

  A. Ascending ramps

    1. Starting position—Lean forward in the wheelchair to bring the center of gravity forward in the chair.

    2. Action—The forward strokes are short and quick.

      a. Begin at the 12 o'clock and end at the 2 o'clock position on the hand-rim.

      b. Repeat the motion rapidly until the top of the incline has been reached.

        Note. If a railing has been installed use the rail by pulling with the upper limb on the railing while pushing forward with the other hand on the handrim of the wheelchair.

  B. Descending ramps

    1. Starting position—Lean the trunk back to place the center of gravity over the rear wheels.

2. Action—Apply pressure to the tires and handrims to control the speed with which one descends the ramp.
3. Tip: Making slight turns to the right and left will slow down the speed of descent.
    a. Turns on the decline are accomplished by alternately shifting the pressure applied to the handrims and tires.
    b. If the decline is steep, one should traverse the ramp making sharp 90-degree turns in either direction during the descent.
IV. Curbs
    A. Ascending curbs
        1. Starting position—Perform a wheelie close to the curb.
        2. Action—In the wheelie position place front casters onto the curb, flex trunk forward to shift weight over the casters, using a power stroke bring the large wheels onto the sidewalk.

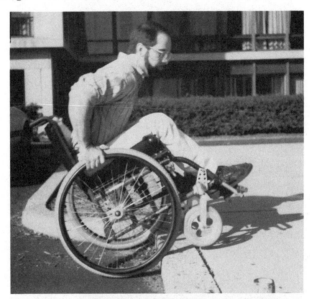

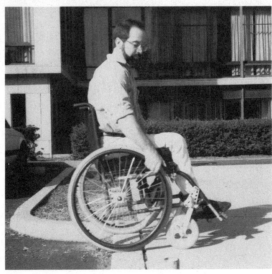

3. Use momentum to help project the chair onto the sidewalk.
B. Descending curbs—forward
    1. Starting position—Perform a wheelie and bring chair forward until the front casters are beyond the curb.
    2. Action
       a. Propel wheelchair forward from the wheelie position.
       b. Ease the large wheels off the curb while maintaining a wheelie position.
       c. Once on the flat surface, lower the front casters.

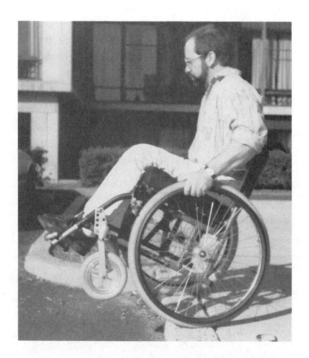

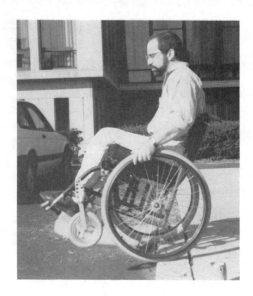

V. Curb Cuts

Curb cuts are provided to minimize the need for ascending or descending curbs in the full wheelie position. The width of the cut and the degree of incline with the street and curb should be studied to determine the practicality of using the curb cut. Plan the route ahead of time to determine the best approach. In the beginning, it may be best to wear a lap belt so that, in case of a fall, one would not be separated from the wheelchair.

A. Ascending curb cuts
1. Starting position — timing and momentum are essential for ease of achieving the top of the cut. Approach the cut squarely.
2. Action — Control speed at the entry of the cut with the upper limbs in the power stroke at the 10 o'clock position.
   a. Perform a low wheelie to raise the casters to avoid dragging the foot pedals.
   b. Gain the top of the cut with minimal effort and maximum control.

B. Descending curb cuts
1. Starting position — Approach the entrance to the cut squarely.
2. Action — Use a low wheelie to avoid hitting the foot pedals on the decline. Apply pressure to the tires and rims to control speed of descent.
3. Tip: A low wheelie may also be necessary to provide additional clearance to ascend onto the surface of the street.

VI. Stairs and Steps

A. Ascend — two-person assist
1. Starting position
   a. Back the wheelchair to the base of the stairs.
   b. One person should be above and one behind the wheelchair to assist.
   c. The person in front at the feet should guard against slipping.
   d. Each assistant should hold the wheelchair on a fixed part of the frame.
2. Action
   a. The assistant standing behind the chair will pull up.
   b. The wheelchair user will pull back on the handrims.
   c. If a rail is available:
      (1) The wheelchair user grips the rail with one hand and crosses the other hand to grasp the handrim closest to the rail.
      (2) The wheelchair user pushes down against the rail pulls up on the tire and handrim while the assistant lifts up on the chair.

B. Descend — one-person assist
1. Starting position — Approach the steps backward, tires squared off with the edge of the steps. The assistant stands behind, at the back of the chair to support the wheelchair and help control the speed of descent.
2. Action
   a. Lean forward, grasp the handrims.
   b. Control the descent by pressure on the handrims.
3. If a rail is available reach back with one hand and grasp the handrim and grip the rail with the other hand.

C. Unassisted stairs forward — This advanced activity may be beyond the expectation of many wheelchair users.
1. Starting position — Descending stairs may be performed in the same position as descending a curb.
2. Action — Descend each stair while maintaining a wheelie position.

   D. Entering a bus
      1. Starting position—Position the wheelchair facing backward to the elevating platform.
      2. Action
         a. Back onto the platform
         b. Propel backward into the bus.
         c. Use wheel locks to secure the wheelchair.
 VII. Transfers
   The more forward the body weight or center of gravity, the higher the buttocks and easier the transfer. This is accomplished by keeping the head forward and down. Hamstring range is so important because without it, the patient will stretch out the low back in order to get the body weight forward. When one depresses against the bed, part of the motion is absorbed in back motion and what is left lifts the buttocks. Therefore, the tighter the back the better. Patients with adequate quadriceps strength or other muscle power may be able to do a standing transfer.
   A. To and from wheelchair and bed or mat.
      Patient may do a sitting transfer, depressing the shoulder girdle and weight-bearing on the hands. At first a sliding board may be necessary, but it should eventually be eliminated.
      1. To the side, using removable armrest. This method is best if hamstring range is less than 100 degrees.
         a. Lock wheelchair.
         b. Transfer legs to bed first. On return, leave them on bed until last.
         c. Place feet on floor before transfer to or from bed.

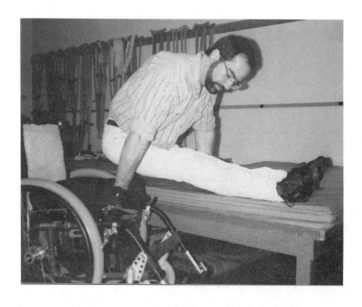

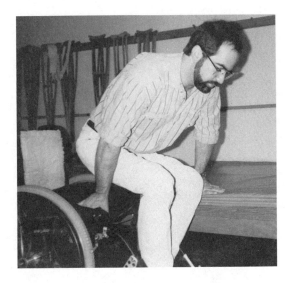

2. Forward with wheelchair facing side of bed; patient must have at least 100 degrees hamstring range and swing away legrests.
    a. Lock wheelchair.
    b. Patient places feet on bed first.
    c. Swing away legrest, unlock chair, and wheel closer until touching bed.
    d. Lock the chair, depress, and slide forward.
3. Backward using a zippered backrest
    a. The patient backs up to side of bed.
    b. Lock wheelchair, unzip back, depress, and slide back.
B. To and from wheelchair and toilet
  1. Facing the front of toilet
    a. Lock wheelchair.
    b. Place feet on floor and swing away legrests.
    c. Position clothing to just above the knees or remove clothing from one leg.
    d. Unlock wheelchair.
    e. Approach toilet as closely as possible.
    f. Lock wheelchair.
    g. Depress shoulders and slide forward, while straddling toilet seat.
    h. Return to chair by reversing procedure.

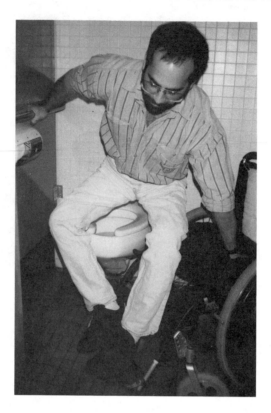

2. Facing the side of the toilet
   a. Approach toilet from the side.
   b. Lock wheelchair, leaving room to swing legrest away on side closest to toilet.
   c. Place feet on floor, swing away legrests.
   d. Unlock wheelchair, approach toilet as closely as possible, lower clothing.
   e. Lock wheelchair; remove armrest closest to toilet.
   f. Hang armrest over wheelchair handle.
   g. Depress shoulders until sitting forward on wheelchair seat.
   h. Depress shoulders, lower self to toilet seat, sit facing forward.
   i. Reverse procedure to return.
3. Backward
   a. Back wheelchair up to toilet as far as possible, lock wheelchair.
   b. Lower clothing.
   c. Unzip or open turnbuckles of backrest.
   d. Place hands as far back on armrests as possible, depress shoulders, slide back onto toilet seat.
   e. Reverse procedure to return to chair.

C. To and from wheelchair and bathtub

This transfer should be made in the sitting position from a chair onto a chair or stool placed in the tub. If the patient has sufficient upper limb strength to get up from the bottom of the tub, the stool or chair may be eliminated. For the ease of transfer and safety, grab bars may be installed. Water temperature must be checked to avoid any danger of burning. All clothing should be removed prior to performing the transfer.

1. Forward, facing side of tub
   a. Approach tub, leaving enough room to swing legrests away.
   b. Lock wheelchair, place legs over edge of tub.
   c. Swing away legrests.
   d. Unlock chair, move chair as close to tub as possible.
   e. Lock wheelchair, place one hand on each armrest, depress shoulders, and slide forward until sitting on rim of tub.
   f. Position legs so that knees are extended and feet are pointing toward end of tub.
   g. Place hands on rims of tub or grab bar, twist, and slowly lower body into tub.
   h. Reverse procedure from tub to chair.
2. Forward, facing end of tub (same procedure as in 1, except approach will be made from end of tub: patient will not have to twist as body is lowered)
   Note. See Chapter 6 for construction of bathtub chair.

D. To and from wheelchair and floor

The ability to transfer from the floor to the wheelchair is an essential activity for the safety and independence of patients with paraplegia. The ability to return to the wheelchair is necessary if the patient falls out of the chair or wishes to transfer to the ground. This activity requires maximum upper limb strength. Preliminary to independent transfer from floor to wheelchair (or wheelchair to floor), the patient should begin with the use of benches or stools of various heights placed in front of the wheelchair seat or one stool placed at right angles to the seat of the wheelchair.

1. Wheelchair to floor—forward
   a. Position feet on the floor off to one side.
   b. Scoot to one side of the chair.
   c. Reach for the floor with one hand; the other remains on the seat of the wheelchair.

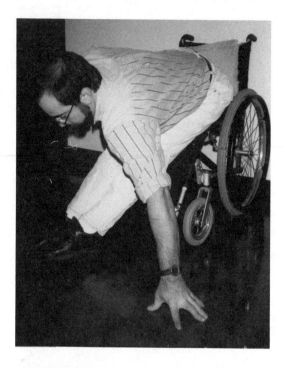

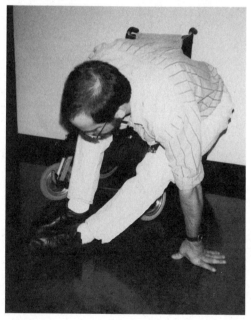

    d. Shift body weight to the hand on the floor.
    e. Slowly lower the body to the floor.
  2. Floor to wheelchair-backward, without use of stools or benches
     a. Lock both large wheels, turn heel loops up, lift foot pedals. Turn
       caster wheels forward to give a wider base of support.
     b. Place front edge of the seat cushion even with front edge of the

deskarm skirt guard or approximately one handwidth from the front edge of the seat.

  Note. Because the seat cushion makes the transfer difficult to learn, this step may be taught after the patient learns the transfer easily without a seat cushion.

c. Sit between the footrests with hips even with the front of the caster wheels.

  Note. If patient's hips do not fit between foot pedals, one can be unlocked and swung away.

d. Place both hands on the upper part of the footrest hanger brackets.

e. Lean the head and trunk slightly forward and lift the body by depressing the shoulders and extending the elbows.

f. Shift body weight slightly backward and over the left arm, keeping the elbow locked in extension, if possible.

g. Quickly place the right hand on the lower level of the deskarm or seat. Left elbow must be kept locked in extension to support the body.

  Note. Some patients may prefer to place their hand on the seat.

h. Shift body weight slightly backward and toward the right arm.

i. Quickly place the left hand on the lower level of the deskarm or seat.

j. Elevate the body by depressing shoulders and extending elbows.

  Note. Many patients are able to eliminate the next four steps. If they are able to rest their hips on the seat, they place their hands on the padded deskarm and continue with step o.

k. Shift weight slightly backward and over the right arm, keeping the elbow locked in extension, if possible.

l. Quickly place left hand on the padded level of the armrest.

m. Shift body weight slightly backward and toward the left arm.

n. Quickly place right hand on the padded level of the deskarm.

o. Elevate the body by leaning slightly forward and depressing the shoulders and extending the elbows until the hips are above the seat and near the back rest.

p. Lower the body gently onto the seat by gradually relaxing the shoulders and elbows. The seat cushions should slide into place as the trunk is lowered. However, steps o and p may need to be repeated several times, or other adjustments made for proper placement of the cushion.

q. Lower the foot pedals, pull heel loops back, and place the feet on the pedals.

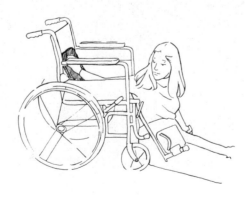

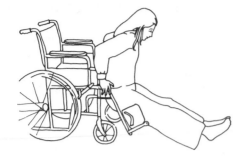
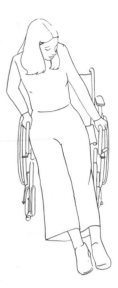

3. Backward approach—with stool at right angle to wheelchair.
   a. From a sitting position on the floor with back toward wheelchair seat, place one hand on the stool, the other hand on wheelchair seat.
   b. Shift weight to arms, depressing shoulders, raise body from floor onto seat of wheelchair.
   c. Shift weight back into wheelchair and adjust legs.
   d. From wheelchair to floor, reverse aforementioned procedure
4. Sideways approach—from floor
   a. Lock wheelchair.
   b. Position in front of wheelchair off to one side.
   c. Flex hips and knees.

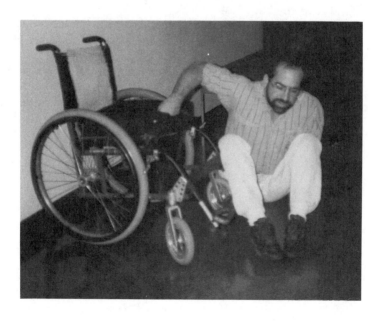

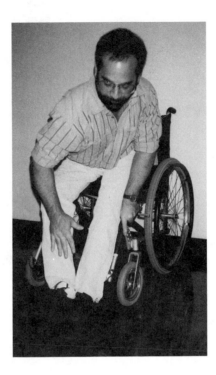

d. Place one hand on the wheelchair seat and the other close to the hips.
e. Push down, depressing the shoulder girdle and shifting the body weight toward upper limb on the seat of the wheelchair.
f. Quickly shift weight onto the seat and remove the hand on the seat.
g. Position self comfortably into the chair.
   Note. Fluid motion and momentum increase the ability to perform this transfer.
5. Forward approach—from floor to wheelchair
   a. Lock wheelchair, place casters forward, and swing footrests to sides. Sit diagonally to the front and left side of wheelchair.
   b. Place both hands on the front part of the deskarms, (right hand on left deskarm, left hand on right deskarm).
   c. Pull self to kneeling, facing the wheelchair.
   d. Push down on both hands until elbows are extended and body is raised, while twisting trunk to the right.
   e. Lean left hip onto the wheelchair seat. Must be stable enough to be able to momentarily move hands to change their position.
   f. Place left hand on wheelchair seat and right hand on right armrest.
   g. Place left hand on left armrest.
   h. Push down on hands until elbows are straight and hips are well back in the wheelchair.

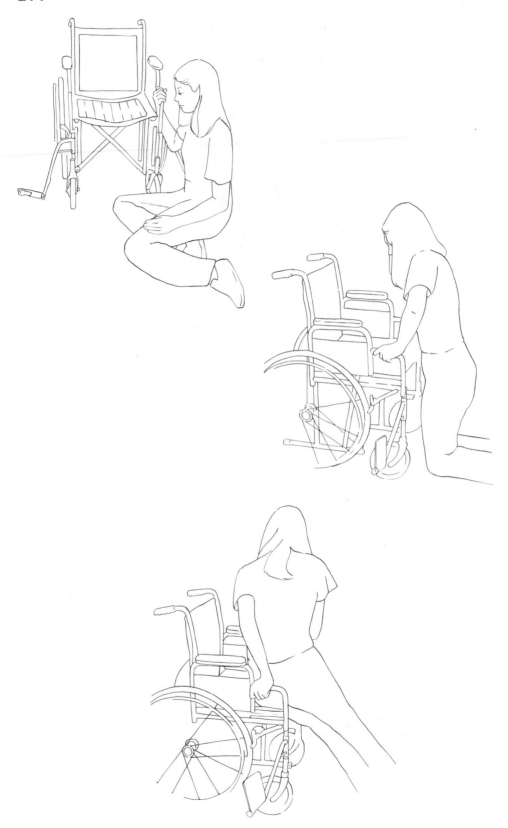

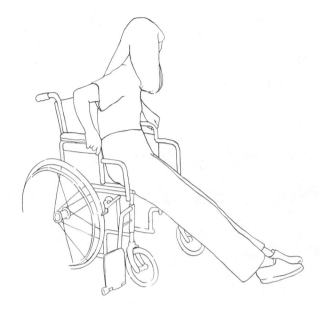

       i. Ease into the sitting position, swing the footrests back into position, and place feet on the footrests.

E. To and from wheelchair and automobile—side approach

Using a sliding board may be a preliminary to independent transfer from wheelchair to car.

  1. Approach front seat of car, lock wheelchair, and remove legrest on side closest to car.

  2. Approach as closely as possible to carseat; lock brakes.

  3. Remove armrest on side closest to carseat; place armrest and legrest on back seat of car.

  4. Slide to the edge of wheelchair by depressing shoulders.

  5. Place one hand on seat of wheelchair and one hand on seat of car; depress shoulders, transferring to carseat.

  6. Place legs in car.

  7. Reverse procedure for car to wheelchair.

F. Placing wheelchair into back seat of automobile

  Note. In order for a person to transfer the wheelchair into an automobile, the car must be a two-door model.

  1. Move front seat as far forward as possible.

  2. Sit as far to edge of right front carseat as possible.

  3. Unlock wheelchair brakes.

  4. Brace one hand against dashboard while folding wheelchair with other hand.

  5. Grasp chair by both front vertical bars, and turn chair until it is facing the back seat.

  6. Tip chair until casters rest on edge of floor.

  7. Shift body toward far side of the car; pull back of front seat forward.

  8. Lift wheelchair into car, and lock wheelchair brake to keep it from rolling.

  9. Adjust front seat for driving position.

G. Placing wheelchair into front seat of the automobile

  1. Transfer into the automobile and fold wheelchair.

2. Hold onto a sturdy portion of the car with one hand.
3. Lean to one side to grasp the front portion of the frame of the chair and lift the casters into the front of the automobile.
4. Pull the large wheels into the floor of the front seat.
5. Reach over the wheelchair to close the car door.

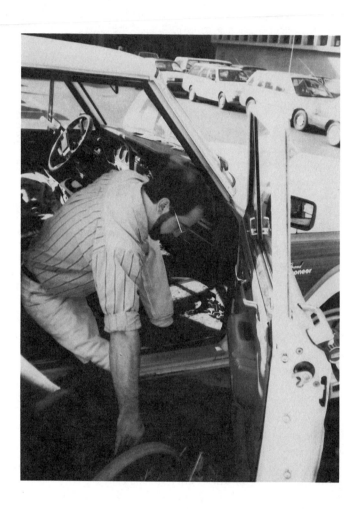

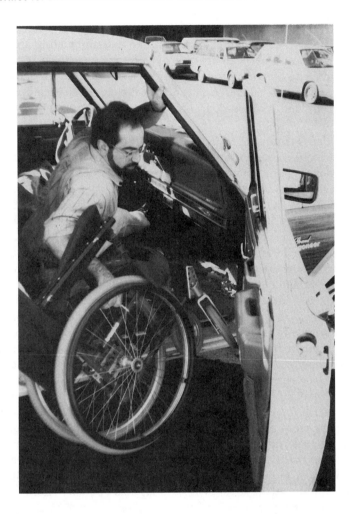

UPRIGHT ACTIVITIES

The activities described in this section are all explained with the understanding that the patient is wearing splints or bilateral long leg braces. A critical factor in the success of an individual's rehabilitation program is the individual's tolerance for gadgetry. The patient has to cope with many pieces of equipment and may view orthoses as overwhelming. Orthoses take time to don, are conspicuous, and, if not well fitted, can cause serious damage to the skin and underlying tissue. Orthoses can be assumed to fit properly when delivered to the patient, and deficiencies can be detected in the assessment process. Subsequently, the patient may gain or lose weight, thereby disturbing orthotic fit. The young adult with paraplegia may resent orthoses because they are a visible indication of disability.

Orthotics

Individuals with high thoracic lesions need assistance to sit securely and may also need a respiratory aid, both of which can be provided by appropriate spinal orthoses.

Standing may be a therapeutic goal, in order to prevent the deleterious effects of disuse osteoporosis. For some patients, standing and ambulating are realistic goals. Ambulation requires stance stability and some means of advancing the lower limbs. The patient must be able to proceed from the seated to the upright position easily. Community ambulation entails the need to maneuver over irregular sidewalks and curbs. Many indoor and outdoor environments also present stairs and other obstacles.

Trunk orthoses is prescribed for patients with paraplegia, include a lumbosacral corset that increases intra-abdominal pressure in order to assist respiration. If sitting stability is poor, a thoracolumbosacral corset may be desirable. The thoracolumbar flexion control orthosis helps the wearer maintain an erect sitting posture. The frame exposes most of the skin, thus minimizing risk of decubitus ulceration.

Craig-Scott orthosis is a special version of a knee-ankle-foot orthosis designed for individuals with thoracic injury. The orthosis includes metal limited motion ankle joints or a plastic solid ankle. The limited motion joints, although heavy, permit the orthotist to determine the optimum ankle angle to enable the patient to have the most stability. Patients differ in height and body composition; consequently, a standard angle does not provide everyone with the best alignment. Knee locks are required; ordinarily the pawl lock with bail release provides simultaneous locking of medial and lateral uprights for maximum stability. A pretibial band is faster to don than is the leather knee cap; the band does not interfere with the patient's proceeding from sitting to standing or the reverse. A single thigh band is used on proximal uprights, which are somewhat shorter than other knee-ankle-foot orthoses. The shorter uprights eliminate any risk of perineal impingement; in addition, they minimize the anteriorly directed force that tends to force the thigh forward into flexion. Craig-Scott orthoses can be worn only by those who do not have hip flexion contractures.

The individual with paralyzed hip musculature can stand securely by leaning slightly backward at the hip joints; the iliofemoral ligaments resist backward movement. Ambulation requires forearm or axillary crutches so that the patient can perform the drag-to, swing-to, or swing-through gait patterns. Forceful elbow extension enables the patient to accomplish swing phase of gait. Strategic orthotic alignment provides stance phase stability.

If the patient is troubled by severe adductor muscle spasticity, then hip-knee-ankle-foot orthoses are required. Sometimes a bar must be added to connect the medial uprights of the orthoses to prevent adduction at the hip joints.

Another option for individuals with paraplegia is the reciprocating gait orthosis, a special type of trunk-hip-knee-ankle-foot orthosis. This orthosis gives the patient sufficient stability so that he or she can advance a single limb during the swing phase with the aid of crutches. The four-point gait involves the wearer extending the elbows forcefully after shifting weight to the stance limb and leaning the upper trunk posteriorly. After the swinging limb strikes the floor, the process is repeated with weight shifted to the opposite side.

Paraplegia Secondary to Spina Bifida

Patients with spinal cord injuries are usually young adults, but those with spina bifida who are treated in a rehabilitation center are usually children. Consequently, management must take into account growth and development. Children learn with their hands, making crutchless standing and walking imperative for youngsters. The lesion itself involves defects in one or more vertebrae; thus, scoliosis is a prominent orthopedic problem. Other common skeletal disorders are dislocated hip joints and talipes equinovarus.

Skeletal development requires that the youngster have some means of standing. Ideally, the upright posture should leave the hands free to explore the environment. Orthoses should also be readily adjustable to accommodate the child's longitudinal and circumferential growth. Scoliosis orthoses will probably be worn, especially by those with thoracic lesions. Although many children with severe scoliosis require surgical stability, they may be fitted with an orthosis to minimize curve progression until surgery is performed. The upright position also helps the femurs to seat themselves more satisfactorily in the acetabula. Often the hip joints present abnormal anteversion that can interfere with forward progression in gait. If the feet are not treated surgically, then orthoses are needed to obtain and maintain a plantigrade position. The child also needs one or more means of moving from place to place.

Standing Frame

Very young children are often fitted with a standing frame to enable standing without need to clutch a walker or other aid. Because the mass-produced standing frame does not depend on precise fit, it remains satisfactory as the child grows. The shoes are not attached permanently to the frame, so foot growth requires only purchasing larger shoes, without any additional expense of constructing new inserts or transferring stirrups. Standing also aids urinary drainage and skeletal development. Well-coordinated children are able to ambulate in a standing frame by shifting weight to one side, then rotating the trunk to cause the base of the frame to pivot diagonally forward. Weight shift to the opposite side results in further progression.

Parapodium

The parapodium is another crutchless standing appliance. The child can maneuver in the same pivoting fashion. The parapodium is particularly satisfactory for nursery school, because the wearer can go from the standing to sitting independently. Both the standing frame and the parapodium accommodate scoliosis bracing, because the chest and dorsolumbar pads simply fit over the Milwaukee or similar orthosis.

By the time the child reaches kindergarten or first grade, especially if mainstreamed into the school system, peer pressure may force abandonment of the parapodium which must be worn on the outside of one's clothing. Custom-made orthoses are then the only option for continued standing and walking. Plastic and metal knee-ankle-foot orthoses are especially satisfactory for patients with lumbar lesions. The solid ankle portion control deformed feet adequately. Drop ring knee locks are usual; the lightweight child usually does not require the stability of medial and lateral locks. Plastic thigh and calf shells are impervious to urine. Avoidance of a pelvic band on the lower-limb orthoses is desirable if the child must also wear a scoliosis orthosis. A webbing strap can be used to control excessive hip medial rotation, in the manner of bilateral Silesian bandages used on above-knee prostheses.

Orthoses can be adjusted for growth by simple means. Longitudinal growth requires that the shells be detached from the uprights, two new holes drilled into the plastic, and the uprights rescrewed into the new holes. Circumferential growth is accommodated by heating the thermoplastic shells and reshaping them. Foot growth is anticipated by the initial construction of the orthosis. Unlike the adult's brace, the child's insert may be made full length, terminating at the toe tips. The foot will grow beyond the margin of the insert, which can be trimmed for best fit. Leather and metal orthoses can be lengthened by changing the position of the overlapping uprights and by hammering the calf and thigh bands into shallower configuration. Stirrups must be transferred to new shoes.

School-age children can manage with the reciprocating gait orthosis; by adolescence many patients with thoracic lesions abandon bracing, preferring to speed about in a wheelchair wearing clothes sanctioned by their peers. A spinal orthosis, such as a plastic thoracolumbosacral jacket, may be required to ensure symmetrical sitting posture.

I. Measuring for Axillary Crutches
   A. *Supine:* From anterior fold of axilla to a point 6 inches out from lateral border of foot

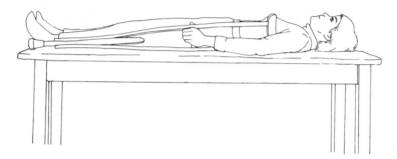

   B. *Standing:* From two fingers below anterior fold of axilla to a point 6 to 8 inches to the side of foot
   C. *Handpiece (standing):* From two fingers below anterior fold of axilla to center of hand when elbow is flexed 15 to 30 degrees, shoulders relaxed, wrist dorsiflexed
II. Parallel Bar Activities
   Balance exercises help the patient locate his or her point of balance, learn control of body segments, and master body weight shifting.
   A. Parallel bar stance
      1. *Position:* Head up; pelvis forward and rolled under trunk
      2. *Principles*
         a. Bars raised to permit slight elbow flexion
         b. Feet apart (approximately 4 inches) for a firm base of support
         c. Pelvis over feet
         d. Hands about 4 inches in front of hips, weight equally distributed between palms of the hands and feet
         e. Head erect and shoulders relaxed with shoulders balanced directly over the ankles

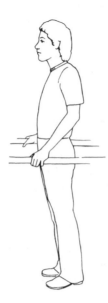

B. Weight shifter, side to side
   1. *Position:* Parallel bar stance
   2. *Action:* Shift the weight of the body from side to side by alternately pushing off from one bar and then the other. Repeat at a moderate rate.
C. Weight shifter, forward and back
   1. *Position:* Parallel bar stance
   2. *Action:* Transfer body weight onto the hands and flex elbows slightly. Return to starting position. Repeat.
D. Arm raiser, forward
   1. *Position:* Parallel bar stance
   2. *Action:* Body weight distributed over both feet equally. Raise either arm directly forward to shoulder level, without disturbing balance. Lower arm and grasp the bar. Repeat with opposite arm. Progression: Raise both arms forward simultaneously. Repeat.
E. Arm raiser, sideward
   1. *Position:* Parallel bar stance
   2. *Action:* With body weight distributed equally over both feet, raise either arm sideward to shoulder level. Lower and repeat with opposite arm. Progression: Raise both arms sideward. Repeat.
F. Arm swinging
   1. *Position:* Parallel bar stance
   2. *Action:* Remove the hands from the parallel bars and lower the arms to the sides. Swing arms freely forward and backward without disturbing balance. Swing either reciprocally or simultaneously. When balance is upset, the patient should regrasp the bars, reestablish the point of balance, and begin exercise again.
G. Hand clapping
   1. *Position:* Parallel bar stance
   2. *Action:* Remove hands from bars and lower to the sides. Raise both arms overhead and clap the hands together several times. Lower arms and

repeat. (This exercise may be performed in front of body and behind body.)

III. Strengthening Exercises (to continue development of essential crutch-walking muscles)

   A. Push-ups
      1. *Position:* Parallel bar stance with hands in line with hips
      2. *Action:* Push down on bars simultaneously with both hands, straighten elbows, and depress the shoulders, lifting the body so that the feet clear the floor. Lower feet to the floor and reestablish point of balance. Repeat and increase number of repetitions.

   B. Double push-ups—same as 1, except feet may not return to floor between push-ups.

   C. Jack-knife
      1. *Position:* Parallel bar stance with hands in line with hips
      2. *Action:* Push off the parallel bars with both hands simultaneously and place them backwards about 8 to 10 inches to the rear of the hips. Shift body weight backward onto the hands and allow hips to jack-knife. With the shoulders stabilized, use the latissimus and lower third of the trapezius muscles to pull the trunk forward and upward, extending the hips. Bring hands forward to the starting position. Repeat.

   D. Dipper
      1. *Position:* Parallel bar stance with hands placed forward well ahead of hips
      2. *Action:* Shift body weight forward onto hands and allow elbows and hips to flex until trunk is parallel to the floor. Straighten elbows and return to starting position. Repeat.

   E. Knee-lock toucher
      1. *Position:* Parallel bar stance
      2. *Action:* Shift body weight forward onto hands and allow elbows and hips to flex "semijacked." Balance body weight with one hand. Reach down and back with the opposite hand and touch knee-lock on the same side. Return body to an erect position. Repeat. Variation: Touch free hand to the floor.

IV. Coordination Exercises (to develop elements or certain patterns of movement transferable to ambulation and functional activities)

   A. Four-count coordinator
      1. *Position:* Parallel bar stance
      2. *Action:* Raise both arms forward simultaneously to shoulder height. Move arms out to sides. Move arms forward. Lower arms to starting position. Repeat.

   B. Six-count coordinator
      1. *Position:* Parallel bar stance
      2. *Action:* Move arms forward. Move arms out to side. Raise arms upward overhead. Lower arms down to shoulder level. Return arms forward. Lower arms to starting position. Repeat.

   C. Hip hiker
      1. *Position:* Parallel bar stance
      2. *Action:* Shift body weight to one side and raise the hip on the opposite side by pushing down forcefully on the bar on the same side. Return to starting position.

D. Leg swinger
   1. *Position:* Parallel bar stance
   2. *Action:* Shift body weight onto one side and raise the opposite hip. Swing the raised leg back and forth for several counts. Repeat at a slow rate. Swinging of the leg should be stopped and started again at frequent intervals. Do not use momentum.

V. Gait Training (to teach beginning of basic gait fundamentals and skills and to develop proper gait patterns and habits)
   A. Four-point gait drill
      1. *Position:* Parallel bar stance
      2. *Action:* Place right hand forward and shift the body weight to that side. Hike the left hip and move the leg forward. Place the left hand forward; shift weight. Hike the right hip and move leg forward. Repeat until entire distance of the parallel bars has been traversed.
         Note. Push off the bars with the hand on the same side. Do not pull with opposite hand.
   B. Drag-to gait drill
      1. *Position:* Parallel bar stance
      2. *Action:* Place hands forward simultaneously. Shift body weight forward onto hands, allowing elbows to flex slightly. Forcefully push down on the bars, extend elbows, depress shoulders, and drag feet along the floor in line with hands. Repeat the distance of the bars.
   C. Swing-to gait drill
      1. *Position:* Parallel bar stance
      2. *Action:* Same as for drag-to gait, except lift body clear of the floor and swing forward, placing feet in line with hands. Repeat.
   D. Swing-through gait drill (see illustrations in following section on pre-elevation exercises)
      1. *Position:* Parallel bar stance
      2. *Action:* Same as for drag-to gait, except swing forward through the hands, placing feet beyond them. As the feet hit the floor, lift head and roll the pelvis forward under the trunk. Use forward momentum of the body and maintain hyperextended position. Repeat.
   E. Sideward gait drill
      1. *Position:* Parallel bar stance, facing one bar with both hands on the same bar
      2. *Action:* Move right hand to the right and shift body weight over the left leg. Hike the right hip and move the leg to the right. Shift weight to the right leg. Repeat with left leg. Repeat to the left. Legs may be moved simultaneously.
   F. Backward four-point gait drill
      1. *Position:* Parallel bar stance
      2. *Action:* Shift body weight to the right. Hike the left hip and move leg backward. Shift the weight of the body slightly to the left and place right hand backward. Hike the right hip and place leg backward. Repeat.
   G. Backward swing-through gait drill
      1. *Position:* Parallel bar stance, placing both hands to the rear of the hips
      2. *Action:* Shift body weight onto hands, allowing elbows to flex slightly. Push down forcefully on the bars, extend elbows, and raise the body off

the floor; swing backward through the hands, placing the feet behind them. Repeat.

VI. Pre-elevation Exercises (to teach certain fundamental movements involved in the performance of elevation activities, which, if properly used, will lead to increased ability to perform the same movement with crutches) Equipment needed: stools or benches 2 to 6 inches in height.

A. Ascending drill forward (leg swing)
1. *Position:* Parallel bar stance, facing stool at a slight angle
2. *Action:* Shift body weight to one side, hike the opposite hip, and swing leg forward and backward until enough momentum is gained so that the leg will clear the height of the apparatus to be ascended. With the foot firmly placed on the bench, shift weight forward onto the hands. Push up, straighten the elbows, and transfer weight onto the forward leg. As weight is displaced forward, hike the opposite hip and swing the hanging limb forward onto apparatus. Repeat.

B. Ascending drill forward (swing up)
1. *Position:* Parallel bar stance, directly facing apparatus at a distance permitting a full swing-through of the body
2. *Action:* Shift body weight onto hands, allowing elbows to flex slightly. Push down forcefully on the bars, extend elbows, depress shoulder, and raise body off the floor, swinging lower limbs onto the stool. As forward momentum of the body continues, push off from the bars and place the hands in front of the body. Repeat.
   a. Parallel bar stance (resting position). Gravity is posterior to the hips and anterior to the ankles.

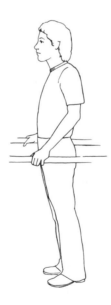

   b. Place hands forward and lean on them. Gravity is anterior to both hips and ankles.

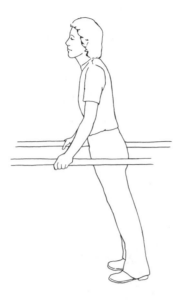

c. Push down against bars and hike the hips.

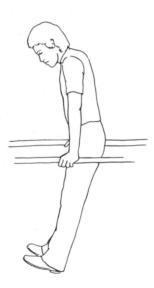

d. Swing lower limbs forward.

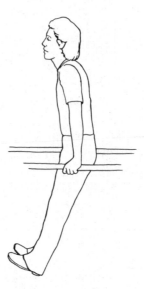

e. Set the feet down anterior to the hands. As soon as the heels contact the ground, push hips forward.

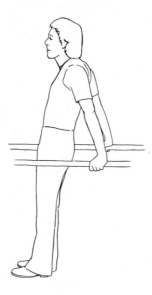

f. Push hands down against the bars, then lift them as momentum carries the body forward. Placing the hands on the bars stops the forward momentum of the body.

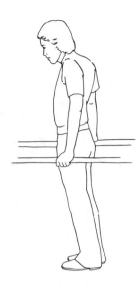

C. Ascending drill backward (leg swing)
   1. *Position:* Parallel bar stance with back to the apparatus
   2. *Action:* Shift the weight of body over onto one leg. Hike the opposite hip, swing leg backward and up onto the stool. Walk hands backward until the weight is over the extremity on the bench and the opposite limb is hanging freely. Hike and swing the limb onto the apparatus. Continue walking the hands backward until as much weight as possible is over the limbs.
D. Ascending drill backward (back jack)
   1. *Position:* Parallel bar stance with back to the apparatus, hands in line with hips
   2. *Action:* Quickly lower head, push down forcefully on the bars, extend the elbows, and "jack" the hips up and backward, lifting feet onto stool. Repeat.
E. Descending drill forward (hip hiking)
   1. *Position:* Parallel bar stance, standing on top of the stool with the body slightly flexed at the hips
   2. *Action:* Placing hands well ahead of hips, shift weight onto hands. Advance either foot forward so that the heel rests on the stool with the forefront over the edge. Advance the other foot forward and off the stool. Push down forcefully and equally on the bars and lift the foot that is on the bench. Lower body to the floor between the hands. Keep the pelvis well ahead of the body, place hands ahead of the hips, and assume the parallel bar stance. Repeat.
F. Descending drill forward (stepping off)
   1. *Position:* Parallel bar stance on top of stool with body slightly flexed at the hips
   2. *Action:* Placing hands well ahead of hips, shift body weight to either side, and hike the hip on the opposite side. Swing the leg forward off the stool and lower to the floor. While bearing down forcefully on the hands, hike the opposite hip and lower leg to the floor. Repeat.

G. Descending drill forward (swing off)

   1. *Position:* Parallel bar stance on top of stool with body slightly flexed at the hips

   2. *Action:* Placing hands well ahead of hips, shift weight onto hands. Advance feet down equally so that the heels rest on the bench. Push down equally on the bars, lift body clear of the stool, and swing forward through the hands. Place the feet beyond them. As the feet hit the floor, lift the head and roll the pelvis under the trunk. Push off bars and place hands ahead of hips. Repeat.

VII. Lead-up Crutch Exercises (an intermediate level between parallel bars and crutches)

   A. Crutch-bar stance

      1. *Position:* Identical to that of parallel bar stance except that one bar and one crutch are used

   B. Crutch-bar shifter

      1. *Position:* Crutch-bar stance

      2. *Action:* Shift body weight forward onto hands. Return to starting position by pushing down forcefully on the bar and handpiece. Repeat. Variation: Shift body weight from side to side.

   C. Arm-crutch raiser

      1. *Position:* Crutch bar stance

      2. *Action:* Shift weight onto hands. Push down forcefully on the bar and crutch simultaneously and push off, thrusting the body weight backward. As the body weight is shifted backward, raise either the crutch or the hand. Sway forward, regain balance and stance, and repeat. *Variation:* Raise crutch or arm sideward. Raise arm and crutch simultaneously.

   D. Arm-crutch placer

      1. *Position:* Crutch-bar stance

      2. *Action:* Shift body weight over onto the crutch and advance the opposite hand forward about 4 inches. Transfer body weight onto hand and move crutch forward in line with the hand on the bar. Return to starting position by alternately placing the hand and crutch backward. Repeat. Variation: Simultaneously moving hand and crutch forward, place hand and crutch backward about 6 inches to the rear of the hips, first alternately and then simultaneously.

   E. Crutch-bar latissimus

      1. *Position:* Crutch-bar stance

      2. *Action:* Push off both the hand and crutch simultaneously and place them backward about 8 to 10 inches to the rear of the hips. Shift body weight backward over hands and crutch and then jack-knife. With the shoulders stabilized, use the latissimus and lower third of the trapezius muscles to pull the trunk forward and upward, extending the hips. Continue until hips are ahead of the body. Bring the hands forward simultaneously. Repeat.

   F. Crutch remover

      1. *Position:* Crutch-bar stance

      2. *Action:* Shift weight to hand on the bar. Reverse the grip on the crutch. Remove the crutch from the axilla and place it cane style with the

upright braced between elbow and shoulder. Return to starting position. Repeat.

    G. Crutch-bar dipper
       1. *Position:* Crutch-bar stance, with crutch held cane style
       2. *Action:* Shift body weight onto hand and crutch. With arm abducted, allow the elbows and the hips to flex until the trunk is almost parallel with the bar. Straighten the elbows and assume the starting position. Repeat.

    H. Crutch placer
       1. *Position:* Crutch-bar stance, crutch cane style
       2. *Action:* Flex elbows and hips until trunk is parallel to floor. Shift weight to the hand on the bar. Supinate the forearm and place the crutch flat on the floor with the handpiece in line with the tip of the foot. Return to starting position.

    I. Pushing up on crutch and bar
       1. *Position:* Crutch-bar stance
       2. *Action:* Push on crutch, extending elbows until feet are off floor. Lower body by flexing elbows slowly, landing heels first. Return to starting position. Move crutch forward quickly when heels touch floor to maintain balance.

VIII. Ambulation Activities

Axillary crutches will be used. Forearm crutches are preferable for ambulatory patients with bilateral lower limb and trunk weakness. Use of forearm crutches requires good balance and coordination. This is a prerequisite for ambulation for patients with bilateral lower limb and trunk weakness. Forearm crutches are also an advantage on stairs, curbs, and transfers from floor to sitting. Activities described in the preceding section on parallel bar activities should be practiced with crutches prior to ambulation and transfer activities.

    Level ambulation: Follow procedures described in gait training ambulation on level surface.

    Energy costs in paraplegic ambulation are as follows:

- Cost decreases the lower the level of injury (cost/distance)
- Cost/time decreases the lower the level of injury
- Cost/distance decreases as rate increases
- Cost decreases with training
- Oxygen requirement four to six times that of resting state (this requirement is similar to that noted in normal walking at a rate of 90 to 130 meters/minute—fast walking).

IX. Transferring Activities
    A. From wheelchair to standing position
    Always have wheelchair locked, casters forward and locked, and footrest swung away to side. If possible, place wheelchair against a wall.
       1. Facing chair, both knees of braces locked
          a. Place crutches on each side of wheelchair.
          b. Sit as near to right side as possible. Place right foot slightly forward and away from the left foot.
          c. Place left hand behind on right armrest, grasp left armrest with right hand.

d. Shift weight to hands, lifting body off seat, twisting and turning body and feet until facing the wall.
e. Distribute weight over hands and feet in jack-knife position.
f. Straighten up, tucking hips under, shifting weight to right hand and feet.
g. Pick up left crutch and place under arm.
h. Shift weight to left crutch and pick up right crutch. Place it under the arm.
i. Step sideways or back, as necessary.

Alternate method, facing chair: Cross right foot over left before standing.

2. Facing sideways, both knees of braces locked (this method is easiest with forearm crutches)
   a. Place both crutches on left side of wheelchair.
   b. Sit as near to right as possible. Place right foot slightly forward and away from left foot.
   c. Place left hand on left armrest and hold crutch in right hand, cane style. Place crutch to side of right thigh.
   d. Lean forward at hips, shift weight to hands, and lift body off seat, pulling feet backwards to assume standing in jack-knife position. *Be sure that right crutch and left hand are anterior to feet.*
   e. Straighten up, tucking hips under, shifting weight to left hand and feet.
   f. Place right crutch under arm, crutch style.
   g. Shift weight to right, pick up left crutch and place it under arm. Resume crutch stance.

3. Forward, "muscling up," both knees of braces locked. Use forearm crutches for this activity. Athletes can do this but need a great deal of working area.
   a. Do not swing legrest to side.
   b. Place crutches (in hands) at side of wheelchair forward to hips. Lean forward at hips.
   c. Push down on crutches until feet are flat. Immediately place crutches forward to stop forward momentum of body.
   d. Catch weight on hands, tuck hips under.

B. From standing to wheelchair

Always have wheelchair locked, casters forward and locked, and footrests swung away to sides. Have wheelchair against wall if possible.

1. Facing chair, both knees of braces locked
   a. Approach chair from front, close enough to be able to position crutches at side of wheelchair.
   b. Shift weight to left, remove right crutch and place it on right side of handgrip of wheelchair (use wall if wheelchair is against wall). Grasp right armrest.
   c. Shift weight to right, place left crutch as above.
   d. Flex forward at hips into jack-knife position. Gain balance, be sure feet are far enough back so that there will be no danger of tripping while turning.
   e. Lean on hands, twist and turn body and feet to right, lower body onto seat until sitting.

f. Reverse arms, straighten self in chair, unlock braces, place feet on footrests.
2. Facing sideways, both knees of braces locked.
   a. Approach wheelchair to the left side in front of seat, close enough to be able to grasp left armrest. Have left crutch at left side of wheelchair.
   b. Switch right crutch to cane position (not with forearm crutches).
   c. Shift weight to right, place left crutch against left side of chair, and grasp left armrest.
   d. Lower body to left until sitting. Place right crutch to right of wheelchair, and grasp right armrest.
   e. Push on armrests to straighten self in chair.
   f. If using forearm crutches, merely let go of handle and keep cuffs on forearm until sitting.
C. From standing to straight chair without arms
   1. Facing side of chair, both knees of braces locked. Use same method as facing front of wheelchair except use chair back and seat of chair instead of armrests.
   2. Facing sideways to front of chair, both knees of braces locked. Use same method as facing side of wheelchair except use chair back for armrest.
D. From straight chair without arms to standing
   1. Facing side of chair (use back and seat of chair).
      a. Slide forward to side of the chair until feet are touching the floor.
      b. Slide to one side of the chair seat.
      c. Place hands as close as possible to the middle of the chair seat and back.
      d. Push down onto chair twisting and raising the buttocks until standing on both feet.
      e. Shift weight to one side and place the opposite crutch under axilla.
      f. Shift weight to crutch and feet and place the other crutch under axilla.
      g. Pushing on crutches, assume a balance position with hips in extension.
   2. Facing sideways to side of chair, both knees of braces locked
      a. Slide forward to side of the chair until feet are touching the floor.
      b. Twist trunk placing hand as close to the middle chair back as possible.
      c. Pick up one crutch and hold it cane style (forearm crutch put cuff on).
      d. Push down on crutch and chair, quickly lifting buttocks.
      e. Shift weight to feet and crutch.
      f. Assume a balanced position.
      g. Place other crutch under axilla.
      Note. This method requires agility and considerable upper limb muscle strength.
E. From standing to and from toilet
   1. Approach forward, facing side or side to front depending on bathroom layout.
   2. Use methods in steps C1 and C2.
   3. Grab bars would be of great assistance but be sure that they will not hinder wheelchair transfer if patient also uses wheelchair.

F. From bed to standing
  1. Assume sitting position on the bed with the legs over the side of the bed (short sitting).
  2. Lock both braces.
  3. Take both crutches as one, grasping the handpieces, palm up.
  4. Quickly twist body until facing the side of the bed, and bring crutches over to the other side of the feet.
  5. Place free hand on the bed, push down with both hands, and lift the body up off the bed.
  6. Body weight is transferred to both feet, placing crutches under the arms, keeping the pelvis well forward.
G. From standing to bed
  Reverse of IX. F.
H. Falling forward to the floor
  This technique is taught to protect oneself in an emergency; use mats.
  1. Lean forward until balance is disturbed.
  2. Discard crutches by supinating forearms, extending elbows, and abducting shoulders.
  3. If forearm crutches are used, merely release handgrips.
  4. Catch the fall of your body on your hands, roll onto forearms, and let your body down easily.
I. Falling backward to floor
  Teach patient to twist body and catch weight on hands.
  1. Lean backward until balance is disturbed.
  2. Discard crutches forward, twist body in direction of fall, breaking the fall with your hands.
  3. Let the body down easily.
J. From floor to standing
  1. Come to position of balancing on hands and feet that requires good hamstring range. Use either of the following two methods:
    a. Prone with crutches placed on each side of body with the tops toward the feet at ankles or both crutches on same side of body. Patient pushes up on hands, tucking head under and rounding back. Walk hands back until hips flex and some weight is on feet.
    b. Sitting with crutches far to one side (left) of body. Have axillary crutches one on top of other. Cross leg (locked braces) farthest from crutches. Place hands on mat between body and crutches. Push up on hands and twist body, keeping head tucked under and back arched, until hips flex. Continue as previously described.
  2. Adjust weight on hands and feet so that feet bear more of the weight and feet are apart. There are three methods:
    a. Climbing up axillary crutches with crutches at side
      (1) Grasp both crutch handgrips together with closest hand, palm facing forward (supinated). Lift crutches to vertical position by pronating forearm, medially rotating and abducting shoulder, flexing elbow.
      (2) Brace crutches (held in cane fashion) against shoulder. Shift weight from opposite hand and place hand on lower shaft of the crutches.

(3) Gradually move the lower hand up the shaft of the crutches, tucking the hips under as the standing position is approached.

(4) Reestablish balance on feet and crutches.

(5) Remove the top crutch and place it under axilla.

(6) Shift body weight to crutch under axilla. Reverse grip on the other crutch and place it under the axilla.

(7) Reestablish balance.

   b. Using one crutch in each hand, axillary crutches

(1) Grasp the handpiece of one crutch, palm forward.

(2) Place the crutch on the floor by pronating the hand, medially rotating and abducting shoulder, and lifting crutch to semivertical position.

(3) Balance with the crutch held cane style, braced firmly against the arm and shoulder.

(4) Bring other crutch to same position.

(5) Push up to erect position, rolling the hips forward under the body.

(6) Walk crutches back to resume crutch stance.

   c. Using one crutch in each hand, forearm crutches

(1) Use same method as above except place hands through cuffs on both sides before grasping one handgrip.

(2) Side opening cuffs are the best for this: Pressure tends to force forearm out of front opening cuff.

  K. From standing to floor

Reverse methods in IX. J. These methods should be used rather than falling techniques unless an emergency arises.

X. Elevation Activities

  A. Ascending stairs with a handrail

    1. *Position:* Crutch balance stance facing the stairs and near the handrail

    2. *Action:* With the hand nearest the handrail grasp the handrail, and with the other hand reach across the body and remove the crutch from under the arm at the side of the handrail. Place the crutch along with the other crutch, to be used as one, under the arm farthest from the handrail. Adjust the crutches in position next to the feet. Shift the body weight from the feet directly over the crutches and the arm of the hand on the handrail. With the arm of the hand on the handrail held in extension, push down on the handgrips and lift both feet and the body up onto the step above. The head is kept forward so that the weight of the body will be distributed over the arms and the crutches, permitting a slight bending of the hips, if possible. As the feet land on the step above, the hips are rotated forward so that the pelvis is well ahead of the body, thus eliminating the danger of jack-knifing before the crutches can be advanced. Once balance has been reestablished on the legs, the crutches are advanced to the same step as the feet, and a crutch balance stance is assumed with both crutches under the arm farther from the handrail and the other hand grasping the handrail.

  B. Stair climbing — second method: arm between crutch struts

Same as method X. A but with arm between crutch struts

  C. Ascending stairs backward

1. *Position:* Crutch balance stance with back facing the stairs.
2. *Action:* Same as X. A.

D. Descending stairs with handrail — first method: Crutches under the arms
   1. *Position:* Crutch balance stance near the handrail at the top of the staircase directly facing the stairs
   2. *Action:* Grasp the handrail with the hand nearer to it and remove the crutch from under the arm nearer the handrail. Place the crutches, to be used as one, under the other arm. Lower both crutches to the next step. Move both feet alternately or together to the edge of the step so that half of both feet overlap the edge. With the head forward, shift the weight onto both hands, raise the body off the step, and slowly lower both feet to the step below. When the feet are placed on the step and as balance is being reestablished on both lower limbs, the pelvis is rotated forward to prevent jack-knifing.

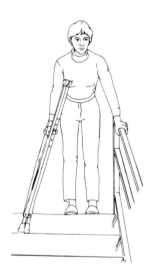

E. Stair descending — second method: using shoulder rests
   If the individual, for any reason, cannot control the tendency to jack-knife, this method may be attempted.
   1. *Position:* Crutch balance stance near the handrail at the top of the staircase directly facing the stairs
   2. *Action:* Grasp the handrail with the hand nearer to it and remove both crutches from under the arms. Holding both crutches to be used as one at the shoulder rests, place crutches two steps below. Move the feet alternately or together to the edge of the step so that both feet are overlapping. With the head lowered, shift the body weight directly over the arms. Bearing down on the crutches and the handrail, extend the arms, lift the body, and lower both feet to the step below. Without moving the crutches, rotate the pelvis ahead of the body and reestablish the body weight onto the legs.

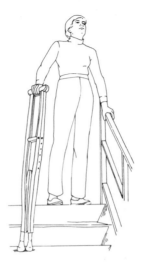

F. Ascending curb-turning maneuver
  1. *Position:* Crutch balance stance facing the curb at a 45-degree angle (Whether the individual angles off to the left or to the right depends on which limb will swing up on the curb. If the individual is going to swing the left leg, it will be necessary to face the curb at a 45-degree angle to the right)
  2. *Action:* Swing one leg up and place the heel on the curb. Shift the body weight over the leg and crutch opposite the limb that has been placed on the curb. Whether the swinging action will be due to muscular power of the lower limb or the trunk, or to the help of the hands and the displacement of body weight, will depend on the individual's musculature and its control. Turn in the direction of the crutch and limb bearing the weight, carry the weight-free crutch over the limb on the curb and replace it on the street level. At the completion of this movement, the individual has completed a quarter turn. Shift the weight equally onto both crutches and the limb on the curb until the other limb is clear of the ground. Swing the limb backward up onto the curb. Shift the weight over onto one crutch and bring the other crutch up on the curb. As the crutch is brought up on the curb, the pelvis is rotated forward and ahead of the body. Shift the weight over onto the crutch which is on the curb and bring up the other crutch. The pelvis should be held ahead of the body to prevent jack-knifing. Adjust the position of the crutches and the feet into a good crutch balance stance, preparatory to ambulating. When approaching the curb the individual should allow enough distance to swing the limb up onto the curb. When the lower limb is swung up and the heel placed on the curb, the limb should be placed sufficiently forward so that the limb will not slip off the curb during the turning maneuver.

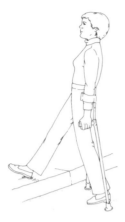

G. Ascending curbs: Leg swing backward
   1. *Position:* Crutch balance stance with the back to the curb at a 45-degree angle (Here again, the direction in which the individual will angle off will depend on which lower limb the individual will use to swing up onto the curb)
   2. *Action:* Shift most of the body weight over onto one crutch and the limb on that side. Swing the other limb back up and place the foot on the curb. Push down, extending the elbow of the arm on the crutch bearing most of the weight, and raise the limb clear of the ground. Swing the free leg back up onto the curb. Shift the weight over onto one crutch and the limbs and place the other crutch on the curb. Repeat the same procedure to place the other crutch up on the curb.
H. Ascending curbs: Forward jack
   1. *Position:* Crutch balance stance facing the curb at a 45-degree angle (the foot of the limb that will be raised up onto the curb first is as close to the curb as possible)
   2. *Action:* Remove the crutch from under the arm on the side of the limb which will be raised onto the curb first. Hold the crutch cane fashion with the forearm firmly braced between the crutch struts and place it up on the curb. With the other crutch still under the shoulder, lean forward, shifting the weight onto both crutches. Lower the head, push down on both crutches, lifting the body and placing the feet up on the curb. With the body weight distributed between the lower limbs and the crutch on the curb, raise the other crutch to the curb. Readjust the position of the crutches and the feet, assuming the proper crutch balance stance.
I. Ascending curbs: Swing-through
   1. *Position:* Crutch balance stance directly facing the curb. The distance from the curb should allow a full swing-through of the body from the starting position onto the curb.
   2. *Action:* With the head lowered, shift the weight over onto both crutches. Continuing the shift of the weight over onto the crutches and as the crutches approach the perpendicular, push down forcefully and equally on the handgrips, lifting the body and swinging through the crutches, landing the feet up onto the curb. If possible, the hips are kept well ahead of the rest of the body throughout the entire swing-through, so that the individual lands in a hyperextended position, and the pelvis

should be rotated forward as soon as the feet land on the curb. Using the forward momentum of the body and maintaining the hyperextended position, lift crutches simultaneously onto the curb, and place them in front of the body.

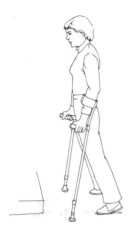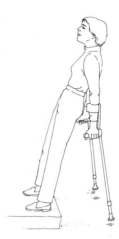

J. Ascending curbs: Backward jack
   1. *Position:* Crutch balance stance with back to the curb and the heels flush up against the curb
   2. *Action:* Maintaining the crutch balance stance, move the crutches back toward the feet so that the crutch tips are in line with the feet. With the head low, push down forcefully on both crutches, jacking the hips up and backward, lifting the feet onto the curb. Once balance has been reestablished on the curb, the crutches are alternately brought from the street level onto the curb. This is accomplished by shifting the weight and simultaneously pushing off from the other crutch, thrusting the body upward and permitting the crutch on that side to be placed on the curb. This is repeated to bring the other crutch up onto the curb.
K. Ascending curbs: Back swing-through
   1. *Position:* Crutch balance stance with the back to the curb (the distance from the curb should allow enough room to permit a full back swing-through of the body from the starting position up onto the curb)
   2. *Action:* Maintain the hyperextended position of the body and place the crutches behind the feet. Shifting the weight back over onto the crutches, push down forcefully and equally on the handgrips, lifting the body, swinging back through the crutches, and landing the feet onto the curb.
L. Descending curbs—hip hiking
   1. *Position:* Crutch balance stance standing near the edge of the curb
   2. *Action:* Shifting the weight directly over the feet, lift both crutches and place them in the street close to the curb. Gradually shifting the weight over onto the crutches, advance one foot forward so that the heel rests on the curb with the forefoot over the edge. Advance the other foot forward and off the curb. Bearing down forcefully and equally on the handgrips of both crutches, lift the foot that is on the curb forward and off the curb, lowering the body to the street between the crutches. Keeping the pelvis well ahead of the body, balance is reestablished in

this position and the crutches are advanced forward to the crutch balance stance.

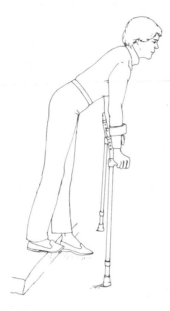

M. Descending curbs—alternate stepping off
   1. *Position:* Crutch balance stance near the edge of the curb
   2. *Action:* Raise both crutches off the curb and place them in the street near the curb. Taking small alternate side steps with the crutches, increase the distance between the crutch tips. Shift the weight onto both crutches and advance one foot forward so that the heel rests on the curb with the forefoot over the edge. Pushing down forcefully on the handgrips, clear the other foot off the curb, and, while shifting the weight over onto the crutch on that side, gradually lower the foot to the street. Lower the other foot to the street with a pushing down motion on the crutches. Reestablish balance and assume the crutch balance stance.
N. Descending curbs—swing-through
   1. *Position:* Crutch balance stance at the edge of the curb
   2. *Action:* Lift both crutches from the curb and place them in the street sufficiently away from the curb so as to permit a swinging of the body through the crutches. Shifting the weight gradually over onto the crutches and pushing down on the handgrips as the crutches approach the perpendicular, lift the body off the curb and swing completely through the crutches, landing in the street ahead of them. Keeping the pelvis well ahead of the body, advance the crutches beyond the feet and assume the crutch balance position.
O. Ascending stairs without a handrail—front jack
   1. *Position:* Crutch balance stance facing the stairs at a 45-degree angle (the position of the feet is as close to the step to be mounted as possible)
   2. *Action:* Remove the crutch from under the arm on the side nearest the stairs. Holding the crutch cane fashion with the elbow flexed and the forearm braced between crutch struts, place the crutch up on the step to be mounted or the step above that if preferred. With the other crutch still

under the shoulder, lean forward while shifting the weight over onto both crutches. Lower the head, push down on both crutches, lift the whole body by jacking at the hips, and place the feet up on the step. Keeping the pelvis ahead of the body, distribute the body weight between the lower limbs and the uppermost crutch, preparatory to raising the other crutch up onto the same step as the feet. Readjust the position of the crutches and the feet and prepare to repeat the procedure for ascending the next step.

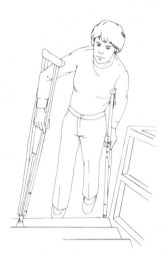

P. Ascending stairs — leg swing backward
  1. *Position:* Crutch balance stance with the back to the stairs at approximately a 45-degree angle (the direction in which to angle-off depends on which limb the individual will use to swing up onto the step)
  2. *Action:* Readjust the crutches and the stance so there will be adequate clearance to swing either lower limb sideward and backward while still maintaining stability on three points of support — one limb and the two crutches. Gradually shift most of the body weight over onto one crutch and the limb on that side. Swing the other limb back and place the foot on the next step. Push down straightening the elbow of the arm on the crutch bearing most of the weight, and raise the limb on the lower step clear of the tread. Swing the free limb back onto the step. Raise crutches to the next step, simultaneously or alternately, according to ability or preference. Readjust the position of the crutches and the feet and prepare to repeat the procedure for ascending the next step.
Q. Descending stairs without a handrail — hip hiking
  1. *Position:* Crutch balance stance at the top of the staircase directly facing the stairs
  2. *Action:* Move the feet forward and as near to the edge of the step as possible without endangering stability or stance (four points of support, both crutches and both feet). Shifting the body weight directly over the feet, lift both crutches simultaneously or alternately, and place them on the tread of the step below. While gradually shifting the weight over onto the crutches, advance one foot forward so that the heel rests on the lip with the forefoot hanging free over the edge. Advance the other foot

forward and completely off the step. Bear down forcefully and equally on the handgrips of both crutches, hike the hip, and lift the foot that is on the step forward and off the tread, lowering the feet between the crutches to the step below. Readjust the crutches and the feet to reestablish balance and stance preparatory to repeating the procedure for descending to the next step.

R. Descending stairs—using shoulder rests
    1. *Position:* Crutch balance stance at the top of the staircase facing the stairs at a slight angle (the direction in which to angle-off depends on the crutch that will be placed on the step below)
    2. *Action:* Shift the body weight over onto the crutch opposite the one to be placed on the step below and remove the other crutch from under the arm. While holding the crutch at the shoulder-rest, place the crutch on the tread, as close to the riser as possible, two steps down. Lower the head and gradually transfer the body weight forward and over onto the lower crutch. Push down on both crutches, lift the entire body clear off the step, and lower the feet onto the tread of the next step. Keeping the pelvis ahead of the body, bring the crutch, which is under the arm, down to the same step as the feet.

S. Descending stairs—alternate stepping off
    1. *Position:* Crutch balance stance at the top of the staircase directly facing the stairs
    2. *Action:* Raise both crutches off the top step, alternately or simultaneously, and place them on the tread of the next lower step. Taking small alternate side steps with the crutches, increase the distance between the crutch tips, assuming as wide a base as possible. Shift the weight over onto both crutches and advance one foot forward so that the heel rests on the tread with the forefoot over the edge of the step. Bearing down forcefully on the handgrips, clear the other foot off the step, shift the weight onto the crutch on that side, and gradually lower the foot to the next step. Lower the other foot to the step by simultaneously pushing down on the crutches and hiking the hip on the same side. Reestablish balance by readjusting the position of the crutches and the feet preparatory to repeating the procedure for descending to the next step.

T. Ramps
Ascend and descend ramps using short steps and any gait except for swing-through.

10

Functional Activities for Involvement of All Four Limbs and Trunk

Quadriplegic patients often spend more time in rehabilitation than do paraplegic or hemiplegic patients. Their extensive loss of motor and sensory functions require relearning any functional activities that were previously automatic. In rehabilitation more emphasis will be placed on bed mobility, dressing, and wheelchair activities, with little or no emphasis on upright activities other than physiologic standing.

Involvement of all four limbs and trunk may be secondary to traumatic spinal cord or head injury, circulatory malfunctions, bone diseases, infections, tumors, or neurologic diseases such as multiple sclerosis or Parkinson's disease.

For the head-injured patient with involvement of all four limbs and trunk, including abnormal tone, weakness, decreased motor control, and so forth, it may be necessary to alter some of the techniques for teaching bed mobility. Those patients with spasticity may require techniques for inhibition and range of motion prior to being able to use the involved limbs functionally. Individuals must be encouraged to use their limbs and trunk to the best of their capability despite the level of involvement. For example, the person with right-sided weakness and increased flexor tone of the left side may need to use the left side as an assist to hold the side of the bed while the weaker right upper limb pushes into extension to assume short sitting. Teaching those with abnormal muscle tone to use their limbs in weight-bearing positions may promote changes in muscle tone and improve overall function. Individuals presenting with increased muscle tone and limitations in range of motion may be unable to "swing their upper limbs and head to carry their body over" in order to roll. This swinging action may be too fast a motion and may cause an actual increase in spasticity, whereas a weight-bearing technique may enhance a decrease in spasticity and improve the person's function.

Head-injured patients may present with various cognitive deficits such as poor memory, judgment, problem solving, frustration tolerance, motor planning, and sequencing. It is important, therefore, to be consistent in the way activities are taught. This is especially true for the person presenting with a level of awareness (LOA) V or lower. (Refer to levels of cognitive awareness Scale in Chapter 12.) These individuals will benefit from repetition and other memory aides and sometimes written cue cards, assuming that the person's reading comprehension is functional for short phrases.

LYING AND SITTING ACTIVITIES

I. Rolling from Supine to Side or Prone Position
    A. No equipment—If possible, cross legs before proceeding (turning to the right).

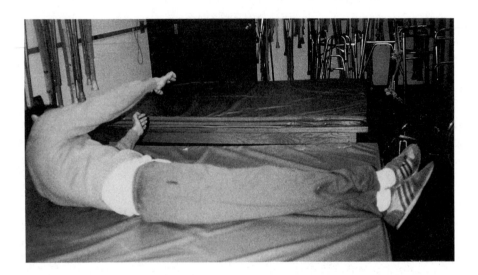

        1. If possible, clasp hands together in front of trunk.
        2. Swing arms and head to right and left until enough force is built up to carry body over to left.
        3. Legs will be carried by momentum.
    B. No equipment—coming to elbows first (turning to the right).
        If the lower limbs cannot be crossed, the hip on the side away from the turn will inhibit the turn. With the limbs crossed, the hips will easily follow.
        1. Come to forearm position (see illustration for Coming to Sitting)
        2. If possible, shift weight onto one elbow to support the trunk, using the free hand to cross one leg over the other.
        3. Swing left arm and head to right while pushing on right forearm.
        4. Legs will be carried by momentum.
    C. No equipment—using side of bed (turning to the right).
        1. Swing left arm over chest.
        2. Hyperextend left wrist and brace against edge of mattress.
        3. Flex elbow forcibly by using biceps.
        4. Pull trunk to side or over to prone position.
        5. To return to supine: Hyperextend left wrist, lock elbow in extension, and force left shoulder back toward mattress.
    D. No equipment—using headboard (turning to the right).
        1. Hyperextend right wrist; raise arm overhead, hooking wrist around headboard.
        2. Swing left arm across chest.
        3. Hyperextend left wrist and brace against mattress.
        4. Pull with both arms, until in the side or prone position.

5. To return to supine: Push against headboard with heel of right hand; swing left arm backward toward mattress.

E. Using an overhead loop or trapeze, if hand function (turning to the right).
1. Throw left arm into loop or grab trapeze with left hand.
2. Flex left elbow, pulling thorax off of bed.
3. Extend and abduct right shoulder until weight-bearing on forearm.
4. Lean body weight forward, balanced on right forearm.
5. Slip left arm out of loop (or release trapeze) and place arm in front of trunk.
6. Flex left hip and knee, if possible, after arm is taken out of loop.
7. Drop weight off right forearm until prone.

F. With equipment—using wheelchair arm or side rail of bed.
Follow procedure described in using edge of bed, hooking wrist on equipment and pulling trunk over.

II. Coming to Sitting*
A. No equipment.
1. Place hands in pants' pockets or under hips for stabilization.
2. Flex neck and elbows until weight is on elbows.

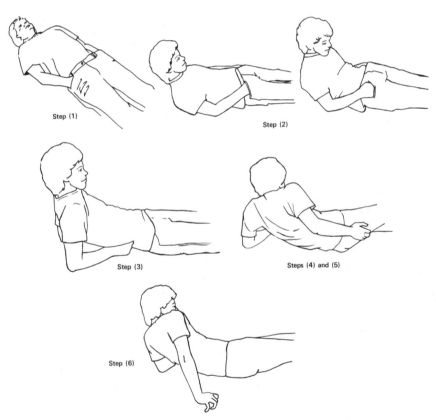

Step (1)   Step (2)

Step (3)   Steps (4) and (5)

Step (6)

Illustration continued on following page

---

*Adapted from Rancho Los Amigos Medical Center, Department of Physical Therapy, Downey, CA.

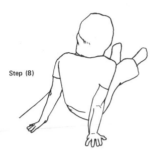

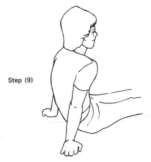

Step (8)   Step (9)

3. Shift elbows backward, one at a time, until weight is on forearms.
4. Roll to one side, shift weight over to one elbow.
5. Fling other arm backward, laterally rotating and extending shoulder and elbow until heel of hand contacts mattress (interphalangeal joints should be flexed).
6. Come to sitting by shifting weight onto extended arm (if hand slips, may need to use an adhesive glove or palmar strap, or merely to lick heel of hand).
7. Repeat step 5 with other arm.
8. Gain balance with weight on both extended arms.
9. Walk hands toward hips.
10. To lie down, reverse procedure.

B. With equipment — using a rope with a loop tied in the end.
1. Hook hyperextended wrist through loop on rope.
2. Pull on rope, bending elbow forcibly, and throw head forward, raising shoulders off bed.
3. Fling opposite arm backward; lock elbow in extension.
4. Push on extended arm and pull with flexed arm until in a sitting position.
5. To lie down, reverse procedure.

C. With equipment — using overhead loops.
The loops attached to an over-the-bed rail are in graduated lengths from the longest near the individual's head while supine to the shortest when the individual is sitting. The lengths and distance must be adjusted for each person's upper limb and trunk length.
1. Place one arm in the longest loop.
2. Flex elbow and pull, lifting head, neck, and thorax.

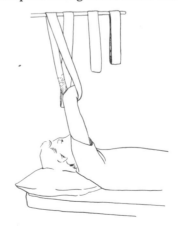

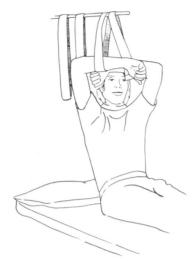

3. Place other arm in the next loop, pull, and continue with arms in loops until sitting.
4. Reverse procedure to lie down.

III. Moving in Bed
   A. Moving toward foot of bed—no equipment, long sitting position.
      1. Place both hands on mattress close to hips; lock elbows.
      2. Throw trunk forward, using momentum to slide toward foot of bed.
   B. Moving toward head of bed—no equipment.
      1. Semisitting, rest on forearms (shoulder hyperextended).
      2. Push against mattress, flexing shoulders.
      3. Pull body toward head of bed.
      Alternate method, moving toward head of bed—no equipment.
      1. Place both hands behind hips; lock elbows.
      2. Shift weight onto arms.
      3. Throw trunk and head forward, using momentum to slide toward head of bed (head should be flexed forward at all times, to prevent falling backward).
   C. Toward side of bed—sitting (to the right) without equipment.
      1. Come to long sitting position.
      2. Place extended right arm in front of right hip and about a foot to the right side.
      3. Place extended left arm in front of left hip and close to left side of hip.
      4. Push against bed, elevating buttocks.
      5. Set buttocks down close to right hand.
      6. Keeping trunk bent forward at hips, use hands to move and realign legs.
IV. Balancing Activities
   A. Long sitting (hamstring range at least 90 degrees).
      1. Maintain sitting balance without use of hands.
      2. Actively shift trunk to front, back, and sides using arms. Use arms and head to control balance when the trunk is shifted.
      3. Practice protective falling when pushed off balance.
      4. Raise arms overhead; abduct.

5. Use upper limbs to shift trunk weight.

6. Throw and catch a ball.

B. Short sitting (hamstring range less than 90 degrees)
   Repeat above activities.

V. Passive Self Range of Motion*

Most patients with quadriplegia who have good muscle power in their shoulders, elbow flexors, and wrist extensors; full elbow extension range; and 110 degrees of straight leg raising, learn to do their own range of motion to the lower limbs. Individual differences in such things as spasticity, balance, weight, and motivation will influence the ability to accomplish this activity. Patients are encouraged to range their lower limbs daily before getting out of bed and several times during the day if contractures develop easily.

Range of motion is performed in the sitting position. To aid in balance, lean against the wall, against the back of the wheelchair with lower limbs supported on bed or mat, or against the headrest of the bed. If the head of the bed is gatched, lean against it. The side-lying position can also be used for hip and knee flexion. Assume the position as described, count to 10 slowly, then slowly replace limb to the resting position. Repeat 10 times.

A. Hip and knee flexion.

1. Lock right elbow and balance on that arm.

2. Place left wrist under left knee and pull the knee toward chest as far as possible.

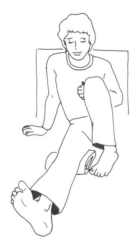

Note. Keep fingers flexed on right hand to maintain tightness in finger flexor tendons.

Hip and knee flexion—Alternate method for patients who have difficulty with procedure A2 (placing left wrist under left knee)

*Adapted from Rancho Los Amigos Medical Center, Department of Physical Therapy, Downey, CA.

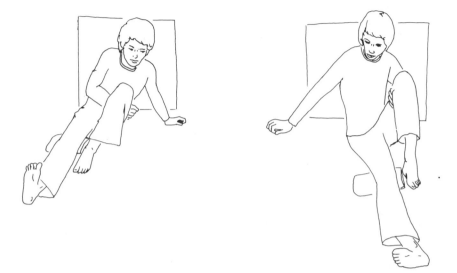

1. Lock left elbow and balance on that arm.
2. Place right wrist under left knee and pull the leg toward chest.
3. Lean against the headboard for balance. Shift weight to the right side and lock right elbow in extension.
4. Place left wrist under the knee and continue to pull knee as close to chest as possible.

B. Hip medial rotation and adduction.
   1. Lower the leg from the hip and knee flexion position until the foot is flat on the bed, leaving the hip and knee partially flexed. Continue to balance on the right arm.

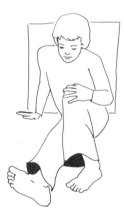

   2. Place the left hand on the lateral (outside) border of the knee and push it across the right leg.
C. Hip lateral rotation and abduction.
   1. Start from the same position as illustrated in B.

   2. Continue to balance on the right arm.
   3. Place the left hand on the medial (inside) border of the knee and gently push the leg into lateral rotation and abduction.

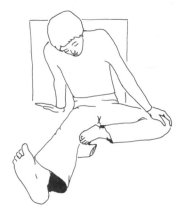

D. Ankle dorsiflexion.
   1. Leave the leg in the position illustrated in C.
   2. Brace left leg by placing left forearm against it. Lean forward and balance over the arm.
   3. Place the dorsal surface (back) of the right hand under the forefoot (ball of the foot).

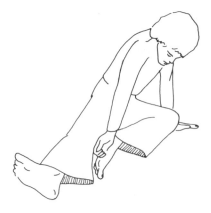

   4. Extend the wrist and push the foot up toward knee.
   5. Repeat entire procedure on opposite leg.
      Note. Dorsiflexion with the knees in extension can be accomplished if the patient has adequate hamstring range (approximately 110 degrees) and the ability to recover from a forward leaning position to the upright position.
VI. Skin Inspection
   A. Refer to section on bilateral lower limb and trunk involvement in Chapter 9. The same principles apply for weakness of all four limbs and trunk.
VII. Dressing Activities*
   The suggested procedures for teaching dressing techniques to the patient with

---

*Adapted from Rancho Los Amigos Medical Center, Department of Physical Therapy, Downey, CA.

spinal cord injury have proved satisfactory for many patients, and total to partial independence has been achieved. Side benefits have also occurred during the dressing practice, such as increased muscle strength and general endurance, increased range of motion in hip flexion and knee extension, plus increase in ability to control body.

A. Minimum criteria for dressing training.
   1. Upper limb dressing (putting on and removing undershirt, bra, blouse, shirt, or sweater, plus fastening and unfastening appropriate fasteners).
      a. Neck stability medically cleared.
      b. Muscle strength of fair to good in shoulder: deltoid, trapezius (upper and middle), serratus anterior, rotators; elbow, biceps.
      c. Range of motion: Shoulder flexion and abduction (0 to 90 degrees), shoulder medial and lateral rotation (0 to 30 degrees), elbow flexion (15 to 140 degrees).
      d. Sitting tolerance and balance in bed and/or wheelchair achieved with assistance of bed side rails or wheelchair safety belt.
      e. Prehension for fastening fasteners achieved with flexor hinge hand splints if patient has wrist extensor power.
   2. Lower limb dressing (putting on and removing undershorts, trouser, shoes, and socks).
      a. Muscle strength: fair to good strength in pectorals, rhomboids, supinators, and radial wrist extensors.
      b. Range of motion: knee, flexion and extension (0 to 120 degrees) to permit sitting with legs fully extended and reaching hands to midcalf area; hip flexion (0 to 110 degrees).
      c. Body control, such as ability to transfer from bed to wheelchair with minimum assistance; ability to roll body from side to side, balance when lying on side, and/or turning prone and returning to supine.
      d. Spasms are used to advantage to flex and extend lower limbs if patient can control them.
   3. *Contraindications* for upper limb and lower limb dressing training.
      a. Breathing ability—vital capacity below 50 percent (patients with this vital capacity can often do upper limb dressing).
      b. Pressure sore or unusual tendency of skin to break down when rolling or transferring.
      c. Continued patient resistance to dressing—maximum patient cooperation necessary for lower limb dressing.
      d. Pain in neck or trunk that persists when attempting dressing training.

B. Type of clothing recommended*:
   1. The clothing used should be loose fitting and have front fastenings to facilitate early training.
   2. Zippers and Velcro fasteners are most easily managed by patients; grippers are the most difficult.
   3. Since patients do many of the fastening processes by using the thumb as a hook, the following adaptations are recommended:
      a. Loops on zipper pulls
      b. Velcro and hook fastenings

    For more information on adaptive clothes for a particular disability or function, contact Judith Sweeney, P.O. Box 4220, Alexandria, VA 22303.

    c. Reinforced belt loops on trousers

    d. Loops on undershorts

4. Socks without elastic cuffs should be used.

5. Shoes should be carefully selected according to patient's needs. If patient transfers, the shoe must provide foot stability, as in a tie oxford. Other considerations include degree of spasticity in feet and edematous legs and feet. Shoe fastenings or closures can be adapted, using Velcro zippers or flip-back tongues. Loops can be stitched at back of shoe heel for additional help in donning shoes.

C. Dressing aids.

Aids to achieve self-dressing are many and varied. Some patients require special adaptations for individual needs. In general, standard aids include bilateral wrist-driven flexor hinge hand splints (used mainly in fastening and unfastening garments and arranging clothing in desired place), dressing sticks, Swedish reaches, overhead wrist straps, knee straps, monkey bars, button hooks, sock cones, and long-handled shoe horns.

1. Dressing stick—¼-inch doweling, 20 inches long, cup hook, wrist strap of 1-inch-wide webbing.

2. Dressing stick—⅝-inch doweling, 20 inches long, ½-inch stainless steel hook, wrist strap of 1-inch-wide webbing.

3. Dressing stick—1-inch doweling, 12 inches long, ½-inch-wide stainless steel hook, wrist strap of 1-inch-wide webbing.

4. Dressing hook—¼-inch plastic covered with moleskin, ½-inch-wide stainless steel hooks.

5. Swedish Reacher—purchased from J. A. Preston Corporation, New York.

6. Monkey bar—standard orthopedic hospital equipment attached to Balkan frame.

7. Knee strap—1½-inch-wide webbing buckled to Balkan frame. Hook at end of strap is made by removing the spring steel catch from a snap fastener. This hook fastens into a D ring partway up the strap.

8. Wrist strap—1½-inch-wide webbing attached to Balkan frame.

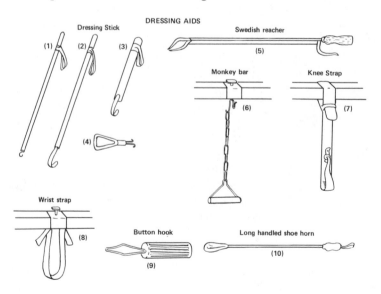

DRESSING AIDS

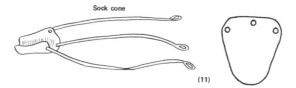

Sock cone

(11)

9. Button hook—purchased from B/K Sales Company, Brookfield, Illinois.
10. Shoe horn—purchased from J. A. Preston Corporation, New York.
D. Sequence recommended for dressing.
1. While patient is in bed, put on undershorts and trousers.
2. Put pants on before the socks.
3. Have patient transfer to wheelchair and put on upper limb garments, shoes, and socks.
4. Reverse this procedure for removing clothing.
5. Sequence may be altered as patients work out unique methods applicable to their individual needs.
6. Those activities in dressing and other self-care that require use of hand splints should be grouped together so that the patient will not have to put on and remove the hand splints frequently. This is not difficult to do as it is not necessary to complete all activities in an exact sequence.
7. Have someone button a shirt or use a button hook and leave it buttoned except for the top one and don it like a cardigan garment.
8. Have someone tie a long tie and leave it tied. Do not untie. Loosen the tie and slip the knot downward enough to take it over your head.
E. Techniques for upper limb dressing.
1. Putting on a cardigan garment.
The method may be adapted for jackets, blouses, sweaters, shirts, and top portion of dresses that open down the front.
a. Patient is sitting in wheelchair. Position shirt on lap with back of shirt up and collar toward knees. The label of the shirt is facing down.
b. Put arms under shirt back starting at shirt tail and into sleeve starting at armhole and working toward cuff. Push shirt past elbows.
c. Using wrist extension, hook hands under shirt back and gather up material.
d. Using shoulder abduction, scapular abduction and adduction, elbow flexion, and slight neck flexion, pass shirt over head.
e. By relaxing wrist and shoulders, and with the aid of gravity, the hands may be removed from shirt back and the arms are now completely through the sleeves. Most of the material of the shirt is gathered up at back of patient's neck across shoulders and underarms.
f. Shirt is worked into place over shoulders and trunk by alternately shrugging shoulders, leaning forward, with aid of wheelchair arms for balance if necessary, and using elbow flexion and wrist extension.
(1) Shrug shoulders to get material down across shoulders.
(2) Hook wrists into sleeves to pull free at axilla.
(3) Leaning forward and/or reaching back and sliding hand against material will aid in pulling shirt down.
(4) Line up shirt fronts for buttoning.

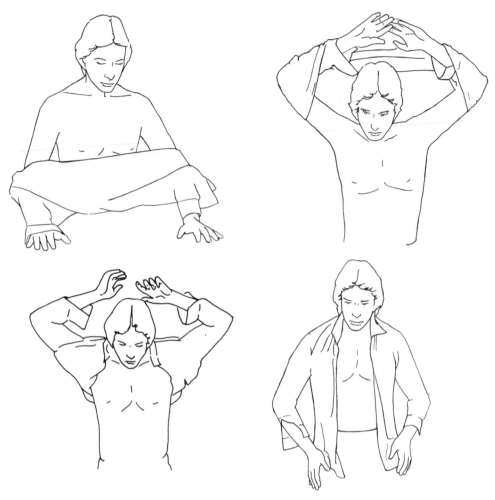

g. Close shirt using buttons, snaps, or Velcro. If the shirt has not been buttoned previously, use a button hook, starting with bottom button, which is easiest to see.

Exceptions to this procedure would be as follows:

a. Arrange shirt on table preparatory to putting on.
b. When trunk stability is a problem, support elbows on table to assist in flipping shirt over head.

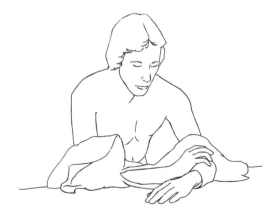

2. Removing a cardigan garment.
   a. Patient is in wheelchair. Unbutton only the necessary buttons. Use a hook, if necessary.
   b. Push one shoulder of cardigan at a time off shoulder. Elevate and depress shoulders, rotate trunk, and use gravity so cardigan will slip down arms as far as possible. Use thumbs alternately in armholes to slip sleeves farther down arms.
   c. Hold one cardigan cuff with opposite thumb and flex elbow to pull arm out of garment. Repeat for other arm. The thumb is used as a "hook" in this step.
3. Putting on bra.
   Ready-made garments may be adapted with Velcro strips, replacing the hooks for greater ease in self-fastening; however, patients with maximum strength and dexterity can master the standard hook fastener. The patient has a choice of a front or back closure.
   a. Patient is sitting in wheelchair. Place bra on lap with straps toward knees and label of bra (inside) facing the ceiling.
   b. Grasp the bra by placing it between the side of the index finger and the thumb.
   c. Position the bra against the trunk by using the thumbs and pressing firmly against the trunk.
   d. Push both ends of the bra together using the thumbs and hook or fasten Velcro by patting in place. An additional thumb loop can be attached to Velcro.
   e. Twist bra around at waist level and place each shoulder strap over the appropriate shoulder.
4. Removing bra (patient sitting in wheelchair).
   a. Unfasten Velcro by placing thumb in thumb loop on Velcro.
   b. Unhook bra by using thumbs and pinching the straps of the bra together.
   c. Lean forward and use thumbs to push straps down arms until bra is removed.
F. Techniques for lower limb dressing.
   1. Putting on trousers (same for undershorts).
      a. Patient is sitting in bed with side rails up. Trousers are positioned at foot of bed with trouser legs over bed end, front side up. Position of trousers can be achieved by throwing or placing trousers with a dressing stick.
      b. Lift one knee at a time by hooking wrist or forearm under thigh and insert foot into pant leg. Use free hand to hold trouser waist as each knee is extended into trouser leg. Proceed until both legs are started into trousers. If patient is unable to maintain knee in flexion by holding with an arm or using spasticity, an overhead strap may be used to maintain knee flexion while pushing trousers over feet.
      c. Work trousers up legs to midcalf (while sitting) by using the palm of the hands with a patting, sliding motion. Try to get trouser cuffs past feet.
      d. Shift weight to one hip, twist trunk so weight is off one hip and with a hand under the waist band pull up over hip, shift weight to the opposite hip and repeat. (A high quadriplegic individual may use an assistive device or use the thumb in a belt loop.)

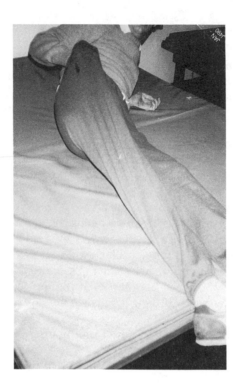

    e. Pull crotch up as far as possible using palms and thumbs.

    f. Straighten trouser legs with palms of hands using a pushing, smoothing motion.

    g. Pull trousers up to buttocks by alternating steps g, h, and i. Insert hands in trouser pockets; pull trousers up. Hook other elbow on monkey bar or side rails for balance.

    h. Lying on side, throw top arm around to back and insert thumb in trousers belt loop at middle of back and pull (elbow flexion, shoulder elevation and adduction).

    i. Roll to other side and repeat step h. These sidelying steps may need to be repeated several times until trousers are in place on hips. Prone position can also be used to pull trousers over buttocks if patient finds it successful.

    j. In supine position, fasten trouser placket by hooking thumb in loop on zipper pull, patting Velcro closed, or using hand splints and button hook for button plackets.

  2. Removing trousers (same for undershorts and pants).

    a. Patient supine in bed with side rails up.

    b. Unfasten fasteners (buttons, snaps, Velcro) using button hook and hand splints or thumbs and side of hands.

    c. Place thumbs in belt loops, pockets, or waistband and work trousers down on the hips. Combine the use of stabilizing arms in partial extension and scooting body toward head of bed.

    d. Continue to use arm as in step c and roll side to side to get trousers down over buttocks.

    e. Patient may sit up and continue pushing trousers down legs by placing each leg alternately in flexion using the opposite arm and pulling one knee at a time into flexion, thus continuing to remove trouser legs.

3. Putting on socks.

Trunk balance is often a problem when sitting in a wheelchair when the patient cannot maintain a crossed leg position while putting on socks and shoes. Some of the methods of dealing with this problem are placing foot on stool, chair, or open drawer; hooking opposite arm around upright wheelchair handle; using wheelchair safety belt; or leaning sideways against wheelchair arm.

Patient ordinarily sits in wheelchair.

a. Use the elbow to support the trunk while raising the foot.

b. Lick the heel of the hand and thumb to provide friction on the sock.

c. Place the thumbs inside the sock and slide the sock over the toes.

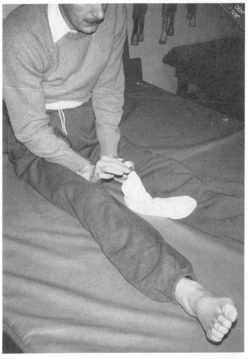

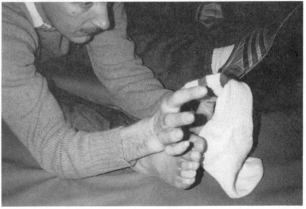

d. Pinch with the thumb and medial side of the hand. Moisten the hand when necessary and slide the sock farther up the heel.
e. Lift the heel and slide the thumb in sock against the heel.
f. Slide the sock over the heel and up over the ankle.

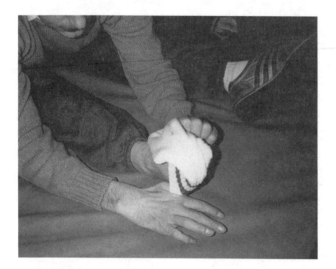

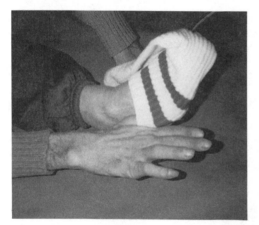

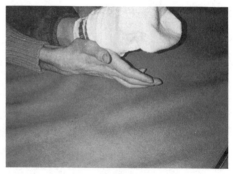

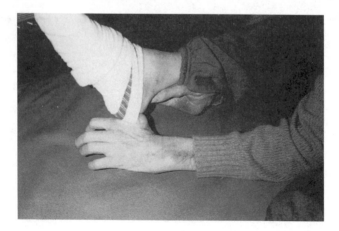

4. Removing socks.
    a. A high quadriplegic may use dressing stick or long shoe horn to push stocking down over heel (cross legs by using wrist extension and elbow flexion if possible).
    b. Use Swedish reacher or dressing hook for prehension on sock toe and pull sock off.
       Note. A high quadriplegic may use a device to aid in saving time and energy.
5. Putting on shoes.
    a. Slide the fingers into the shoe like a shoe horn in reverse. The fingers will be positioned under the tongue of the shoe with the palm up to keep the shoe tongue out of the way.
    b. Using the forearm and the hand lift the heel of the foot and slide the shoe over the toes.
    c. Push the shoe on using the thumb and pull the shoe over the heel.
       Note. A high quadriplegic individual may require assistive devices. If sitting in wheelchair, use an extended handle aid (hook, stick, reacher, or shoe horn) in shoe tongue and place toe into opening of shoe. Remove dressing aid.
    d. Use palm of hand on sole of shoe to pull shoe toward heel of the foot (shoe is dangling on foot). Use one hand to stabilize leg while the other hand is pushing against the sole of the shoe to work it onto the foot. (Use thenar eminence and sides of hand.)

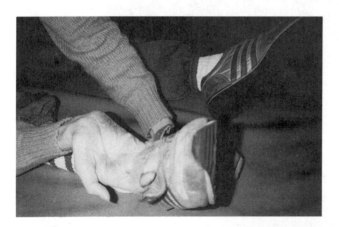

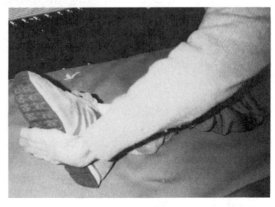

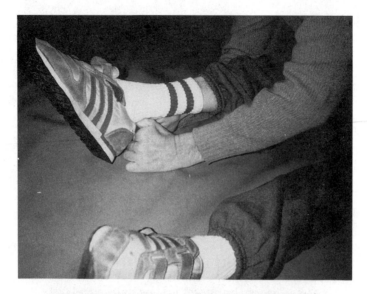

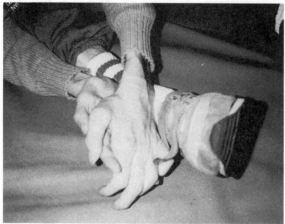

      e. To force foot into shoe, feet need to be flat on floor or wheelchair footrest, knees flexed to 90 degrees. Place shoe horn in heel of shoe and press down on flexed knee.

      f. Fasten fastenings.

  6. Removing shoes (sitting in wheelchair with lower limbs in previous position).

      a. Unfasten fastenings.

      b. Push on heel counter of shoe with shoe horn or extended handle aid until shoe falls to floor.

MAT ACTIVITIES

Mat activities are an important aspect of a functional training program for individuals with involvement of all four limbs and trunk. Mat activities can be conducted in a group or designed for an individual. It is important to remember that the therapist will have to guard the patient closely until trunk balance has been achieved. This may be a major factor in determining when the person would be able to participate in group mat activities. Close guarding may be necessary and may require the attention of a therapist unless the patient has attained trunk balance or the trunk is well supported.

Initial mat activities should emphasize respiratory function and chest mobility, progressing to bed mobility and sitting with support. Progressing to more advanced mat activities, beyond sitting, is not realistic unless the individual demonstrates adequate voluntary motor control. The mat is an ideal place to teach range of motions and dressing activities. (Refer to Chapter 7 for guarding techniques.)

The activities described here assume that the patient has some voluntary control of the shoulder and scapular muscles.

I. Supine Position
   A. Supine on elbows.
      1. *Position:* Supine with upper limbs at side of trunk.
      2. *Action:* Hyperextend head and shoulders until weight is on elbows and "walk" elbows backward.
      3. *Functional carry-over:* Changing bed position and coming to sitting.
   B. Weight shifter.
      1. *Position:* Supine on elbows.
      2. *Action:* Shift weight onto one forearm and reverse.
      3. *Functional carry-over:* Changing bed position and coming to sitting.
   C. Arm raiser.
      1. *Position:* Supine, weight on elbows.
      2. *Action:* Shift weight to one side lifting opposite upper limb off the mat, reverse with the other upper limb.
      3. *Functional carry-over:* Bed mobility and balance.
   D. Rolling to side lying.
      1. *Position:* Supine, assuming forearm weight-bearing.
      2. *Action:* Swing the upper limb and head toward the direction of the turn, the lower limb will follow.
      3. *Functional carry-over:* Changing bed position and coming to sitting.
   E. Moving toward head or feet.
      1. *Position:* Supine, weight-bearing on forearms.
      2. *Action:* (a) Shoulder depression to move toward the head. (b) Shoulder elevation to move toward the feet.
     Note. Unless the lower limbs are well protected it is not good to drag the exposed limbs on the mat.

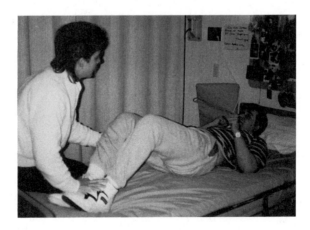

　　　　3. *Functional carry-over:* Coming to sitting.
　　F. Chest raiser.
　　　　1. *Position:* Supine on elbows.
　　　　2. *Action:* Upper back is raised by extending the head and shoulder, while adducting the scapula.
　　　　3. *Functional carry-over:* Changing bed position.
　II. Prone Position
　　A. Assume prone position.
　　　　1. *Position:* Supine or sidelying.
　　　　2. *Action:* Swing free upper limb and head toward the direction of the turn; lower limbs will follow.
　　　　3. *Functional carry-over:* Wheelchair mobility and transfer activties.
　　B. Weight shifter.
　　　　1. *Position:* Prone weight-bearing on forearms.
　　　　2. *Action:* Shift weight from elbow to elbow, lift, and reach with the free upper limb.
　　　　3. *Functional carry-over:* Developing stability in the shoulders and scapula, dressing and transfer activities.
　　C. Prone over.
　　　　1. *Position:* Prone on elbows.
　　　　2. *Action:* Shift weight from elbow to elbow, pulling body forward and pushing body backward.
　　　　3. *Functional carry-over:* Developing shoulder girdle musculature for wheelchair mobility and transfers.
　III. Sitting Position
　　A. Assume sitting (refer to lying and sitting activities for the procedure to come to sitting).
　　B. Sitting balancer.
　　　　1. *Position:* Long sitting with trunk support.
　　　　2. *Action:* Shift weight side to side and forward and back.
　　　　3. *Functional carry-over:* Balancing for dressing and wheelchair activities.
　　C. Sitting reacher.
　　　　1. *Position:* Long sitting with support; upper limbs at side of trunk.
　　　　2. *Action:* Shift weight to one upper limb and reach forward with the other, reach to the side, and return. Repeat with the other upper limb.
　　　　3. *Functional carry-over:* Balancing for dressing and wheelchair mobility and transfers.
　　D. Foot toucher.
　　　　1. *Position:* Long sitting with support (hamstring length will determine whether patient is able to touch the toes).
　　　　2. *Action:* Reach toward feet with both upper limbs and return.
　　　　3. *Functional carry-over:* Dressing and range of motion exercises.
　　E. Trunk twister
　　　　1. *Position:* Long sitting with support.
　　　　2. Action: Use the upper limbs to twist the trunk to the right and left.
　　　　3. *Functional carry-over:* Trunk balance.
　　F. Leg mover.
　　　　1. *Position:* Long sitting with or without support.
　　　　2. *Action:* Flex, extend, abduct, and adduct the lower limb with one or both hands. It may require hooking the wrist under the knee. Repeat with opposite limb.

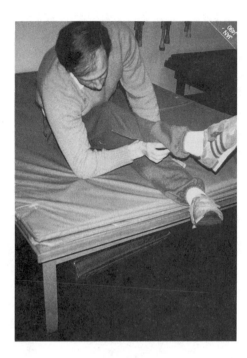

3. *Functional carry-over:* Wheelchair transfers and dressing activities.
G. Short sitting scooter.
   1. *Position:* short sitting weight-bearing on both upper limbs with elbows locked in extension.
   2. *Action:* Depress the shoulders, unweight buttocks and slide or scoot buttocks sideways; repeat procedure in the opposite direction.
   3. *Functional carry-over:* Wheelchair transfers.

WHEELCHAIRS

Wheelchair dimensions and measurements are given in Chapter 6. Individuals with high spinal cord lesions (above C-4) require wheelchair adaptations — because of lack of upper limb function they are unable to propel a wheelchair manually, they may be dependent on a ventilator and they may have limited head control. The power-adapted wheelchair has been designed to provide a means of propelling a wheelchair independently, and it provides a mechanism for pressure relief. An awareness of the basic adaptive components to the power-adapted wheelchair is necessary for those therapists who will be involved in recommending adaptive equipment for their patients with severe involvement of all four limbs and trunk.

Reclining mechanisms are useful so that the individual may remain in the wheelchair and still be able to relieve pressure and take short naps. Inclinator controls operate the reclining backs. These electronic controls have a single speed or adjustable speeds.

Forward propulsion of the power wheelchair can be achieved by several mechanisms: (1) head controls, (2) a puff of air blown into an electronic mechanism, (3) short throw switches, (4) chin controls, (5) sip and puff controls, and in some cases (6) eyebrow control.

High quadriplegic individuals who are ventilator dependent can achieve independent mobility with adaptive wheelchair equipment and recent technology. The following equipment is necessary for ventilator-dependent users: a portable ventilator; a slide-out ventilator and battery tray; a programmable power control accessed by the chin, mouth, lips, or head; a pressure-relieving cushion and a low to zero shear power reclining back for shifting weight; and posture supports. Gutters or troughs are often attached to the arm of the wheelchair to provide support for the upper limbs.

I. Balance Activities
   A. Shoulder girdle depression (push-ups). Use this activity for pressure relief while in wheelchair for extended periods of time.

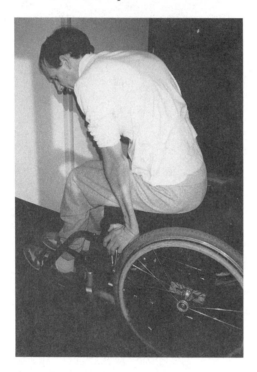

      1. Lean forward in wheelchair, balance trunk without use of arms, regain sitting balance.
      2. Lean forward and touch floor, regain upright sitting—one arm may be hooked behind wheelchair handle if necessary.
      3. Lean to right and left.
   B. Manipulation of wheelchair parts.
      1. Lock and unlock brakes (may require brake extension lever).
      2. Remove feet from foot pedals.
      3. Pull heel loops forward.
      4. Raise foot pedals.
      5. Swing away legrest.
      6. Remove armrests, place on wheelchair handles. (Armrests may have pin-locks to be removed and replaced).
      7. Replace armrests.
      8. Swing legrests into place; pull heel loops back.

9. Lower foot pedal.
10. Place feet on foot pedals.

WHEELCHAIR MOBILITY

Controlled motion of the wheelchair is essential to all other wheelchair activities. Wheelchair techniques performed in a safe and efficient manner allow the individual freedom to participate in many activities with a minimum expenditure of energy. Wheelchair mobility for low (C-6 and below) quadriplegic individuals is similar to that of paraplegic individuals except for the lack of some upper limb strength.

Limitation of the grip is a major factor in developing the necessary skill to use a manual wheelchair. The use of friction tape or surgical tubing on the handrims provides a nonslip surface for the hands. Well-fitting gloves will provide comfort and protection to the hands.

To use a manual wheelchair, a high quadriplegic (C-4 and C-5) individual who lacks the ability to grasp will need projections or lugs spaced at regular intervals on the handrims of the chair. These projections provide a surface against which the user is able to apply force to propel the wheelchair.

I. Level Surfaces
  A. Forward motion.
    1. Starting position: Place hands on the handrims at 10 o'clock, palms facing downward, and lean trunk slightly forward.
    2. Motion.
      a. Flex, then extend, elbows, applying pressure downward.
      b. Snap wrists at the completion of the stroke.
      c. Swing hands in back of hips at the 10 o'clock position on handrims.
      d. Gain momentum, allowing the chair to coast between strokes.

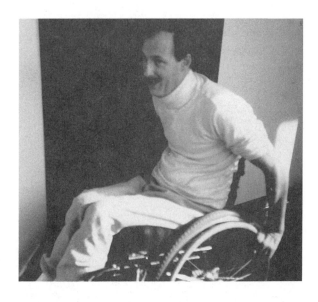

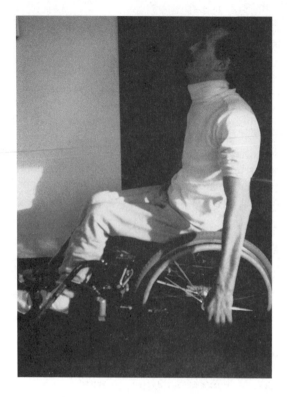

Variation: A high (C-4 or C-5) quadriplegic individual.
    1. Starting position: Elbows slightly flexed, heel of the hand hooked behind lugs at 10 o'clock on the handrims.
    2. Motion.
        a. Flex and extend elbows; lower shoulders.
        b. Snap wrists and swing arms back and up.
        c. Extend head and shoulders with a slight arch to back.
        d. Weight should now be on the rear wheels.

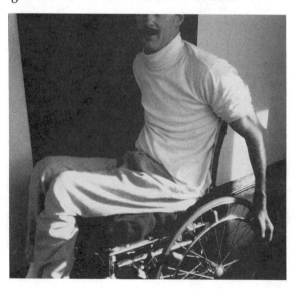

3. Teaching tip—Following complete extension of the elbows let the upper limbs swing back and up, feel the projections with the heel of the hand to know when to make contact with lugs. The speed is maintained by pushing on the projections.

B. Slowing and stopping.
1. Starting position: Wrist in hyperextension, back of the hand under the handrim.
2. Motion: Apply pressure up and in against the handrim.

C. Quick stop.
1. Starting position: Palm up, heel of the hand against the under side of the handrim; use the under side of the forearm and palm.
2. Motion: Apply pressure firmly against the handrim, up and in.

D. Backward motion.
1. Starting position.
   a. Place the heel of hands on handrims forward of lugs or place the thumb between the tire and the projection (C-4 or C-5 quadriplegic individual).
   b. Elbows extended, trunk erect.
2. Motion.
   a. Flex elbows.
   b. Extend neck and trunk to move the center of gravity back to assist with the movement.
   c. Follow through; swing arms forward.
   d. Reposition hands on handrims.
   e. Use the body weight and shoulder muscles to pull back.

E. Slow down backward motion.
1. Starting position—Place the palms in a downward direction under the handrims at the 2 o'clock position.
2. Apply pressure upward, using wrist extensors and shoulder muscles.

F. Turning—stationary.
1. Starting position: One hand placed at the 2 o'clock position, the other at the 10 o'clock position, in the direction of the turn.
2. Motion: Simultaneously use the power stroke forward from the 10 o'clock position with one hand and backward with the other hand at the 2 o'clock position.

G. Turning—in motion.
1. Starting position: Traversing forward.
2. Motion.
   a. Slowly apply pressure on the handrim in the direction of the turn.
   b. Continue to push forward on the other handrim.

H. Cornering, using the wall or object (turning into direction of corner).
1. Starting position: Forward propulsion motion.
2. Motion.
   a. Approach corner.
   b. Swing arm back and out to the side behind the wheelchair axle.
   c. Lean trunk back and toward wall.
   d. Push hand against wall. The drag causes the wheelchair to turn toward corner.

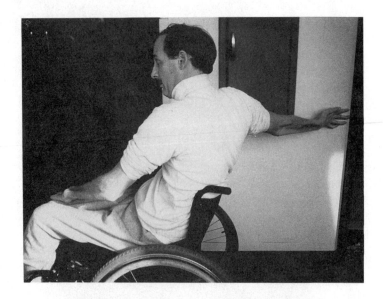

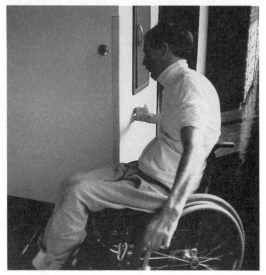

    3. Teaching tip—Maintain momentum as turn is approached and executed.
       Do not start the pressure against the wall until the front wheels are past the
       corner.
I. Cornering (turning outward from corner).
    1. Starting position.
      a. Lean slightly forward.
      b. Place arm about shoulder height in front and to the side of the chair.

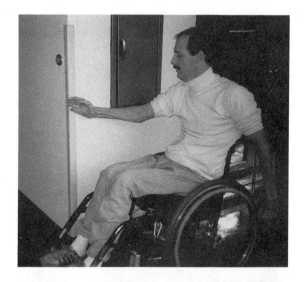

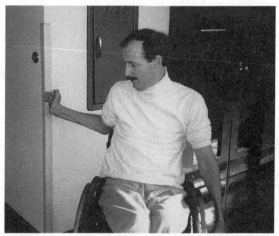

 2. Motion: Place hand on wall pushing away from the wall, causing chair to
    turn away from wall.
J. Through doors (high quadriplegic, C-4 or C-5, pulling door to open).
 1. Starting position: Back chair up to a double or a single door; the handrims
    just clearing the door that will be opened.
 2. Motion.
    a. Place hand in door handle.
    b. Open the door slightly.
    c. Remove hand from door handle.
    d. Using hand against door, push door open until door is past the rim of
       the wheelchair.
    e. Using the rim to block the door open, turn chair toward the door,
       keeping the rim against the door.
    f. Propel chair forward with rim against the door until door is fully open.

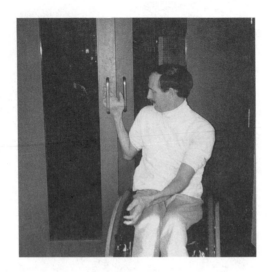

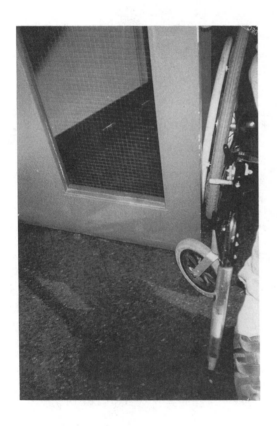

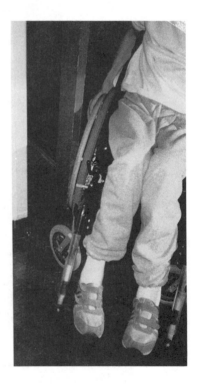

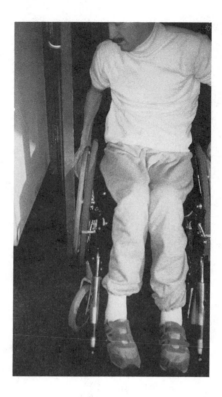

      g. With the wheel continuing to block the door open, back chair with arm that is opposite the door.

      h. Push off from door and propel through doorway backward.

   3. Teaching tip: Because of the tenodesis effect it is important to place hand in door handle before turning the chair completely backward.

K. Through doors (low quadriplegic, C-6 to C-7).

   1. Starting position: Back chair up to a double or a single door; the handrims just clearing the door that will be opened.

   2. Motion.

      a. Push door open far enough so that the door is blocked by the foot pedals.

      b. With the foot pedals against the door, turn wheelchair toward the open door.

Caution. Feet will catch the door as the individual turns toward the door. To avoid injury to the feet let the chair roll back a little as the individual turns through the door.

      c. Hold elbow against the door to keep it open.

      d. Propel through.

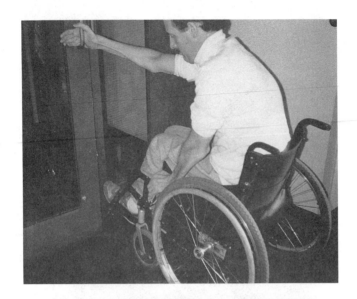

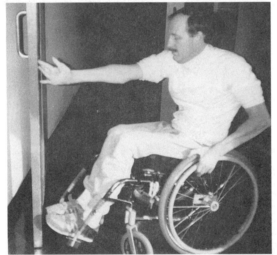

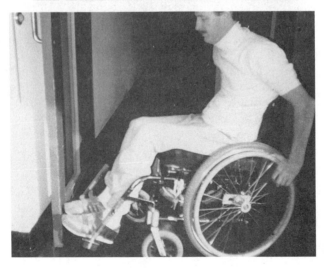

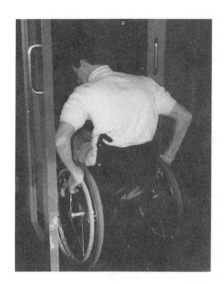
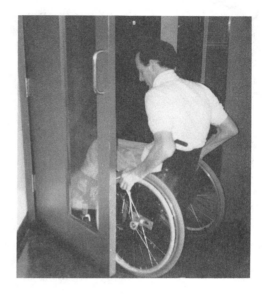

L. Through door (pushing forward).
  1. Starting position: Approach the door to be opened at a slight angle (30 to 40 degrees).
  2. Motion.
     a. Push the door open.
     b. Use toes and foot pedals to brace the door open.
     c. Turn wheelchair toward open door. (See figures on page 270 and top of page 271.)

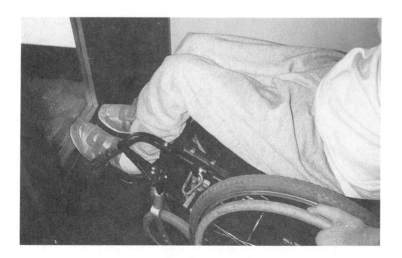

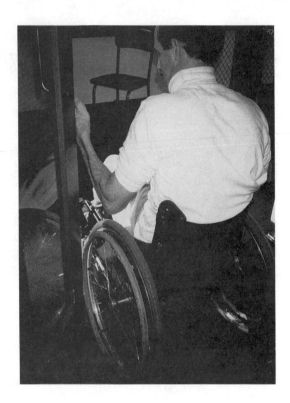

Caution. Do not bang into the door with your toes.

    3. Teaching tip—The weight of the door will straighten out the chair as it goes through.

M. Through two doors (pushing doors open).

    1. Starting position: Center wheelchair between the two doors with one foot pedal against each door.

    2. Motion

        a. Push doors with both feet until wheelchair is through the door past the handrims.

        b. With hands on the doors and elbows flexed, use trunk extension to push doors open.

        c. Propel through the doors. (See figures on bottom of page 271 and top of page 272.)

Caution. If you do not get far enough through the doors, the weight of the doors will push the chair backwards.

N. Wheelies (wheelchair without lugs)—refer to the "Wheelie" section under lower limb and trunk weakness, Chapter 9. This is an advanced technique for a low quadriplegic individual but one that should be mastered. High quadriplegic individuals will probably not be able to master this technique. The static wheelie position is used by resting the wheelchair against a wall. Once positioned, no effort is needed to maintain this position. The dynamic wheelie position is used during activities on uneven surfaces.

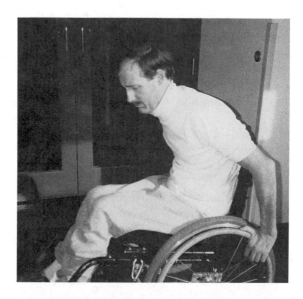

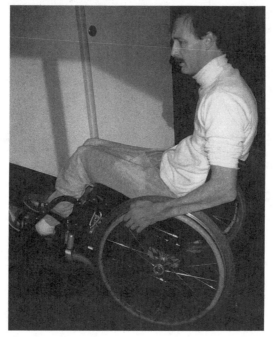

II. Uneven Surfaces
   A. Slanted incline or decline: The chair will tend to follow the slope or slant of the surface.
      1. Starting position: The chair should be positioned in such a way that it is above the line of the slope.
      2. Motion (if the slope is short or incorporates a turn)
         a. Begin forward motion.
         b. Let the chair follow the natural slope of the surface and turn in the direction of the slope.

    Variation: If the slope is long

    a. Push harder on the downhill handrim to keep the chair heading to the high side of the slope.

    Variation: If there is a wall along the high side of the slope

    a. Place your hand on the wall about shoulder height.

    b. Drag your hand along the wall, causing the chair to turn in toward the wall.

    c. Follow the high side of the slope.

    Alternate: Use the wall to push off or direct the chair back toward the wall similar to the cornering technique.

  3. Teaching tip—The secret to propelling across a slanted surface is to understand that the wheelchair will perform similar to a golf ball that is putted across a slanted surface. The speed and degree of slope will influence the roll.

B. Ascending curb cuts.

  1. Starting position: Square off at the entry of curb cut

  2. Motion

    a. Approach with a power stroke.

    b. Perform a low wheelie.

    c. Using a power stroke ascend onto the sidewalk.

C. Descending a curb cut—same as above just described.

D. Ascending a curb cut without using a wheelie.

  1. Starting position.

    a. Square off at the entry.

    b. Come to a complete stop.

  2. Motion: Propel forward.

  3. Teaching tip—A power stroke is used only if it is necessary to elevate the casters to clear the foot pedals.

    Note: Curb cuts—A lap belt may be necessary in the initial phases of training to avoid falling from the wheelchair. Plan ahead for any possible hazards on the street or sidewalk.

E. Ascending ramps.

  1. Starting position.

    a. Hands should be at about 12 o'clock on the handrims.

    b. Trunk should be upright.

  2. Motion.

    a. Lean forward into the ramp.

    b. Quickly extend elbows and snap the wrists.

    c. Follow through; quickly extend trunk.

    d. Swing upper limbs back to the 12 o'clock position on handrims.

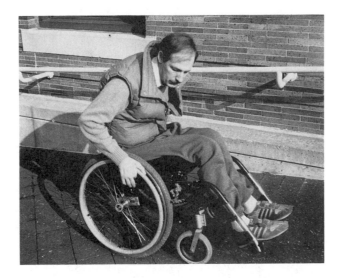

    e. Lean forward and quickly extend elbows.

    f. Repeat forward power stroke.

  3. Teaching tip—Forward flexion of the trunk puts the weight forward, adding momentum, and assists the arms while the chair propels forward. It is important to maintain the head and shoulders in a forward position.

F. Ascending ramps (using hill holders).

The hill holders will automatically engage with gravity and act as a rachet to hold the tire from a backward movement. It holds the wheelchair from rolling while the individual is preparing for the next forward stroke. The hill holders will disengage when the tire is propelled forward. The procedure for ascending ramps using hill holders is the same as previously described.

G. Descending ramps (without using brakes).

  1. Starting position: Trunk leaning slightly back to keep weight over the rear wheels; hands on handrims at 12 o'clock.

  2. Motion: Speed is controlled by pressure on the handrims.

    a. On long steep slopes, apply pressure to the rim with the left hand to turn gradually to the left and pressure with the right hand to turn the chair to the right (the slalom approach); this decreases the forward motion of the chair.

    b. For steeper ramps that are wide enough, traverse the ramp making sharp 90-degree turns in either direction during the descent.

H. Descending ramps (using brakes).

This technique is most often used by high quadriplegic individuals in wheelchairs with brake extensions.

  1. Starting position: Trunk slightly back, body weight over the wheels.

  2. Motion.

    a. Apply the brakes on one side, allowing the chair to turn in that direction.

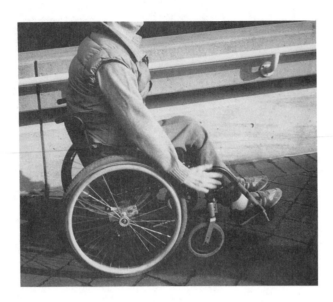

     b. Release that brake handle.
     c. Apply the other brake, turning the chair in the opposite direction.
  I. Ascending curbs: two-step motion forward (pulling up).
    1. Starting position.
      a. Do a wheelie to bring front wheels onto curb.
      b. Position rear wheels next to the curb.
    2. Motion.
      a. Back up, allowing front wheels to turn around.
      b. Approach the edge of the curb to lower the front of the chair.
      c. Throw body weight forward while pushing forward on the handrims.

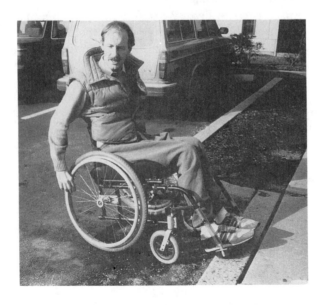

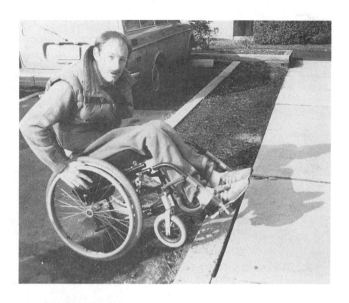

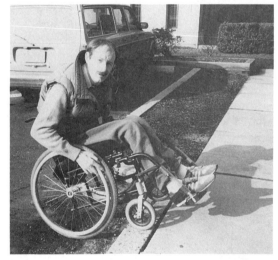

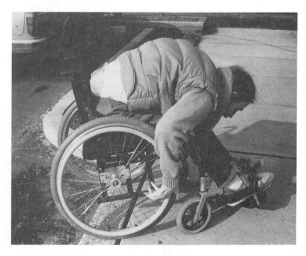

3. Teaching tip—The more weight over the casters the less difficult will be the ascent. Guarding; hands should be in a position to catch the handgrips and prevent the chair from tipping over backward.

J. Ascending curbs: forward—one-motion running start (more advanced).
   1. Starting position: Continue forward motion of the chair. When the footplates are just in front of the curb reach back as far as possible on the handrims.
   2. Motion
      a. Lean backward with the trunk.
      b. Do a low wheelie (just enough to bring the casters to the same level as the curb).
      c. Push forward on the handrims.
      d. Lean forward and bring the chair up onto the curb.
      Caution. If the casters are not raised high enough during the wheelie it will slam the casters into the curb and pitch the trunk forward.

K. Ascending curbs (using projection knobs).
   1. Starting position: Square the casters to the curb, reach back, and place hands on the projection rims at the 10 o'clock position.
   2. Motion
      a. With a quick, hard stroke, elevate the front casters onto the curb.
      b. Bring the rear wheels against the curb.
      c. Roll back slightly to gain momentum.
      d. Use another power stroke.
      f. Lean forward and muscle up the curb.
   3. Guarding: Place one hand forward and near the shoulder to prevent extreme trunk flexion and falling forward out of the chair. The other hand should be near handgrip in the event the chair would tip over backward.

L. Descending curbs (backward)—A high quadriplegic individual will have more control using this method.
   1. Starting position: Position chair with rear wheels at the edge of the curb; casters turned backward.
   2. Motion.
      a. Lean forward.
      b. Pull backward on the handrims.

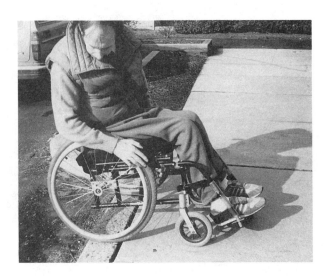

Caution. Footplates may drag on the curb.
3. Teaching tip—Once this procedure is begun, do not stop the motion of the chair. Stopping the motion of the chair will cause the chair to tip over backward.
M. Descending curbs: forward (using projection knobs).
1. Starting position: Square the casters to the curb, reach back, and place hands on the projection rims at the 10 o'clock position.
2. Motion: Carefully lower the front casters onto the street, and slowly lower the back wheels.
N. Descending a *low* curb forward.
1. Starting position: Wheelchair at a slight angle to the curb.
2. Motion.
   a. Shift body weight "uphill," keeping wheels on one side of the chair on the curb.
   b. Propel the chair forward at an angle so the front wheel on one side is over the curb.
   c. Continue the motion until the rear wheel on the same side goes down over the curb.

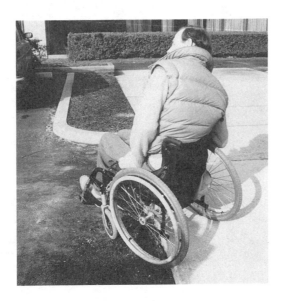

   d. Push forward on handrims to lower the other side of the chair.
O. Descending (forward).
1. Starting position: Square wheelchair to curb.
2. Motion.
   a. Perform a partially controlled wheelie.
   b. As the front wheels near the curb, reach back on the handrims as far as possible, keeping the hands on the handrims.
   c. Propel wheelchair forward.
   d. As the chair comes off the curb, apply pressure on the handrims to prevent the curb from "kicking" the chair forward and over backward.

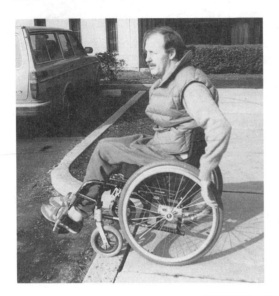

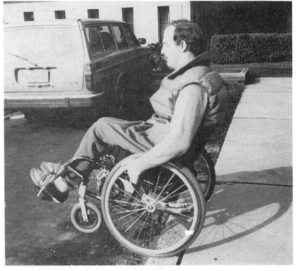

      e. Land on back wheels first.

      F. Lower the front wheels.

P. Stairs

    Stairs are an advanced skill; ascending or descending stairs, one may follow the procedure as stated in Chapter 9.

Q. Entering a bus.

    1. Starting position: Chair is facing backward; square the large wheels against the elevating bus platform.

    2. Motion.

      a. Back onto the platform by reaching back and using the platform railing.

      b. Pull backward onto the platform.

      c. Back onto the bus.

      d. Use wheel locks to secure the chair in position.

      e. If the bus has safety belts the driver should secure the wheelchair.

Transfers

Transfers may require assistance and adaptive equipment such as ropes, sliding board, swivel bars, and loops. Coat the sliding board with a furniture polish to enhance the effectiveness of the board.

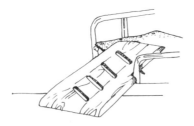

I. To and from wheelchair and bed or mat
  A. Forward (using sliding board).
    1. Starting position.
      a. Front of wheelchair facing side of bed.
      b. Slide board under hips, extending from seat of wheelchair onto bed.
    2. Motion.
      a. Lift both legs onto bed.
      b. Lock wheelchair, bringing wheelchair as close to bed as possible.
      c. Place one hand on each armrest.
      d. Shift most of weight to one side and then to other, scooting opposite leg forward.
      e. Repeat until hands can reach the mattress.
      f. Throw trunk forward, shifting weight from side to side until sitting in the middle of the bed.

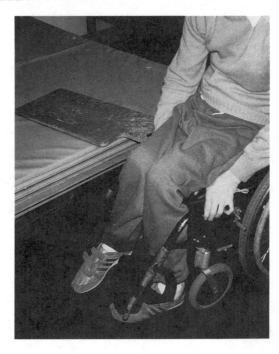

    g. Adjust legs on bed, lean to one side, and lie down.

    h. Adjust position of body on bed by using the headboard.

    i. Reverse procedure to return from bed to wheelchair.

B. Sideways, feet on bed (with or without sliding board).

    1. Starting position: Wheelchair placed at side of bed, facing the foot of the bed; lock brakes.

    2. Motion.

        a. Remove armrest closest to bed.

        b. Place one arm behind backrest of chair.

        c. Lift legs onto bed.

        d. Place one hand on mattress and one hand on armrest or seat of wheelchair.

        e. Push with both hands and throw trunk forward toward the middle of the bed.

        f. Slowly lower trunk and head onto the bed.

        g. When returning from bed to wheelchair, leave legs on bed until last.

C. Sideways, feet on floor (with or without sliding board). This is the most commonly used transfer technique.

    1. Starting position: Wheelchair at side of bed facing foot of bed.

    2. Motion.

        a. Lock brakes, swing away legrest, and remove armrest nearest bed.

        b. Place one hand on armrest or seat of wheelchair, other hand on bed.

        c. Bend trunk forward, pushing strongly on both hands, and scoot sideward onto bed.

        d. bring other hand to the mattress.

        e. Hook one wrist under one knee.

        f. Fall back and pull leg onto bed.

        g. The other leg may be pulled up automatically by momentum or it may need to be pulled onto the bed. Rolling to the side may pull the leg onto the bed.

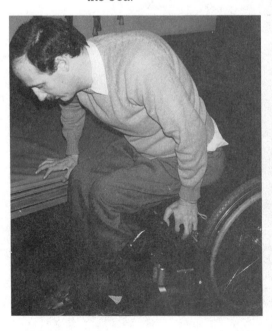
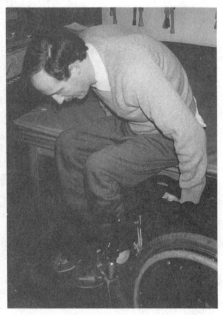

        h. Adjust body in bed using the headboard.

        i. Reverse procedure to return to the wheelchair.

II. To and From Wheelchair and Toilet (an elevated commode seat should be used)

  A. Facing front of toilet.

    1. Starting position: Approach front of toilet.

    2. Motion.

      a. Lock wheelchair.

      b. Place feet on floor and swing away footrests.

      c. Lower or remove clothing.

      d. Unlock wheelchair.

      e. Approach toilet as closely as possible.

      f. Lock wheelchair.

      g. Depress shoulders, slide forward straddling the toilet seat.

      f. Reverse procedure to return to wheelchair.

  B. Facing the side of the toilet (most commonly used technique).

    1. Starting position: Approach toilet from the side, angled slightly toward front of toilet seat.

    2. Motion.

      a. Swing legrest away on the side closest to the toilet.

      b. Place feet on floor; swing away legrest.

      c. Approach toilet as closely as possible, and lower or remove clothing.

      e. Lock wheelchair; remove armrests closest to toilet.

      f. Depress shoulders and slide onto toilet seat.

      g. Reverse procedure to return.

III. To and From Wheelchair and Bathtub or Shower

Patients with weakness of four limbs and trunk do not have sufficient upper limb strength to raise themselves from sitting in the tub. They will need to shower using a tubchair or bench.

  A. Sideward.

    1. Starting position: Wheelchair is placed alongside, facing foot of tub.

    2. Motion.

      a. Lock brakes and remove armrest.

      b. Lift legs into tub or shower stall.

      c. Slide sideward using one hand on bench and the other hand on wheelchair.

      d. Turn to face foot of tub.

      e. Reverse procedure to return.

IV. From Floor to Wheelchair

Most patients with weakness of all four limbs and trunk usually have insufficient strength to perform this transfer independently.

  A. Backward—unassisted.

    1. Starting position: Back to chair, cushion removed, brakes locked.

    2. Motion.

      a. In one motion, throw head and trunk forward, extend elbows, and raise hips up to chair seat.

      b. Push hands against legs to push hips back into chair seat.

      c. To replace cushion, transfer to another surface, place cushion in chair, transfer back to chair.

  B. One-person assist (it is essential to give clear instructions to the person assisting)

    1. Starting position: The wheelchair is placed on its back and locked, cushion is in place.

    2. Motion.

        a. A side-lying position resting on one elbow facing away from the wheelchair is assumed.

        b. The upper trunk is lifted onto the back of the wheelchair.

        c. The legs are lifted onto the legrest by grasping under the knees.

        d. The chair is lifted into the upright position (assistant will support the shoulder and grasp the wheelchair push handles).

  C. Two-person assist.

    1. Starting position: Place wheelchair adjacent to the patient in the normal position, armrest removed, brakes locked.

    2. Motion.

        a. One assistant lifts from under the shoulders, the other from under the knees.

        b. Bring the patient to a sitting position.

        c. Both assistants lift at the same time, bringing the patient toward the chair.

        d. Slowly lower the individual into the chair.

    Caution. When lifting, keep the trunk straight with a slight anterior pelvic tilt. Lift with the legs not with the back.

V. To and From Wheelchair and Automobile

Assistance and the use of a sliding board may be necessary for a safe transfer.

  A. Side approach.

    1. Starting position: Open car door, approach front seat of car at a slight angle to car seat, lock wheelchair, and remove legrest on side closest to car.

    2. Motion

        a. Bring wheelchair as close as possible to side of front seat.

        b. Remove armrest on side closest to carseat.

        c. Adjust sliding board under hip.

        d. Slide to edge of wheelchair seat.

        e. Place one hand on sliding board and the other on seat of wheelchair.

        f. Depress shoulders and slide onto carseat.

        g. Lift legs into a car one at a time.

    Alternate method: Legs may be placed inside of car after step d.

        h. Reverse procedure to return.

VI. Placing Wheelchair into Automobile

Generally, for a person to be independent in the use of an automobile it is better to have a two-door rather than a four-door model. A two-door model is wider than a four-door model, which allows for a greater door width. The front seat should be a split bench style with an armrest; this will provide ease of placing the wheelchair into the back seat area of the automobile.

  A. Starting position.

    1. Move front seat as far forward as possible.

    2. Sit as far to the edge of car seat as possible.

  B. Motion.

    1. Unlock wheelchair brakes.

    2. Brace one hand against dashboard while folding wheelchair with other hand.

3. Hook back of hand around loop* or around the back of the leg rests. Turn chair until it is facing the back seat.
4. Tip chair until casters rest on edge of floor.
5. Shift body toward front side of car, pull back of front seat forward.
6. Lift wheelchair into car, lock wheelchair brake to keep it from rolling.
7. Adjust front seat for driving position.

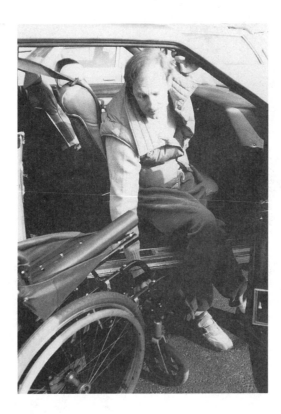

---

*The loop may be necessary because of lack of grasp. The patient hooks the wrist under the loop and pulls the wheelchair into the car. The loop is made of stiff webbing with buckle and rivets. When the wheelchair is folded, the webbing makes a loop in front of the uprights of the footrest units.

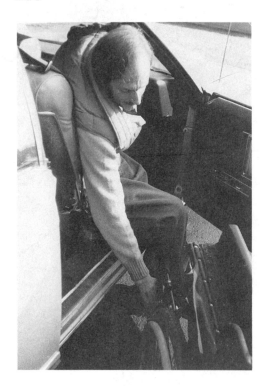

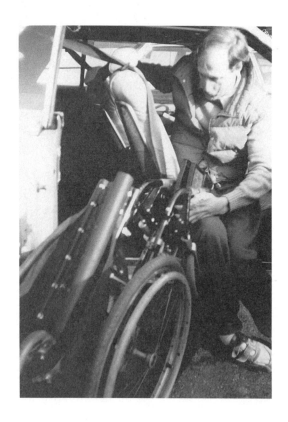

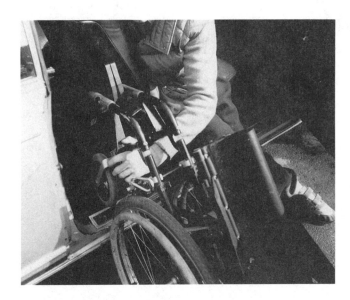

UPRIGHT ACTIVITIES

The feasibility of patients with high spinal cord lesions doing ambulation and elevation activities is remote. If sufficient muscle strength does exist, the procedure for bilateral lower limb and trunk weakness in Chapter 9 should be followed. Variations and modifications may be necessary to fit the needs of the patient. Also see Chapter 6 for methods of standing a patient at home.

It may be possible for individuals with incomplete quadriplegia due to a traumatic brain injury to learn to ambulate using a rolling bedside table or a shopping cart.

Ambulation with Rolling a Bedside Table

Often patients rely too much on their upper limbs to support their weight and do not use their lower limbs as they should. When the wrists are positioned far below the elbows with slight elbow flexion, it is easy to bear most of the weight on the upper limbs. One way to encourage more use of the lower limb is to use a device that is adjustable and can be raised high enough so that the upper limbs are providing less support. Using a raised bedside table can help in achieving this goal. As one raises the height of the table one decreases the amount of upper limb weight-bearing that is possible. It may be necessary to have additional people assisting initially, if the patient is anxious or unsteady. This method is also beneficial for the patient who hyperextends the trunk during ambulation. Trunk flexion and forward weight shift of the trunk can be facilitated if the device is in front of the patient and lowered somewhat, putting the trunk in a position of slight flexion to reach the bedside table. As discussed earlier, weight-bearing is often helpful in decreasing spasticity. For the patient with increased upper limb muscle tone, using a device that has a grasp handle, such as a cane or walker, that requires finger flexion, is not the most beneficial for the patient. With a flat surface such as the table, the patient can be assisted into an open hand position with finger extension to inhibit the flexor tone, as well as work on finger and wrist strength and control in a functional position.

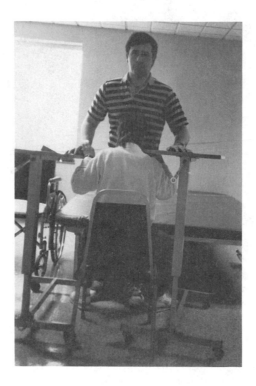

Ambulation with a Shopping Cart

For the patient who presents with forward trunk flexion, thoracic kyphosis, rounded shoulders, and so forth, it is important to encourage a more upright posture during gait activities. One way to achieve this is to attach extension poles to a shopping cart. The patient may then stand with both hands at shoulder height, grasping the poles. This brings the upper limbs into lateral rotation and the scapulae into adduction, facilitating an increase in thoracic trunk extension. This position also brings the shoulder over the hips instead of in front of them. Also, by flexing the shoulders the patient must put more weight on the lower limbs because the upper limbs are no longer in a weight-bearing position.

Initially, when using the shopping cart it is important to have someone at the opposite end of the cart to stabilize and help guide it. One therapist can be behind the patient on a rolling stool in a position to provide facilitation to the lower limbs and trunk. As the patient becomes familiar with the activity and control improves, it may no longer be necessary to have the other therapist stabilizing the cart. Once the patient is able to maintain proper postural alignment and can control the movement of the cart, all assistance may be removed.

Once the patient can maintain the trunk in proper alignment the poles may be removed, using the cart handle for balance. Continue to encourage less upper limb assistance, as the ultimate goal is independent ambulation without any device.

It is beneficial to initiate gait activities with the shopping cart because it offers lateral stability, does not tip or lift off the floor, moves forward easily, and facilitates weight on lower limbs while decreasing weight-bearing on the upper limbs.

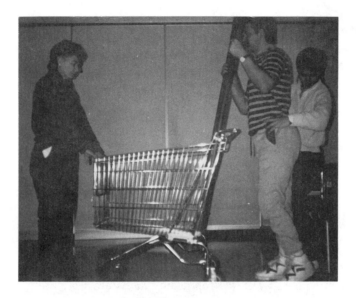

ORTHOTICS

The patient with recent injury needs assistance in maintaining stable neck and trunk posture. Vital capacity is subnormal. Although a complete cervical lesion results in total paralysis of the trunk and lower limbs, as well as partial involvement of the upper limbs, many individuals have incomplete lesions. Those who do may benefit from standing and limited household ambulation.

Orthoses can keep the head balanced securely on the neck, while also improving respiration and enabling safe standing. Cervical orthoses that counteract the tendency of the neck to flex are often needed until the patient regains neck control or until arthrodesis is performed. The Philadelphia collar is especially suitable because its rigid anterior and posterior struts resist flexion and extension, and the resilient collar material avoids skin irritation. A version is manufactured with a hole to accommodate a tracheotomy.

A lumbosacral corset aids respiration. The corset may be the only trunk orthosis needed. Patients who have difficulty sitting may need a thoracolumbosacral flexion control orthosis that stabilizes the trunk but does not aid respiration.

Trunk-hip-knee-ankle-foot orthoses are exceedingly difficult to apply to the patient. It is most unlikely that the individual with incomplete quadriplegia will be able to don such appliances independently. Consequently, standing may be accomplished more readily with the aid of wheelchairs or similar devices, which can be adjusted to the upright position and back again.

≡11
Functional Activities for the Amputee.

To derive the maximum benefit from a prosthesis, an amputee must understand how the prosthesis functions, how to put on the prosthesis, and how to control it. The time required for training depends on the complexity of the device, plus the physical and mental condition of the patient. Medical problems such as cardiac disease, diabetes, multiple amputations, and skin problems can lengthen the training period. Improper fit or malfunction of the prosthesis also impedes training. Prosthetic training can be terminated when the following criteria are met:

1. The amputee has plateaued or reached the highest functional level.
2. The absence of open or irritated areas on the residual limb.
3. The amputee can wear the prosthesis 8 hours a day or is able to tolerate wearing the prosthesis long enough to achieve maximum functional level.
4. The amputee feels comfortable managing the total program.

Without sound training, few persons who have had major amputations will acquire satisfactory use of the prosthesis, and none are likely to achieve optimum functional results. Amputees must learn efficient control of the residual limb and prosthesis as a unit in the activities of daily living and in the demands of their occupation. Many amputees will achieve their highest functional ambulatory levels of independence with the use of canes and crutches. Some amputees will require the use of a wheelchair as a means of ambulation, either part or full time. A wheelchair designed for the amputee has a longer base of support, thereby preventing the tendency of the wheelchair to tip forward. Safety devices especially in the tub and shower area should not be overlooked. Refer to prior chapters for a description of wheelchair mobility and transfers.

MAT ACTIVITIES

The mat activities program for the lower limb amputee should maintain or develop good to normal strength and coordination for the trunk and upper limbs. Some of the patients may have some difficulty with balance in the sitting and standing positions. The remaining lower limb should not be overlooked, it may have developed contractures and weakness owing to inactivity or an ongoing disease process. Special emphasis on the residual limb should include activities to improve or maintain muscle tone, muscle strength, and range of motion. Refer to Chapter 7 for guarding techniques.

I. Supine Position
   A. Bridger.
      1. *Position:* Supine, with the intact lower limb flexed, the residual limb flexed on a low block.

290

2. *Action:* Hyperextend the hips and low back, lifting the hips off the mat.
3. *Functional carry-over:* Transfer off and on a bedpan, dressing, and range of motion for the residual limb.

B. Pelvic tilter (anterior and posterior).
   1. *Position:* Supine with the lower limbs extended and upper limbs at the side.
   2. *Action:* Flatten and arch the low back.
   3. *Functional carry-over:* Erect sanding and ambulation activities

C. Resistive exercises.
   1. *Position:* Supine with maximum weight in each hand.
   2. *Action:* Perform all motions for the shoulder and elbow joints.
   3. *Functional carry-over:* Developing strength for the upper limbs for wheelchair mobility and parallel bar activities.

D. Range of motion.
   1. *Position:* Supine with lower limb and residual limb extended.
   2. *Action:* Perform all motions actively for the hips and knee.
   3. *Functional carry-over:* Maintain or increase range of motion in the lower limbs.

II. Prone Position
   A. Alternating extension.
      1. *Position:* Prone on elbows.
      2. *Action:* Alternately hyperextend the intact and residual limbs.
      3. *Functional carry-over:* Upright mobility and donning of the prosthesis.

   B. Prone push-ups.
      1. *Position:* Prone with hands in line with shoulders.
      2. *Action:* Straighten the elbows, lifting the trunk off the mat.
      3. *Functional carry-over:* Getting up off the floor, standing from a wheelchair, standing transfers, and developing strength in the upper limbs.

   C. Trunk extension.
      1. *Position:* Prone, with arms at the side of trunk.
      2. *Action:* Hyperextend the neck and trunk until upper sternum has cleared mat; repeat.
      3. *Functional carry-over:* Getting up from the floor, developing trunk musculature.

III. Sitting Position
   A. Sit-ups.
      1. *Position:* Supine with lower limbs extended and upper limbs flexed to shoulder level.
      2. *Action:* Flex trunk until scapula clear the mat.
      3. *Functional carry-over:* Development of trunk strength.

   B. Sitting push-ups.
      1. *Position:* Sitting, upper limbs at the side of hips, palms flat on the mat or on blocks.
      2. *Action:* Straighten elbows, depress shoulders, lift the buttocks off the mat.
      3. *Functional carry-over:* Wheelchair transfers.

   C. Resistive upper limb exercises.
      1. *Position:* Sitting, holding maximum weight in one or both hands.
      2. *Action:* Perform all shoulder, elbow, and wrist motions using the weights.
      3. *Functional carry-over:* Developing strength and coordination for the upper limb, useful in transfers.

D. Sitting scooters sideways.
1. *Position:* Short sitting with upper limbs at the side of the trunk with one slightly abducted.
2. *Action:* Depress the shoulders and scoot the pelvis to one side and the other.
3. *Functional carry-over:* Wheelchair transfers and coordination.
E. Scooter forward and backward.
1. *Position:* Long sitting with upper limb slightly ahead of the hips when going forward and slightly behind when going backward.
2. *Action:* Depress the shoulders and swing the buttocks forward or backward. Traverse a distance in one direction then return.
3. *Functional carry-over:* Developing upper limb strength and coordination, wheelchair transfers.
IV. Knee Standing Position (for below-knee amputee)
A. Assume kneeling.
1. *Position:* Hands and knees.
2. *Action:* Walk hands back toward hips, extend neck and trunk. Use support initially with the upper limbs. Reverse procedure to return to the mat.
3. *Functional carry-over:* Getting up from the floor, standing from a wheelchair, and ambulation activities.
B. Kneeling balance.
1. *Position:* Kneel standing, with support.
2. *Action:* Shift weight, forward and sideways, raising upper limbs (flexion, abduction, overhead).
3. *Functional carry-over:* Getting up from the floor, wheelchair transfers, and ambulation activities.
C. Kneeling weight shifter.
1. *Position:* Kneel standing, with or without support.
2. *Action:* Shift body weight left, right, forward, and backward.
3. *Functional carry-over:* Getting up from the floor, and ambulation activities.
D. Leg lifter.
1. *Position:* Kneel standing, with or without support.
2. *Action:* Shift weight to intact limb and raise the residual limb, repeat to the other side.
3. *Functional carry-over:* Balance and ambulation activities.

For satisfactory use of a lower limb prosthesis, gait training and analysis is crucial. Identified are common gait deviations for the amputee with suggested prosthetic or amputee causes.

GAIT ANALYSIS*

I. Lateral bending of the trunk is characterized by excessive bending laterally from the midline, generally to the prosthetic side.
A. Prosthesis causes.
1. Prosthesis may be too short.

*Adapted from Lower Extremity Prosthetics. Orthotics and Prosthetics Center, Northwestern University Medical School, Chicago, IL.

      2. An improperly shaped lateral wall may fail to provide adequate support for the femur.

      3. A high medial wall may cause the amputee to lean away to minimize discomfort.

      4. A prosthesis aligned in abduction may cause a wide-based gait, resulting in this defect.

   B. Amputee causes.

      1. Amputee may not have adequate balance.

      2. Amputee may have abduction contracture.

      3. The limb might be oversensitive and painful.

      4. A very short limb may fail to provide a sufficient lever arm for the pelvis.

      5. Defect may be due to habit pattern.

II. Abducted gait is characterized by a very wide base, with the prosthesis held away from the midline at all times.

   A. Prosthesis causes.

      1. Prosthesis may be too long.

      2. Too much abduction may have been built into the prosthesis.

      3. A high medial wall may cause the amputee to hold prosthesis away to avoid ramus pressure.

      4. An improperly shaped lateral wall can fail to provide adequate support for femur.

      5. Pelvic band may be positioned too far away from the patient's body.

   B. Amputee causes.

      1. Patient may have an abduction contracture.

      2. Defect may be due to habit pattern.

III. Circumducted gait is a swinging of the prosthesis laterally in a wide arc during swing phase.

   A. Prosthesis causes.

      1. Prosthesis may be too long.

      2. Prosthesis may have too much alignment stability or friction in the knee, making it difficult to bend the knee during swing-through.

   B. Amputee causes.

      1. Amputee may have abduction contracture of the residual limb.

      2. Patient may lack confidence for flexing the prosthetic knee.

      3. Defect may be the result of habit pattern.

IV. Vaulting is characterized by a rising on the toe of the normal foot permitting the amputee to swing the prosthesis through with little knee flexion.

   A. Prosthesis causes.

      1. Prosthesis may be too long.

      2. There may be inadequate socket suspension.

      3. Limb discomfort may be a factor.

   B. Amputee causes.

      1. Vaulting is a fairly frequent habit pattern.

      2. Fear of stubbing the toe may cause this defect.

      3. Limb discomfort may be a factor.

V. Rotation of the prosthetic foot on heel strike.

   A. Prosthesis causes.

      1. This defect may be caused by too much resistance to plantarflexion by the plantarflexion bumper or heel wedge.

      2. Too much toe out may have been built into the prosthesis.

   3. Socket may fit too loosely.
  B. Amputee causes.
   1. Patient may extend the residual limb too vigorously at heel strike.
   2. Amputee may have poor muscle control of the residual limb.
 VI. Uneven arm swing is characterized by the arm on the prosthetic side held close
     to the body during locomotion.
  A. Amputee causes.
   1. Amputee may not have developed good balance.
   2. Fear and insecurity accompanied by uneven timing will also contribute to
      this defect.
   3. Defect may be due to habit pattern.
VII. Uneven timing is characterized by steps of unequal duration, usually by a very
     short stance phase on the prosthetic side.
  A. Prosthesis causes.
   1. Improperly fitting socket may cause pain and a desire to shorten the
      stance phase on the prosthetic side.
   2. A weak extension aid or insufficient friction in the prosthetic knee can
      cause excessive heel rise, resulting in uneven timing because of pro-
      longed swing-through.
   3. Alignment stability may be a factor, if the knee buckles too easily.
  B. Amputee causes.
   1. Amputee may have muscle weakness.
   2. Patient may not have developed good balance.
   3. Fear and insecurity may contribute to this defect.
VIII. Uneven heel rise is characterized by the prosthetic heel rising quite markedly
      and rapidly when the knee is flexed at the beginning of swing phase.
  A. Prosthesis causes.
   1. Knee joint may have insufficient friction.
   2. There may be an inadequate extension aid.
  B. Amputee cause: Amputee may be using more power than necessary to force
     the knee into flexion.
 IX. Terminal swing impact is characterized by rapid forward movement of the shin
     piece, allowing the knee to reach maximum extension with too much force
     before heel strike.
  A. Prosthesis causes.
   1. Insufficient knee friction may be a factor.
   2. Knee extension aid may be too strong.
  B. Amputee cause: Amputee may try to be assured that the knee is in full
     extension by deliberately and forcibly extending the residual limb.
  X. Instability of the prosthetic knee creates a danger of falling.
  A. Prosthesis causes.
   1. Knee joint may be too far ahead of the trochanter, knee, ankle line.
   2. Insufficient initial flexion may have been built into socket.
   3. Plantar flexion resistance may be too great, causing the knee to buckle at
      heel strike.
   4. failure to limit dorsiflexion can lead to incomplete knee control.
  B. Amputee causes.
   1. Patient may have hip extensor weakness.
   2. Severe hip flexion contracture may cause instability.

XI. Medial or lateral whips are observed best when the patient walks away from the observer. A medial whip is present when the heel travels medially on initial flexion at the beginning of swing phase; a lateral whip exists when the heel moves laterally.

A. Prosthesis causes.

1. Lateral whips may result from excessive medial rotation of the prosthetic knee.
2. A medial whip may result from excessive lateral rotation of the knee.
3. Socket may fit too tightly, thus reflecting residual limb rotation.
4. Excessive valgus or "knock" in the prosthetic knee may contribute to this defect.
5. A badly aligned toe-break in a conventional foot may cause twisting on toe-off.

B. Amputee cause: Faulty walking habits may result in whips.

XII. Foot slap is a too rapid descent on the anterior portion of the prosthetic foot.

A. Prosthesis cause: Plantar flexion resistance is usually too soft.

B. Amputee cause: Amputee may be driving the prosthesis into the walking surface too forcibly to ensure extension of the knee.

XIII. Drop-off at the end of stance phase is characterized by a downward movement of the trunk as the body moves forward over the prosthesis.

A. Prosthesis causes.

1. The keel of a solid ankle cushioned heel (SACH) type foot may be too short, or the toe-break of a conventional foot may be too far posterior.
2. The socket may have been placed too far anterior in relation to the foot.

B. Amputee cause: There are no specific medical causes of this defect.

XIV. Long prosthetic step is seen when the amputee takes a longer step with the prosthesis than with the normal leg.

A. Prosthesis cause: Insufficient initial flexion in the socket can cause this defect.

B. Amputee cause: Amputee may have flexion contractures, which cannot be accommodated prosthetically.

XV. Excessive trunk extension during stance phase in which the amputee creates an active lumbar lordoisis.

A. Prosthesis causes.

1. Improperly shaped posterior wall may cause forward rotation of the pelvis to avoid full weight-bearing on the ischium.
2. Insufficient initial flexion may have been built into the socket.

B. Amputee causes.

1. Amputee may have hip flexor tightness.
2. Amputee may have weak hip extensors and may be substituting lumbar erector spinae.
3. Weak abdominal muscles.
4. Deviation may be due to habit pattern.
5. Patient may be moving the shoulders backward in an effort to obtain better balance.

Refer to Chapter 12 for Prosthetic Assessment Forms.

EXERCISES FOR THE PATIENT WITH AN
ABOVE-KNEE PROSTHESIS

These exercises are described with the understanding that the patient is wearing an above-knee prosthesis.

I. Transfer activities
   A. Rising from a chair.
      1. Place sound foot behind the prosthetic foot.
      2. Bend body forward.
      3. With hip and knee extension, force the body out of the chair using the prosthesis for balance.

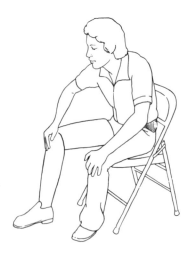

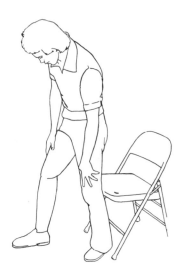

      4. Rise to a standing position by extending the sound knee.
   B. Sitting down in a chair.
      1. Approach chair.
      2. Transfer weight to the normal leg.
      3. Pivot on the ball of the normal foot and bring the prosthetic foot around into position for sitting.
      4. Flex the prosthetic knee slightly.
      5. Lower self into chair with the normal leg, maintaining trunk flexion.

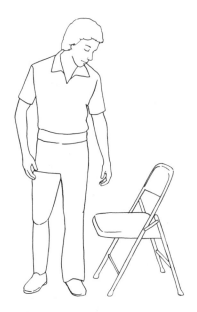
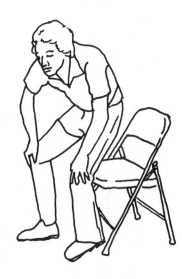

C. Self-protection in falling.

This should be practiced on one or preferably two gymnasium mats or on a soft grassy area. There are two common causes of falling: knee buckling on prosthetic side and feet slipping out from under patient.

    1. Falling forward.

        a. Toes against mat. Relax completely. Pitch forward, breaking the fall with the arms outstretched and absorbing the shock with slightly flexed elbows and shoulders. Partial weight is then transferred to both knees.

        b. Toes against mat—alternate. Relax completely. Pitch forward breaking the fall, as in 1a, with arms outstretched. As the hands hit the floor, roll onto the unaffected hip, then onto the shoulder on that side.

    2. Falling backward.

Attempt to jack-knife at the waist so that the buttocks will strike the mat first, then roll backward onto the rounded back and shoulders.

D. Rising from the floor.

    1. From sitting position roll over onto the hands and knees toward the sound side.

    2. Balance on the prosthetic knee and hands and place sound leg forward well under the trunk with the foot flat on the floor.

    3. Extend the sound knee while maintaining the weight forward on the hands.

    4. Move into the erect position by pushing up strongly with arms and sound leg, and bring the prosthesis forward.

E. Sitting on the floor.

This sequence is done in one continuous movement with the body weight borne progressively by the sound upper and lower limbs and gluteal region.

    1. Place the prosthesis a half-step behind the sound foot, body weight on normal foot.

    2. Bend from waist and flex knees and hips.

       3. Reach for the floor with both hands with arms outstretched; pivot to the sound side.

       4. Gently lower body to floor.

   F. Kneeling on prosthetic knee.

       1. The sound foot is advanced well ahead of the prosthetic foot.

       2. With the major portion of the weight on the normal limb, the trunk, hip, and knees are flexed, and the prosthetic knee is gently placed on the ground.

       3. With maximum knee flexion, maintain body weight posterior on the socket. (A tendency to fall forward may be due to insufficient knee flexion.)

       4. The forearm or hand on the sound side may then be placed on the sound thigh, as a resting position.

   G. Rising from kneeling position.

       1. Place body weight on sound limb.

       2. Bend at the waist.

       3. Extend hip and knee of sound limb. (If necessary, the hand may be placed on the thigh of the sound limb to aid in obtaining hip and knee extension.)

       4. Bring prosthesis forward by hip flexion to a position where the prosthetic foot is slightly behind the normal foot. Lock the prosthetic knee by using amputation limb extension, and stand erect.

   As amputees advance with the training program, they should be taught when rising from a kneeling position to step off on the prosthesis. The procedure is the same, except instead of placing the prostheses behind the sound foot and then extending the knee, the hip flexes bringing the prosthesis in front of the sound lower limb with the amputation limb extended at heel contact to maintain knee stability and progress forward.

II. Parallel Bar Activities.

   A. Weight shifting.

       1. Stand between the parallel bars.

       2. Shift weight laterally from the normal limb to the prosthesis. The shift in weight is accomplished by moving the hips rather than the shoulders, and the weight is thrown alternately over the lateral border of each shoe. The shoulders and the pelvis remain level. Do not flex the normal knee. Do not allow balance to occur by trunk movement, which may cause lateral bending of the trunk on the prosthetic side.

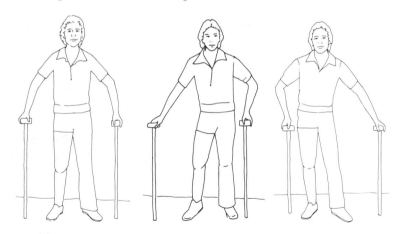

B. Alternate knee bending.
  1. Stand between the parallel bars.
  2. Alternately bend the normal and the prosthetic knee just enough to raise the heel from the floor. This teaches the amputee how to break the prosthetic knee.
  3. Reciprocally flex and extend the knees, starting with the sound knee.

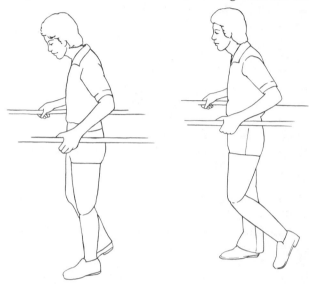

C. Gait training.
  1. Forward and backward stepping on sound leg.
    a. Stand between parallel bars.
    b. Stand with weight on the prosthesis.
    c. Keeping the prosthesis in place on that spot, rhythmically step forward and back with the normal lower limb.
    d. Put full weight on the normal limb at the beginning and end of each step.

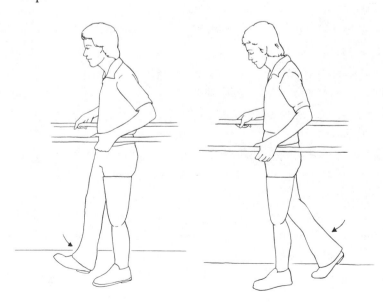

e. The normal foot should pass close to the prosthetic foot to facilitate body weight shift over the prosthesis.

Caution. Warn amputee about knee instability when sound limb is posterior to prosthetic limb.

2. Forward and backward stepping on prosthetic limb
   a. Stand between parallel bars.
   b. Stand with weight on normal limb.
   c. Break the prosthetic knee.
   d. Keeping the normal limb in one place, step forward and back with the prosthetic limb.
   e. Place full weight on the prosthesis at the end of the forward and backward step. Keep the knee in full extension by pressing back with the amputation limb, particularly when the prosthetic limb is forward.

3. Forward and backward stepping—alternating.
   a. Stand between parallel bars.
   b. Keeping the prosthetic foot in place, step forward and back three times with the normal limb.
   c. On the third step, step forward with the prosthesis.
   d. Keeping the normal foot in place, step forward and back three times with the prosthesis.
   e. On the third step, complete the step by coming forward with the normal foot.
   f. Repeat the sequence.

D. Forward walking within the parallel bars
   1. Step off with the sound foot.
   2. Shift the weight forward over the sound leg.
   3. Flex the hip, allowing the prosthetic knee to flex and the shin to follow through into extension.

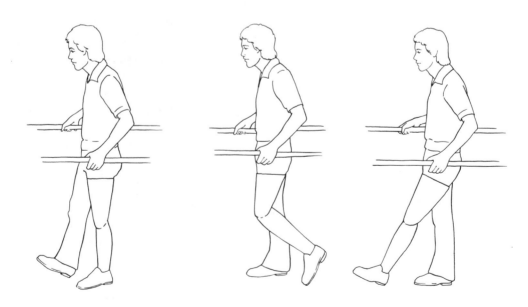

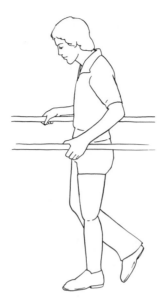

4. Place the prosthetic heel ahead of the toe of the normal foot. Heel contact is made at the time the prosthetic knee goes into full extension.
5. On heel contact, press back with the amputation limb against the posterior wall of the socket. This will maintain the knee in full extension and overcome instability. Simultaneously shift weight to the prosthesis.

E. Side-stepping on normal limb.
   1. Balance on prosthesis; socket should be in adduction.
   2. Swing the normal limb into abduction.
   3. Shift weight to the normal limb.
   4. Adduct the prosthesis and place the prosthetic foot next to the normal foot.
   5. Repeat the sequence.

F. Side-stepping on prosthesis.
   1. Balance on the normal limb.
   2. Swing the prosthesis into abduction.

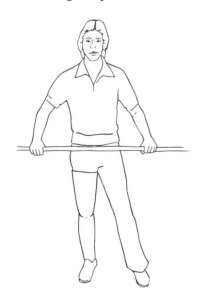
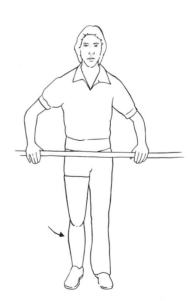

    3. Shift weight to the prosthesis, making sure socket is in adduction.

    4. Adduct the normal leg and place the foot next to the prosthetic foot.

    5. Repeat the sequence.

III. Elevation Activities

  A. Ascending inclines.

    1. Lead with sound leg, taking a step a little longer than usual to avoid catching toe of prosthesis when bringing it forward.

    2. Flex prosthetic hip sufficiently to prevent toe from catching, and swing prosthesis through, avoiding abduction.

    3. Place prosthetic foot down, taking a shorter step than usual. Press back with amputation limb against posterior wall of prosthesis to maintain stability of the knee. The trunk may need to be flexed slightly to overcome the angle of the hill.

    4. Continue up the incline, facing in the line of progression. The shorter prosthetic step compensates for the limited dorsiflexion on the prosthetic ankle and permits the amputee to shift the weight directly over the prosthesis with minimum trunk flexion. In some cases (elderly amputees, those with short or weak amputation limbs, slippery terrain) the following technique may be the method of choice:

      a. Ascend on a diagonal leading with the sound leg; take a longer step with the sound leg than with the prosthesis. Keep prosthetic foot slightly behind the sound foot.

      b. On very difficult inclines, a side-stepping technique may be used. Lead with the sound limb and bring the prosthesis up to it.

  B. Descending inclines.

    1. Lead with prosthetic foot, taking a somewhat shorter step than usual, and press back with amputation limb harder than usual on heel contact. This is necessary to maintain knee stability and to control the rate of descent by using the heel impact as a braking force.

    2. Shift the weight over the prosthesis and, as the sound foot is in a position to recover, voluntarily flex the knee by flexing the hip. Catch the body weight on the sound leg. This is commonly called jack-knifing.

    3. Develop a rhythmic pattern of progression while moving directly forward. In certain cases, depending on the amputee's age, amputation limb length, or musculature, and the terrain (wet, stony, slippery), a modified technique may be necessary, such as:

      a. Using unusually short steps.

      b. Using repeated single steps.

      c. Descending sideways.

  C. Ascending stairs.

    1. Maintain weight instantaneously on the prosthesis and then lead with the sound foot. Advance one or two stairs at a time.

    2. Extend the hip on the amputated side, with slight abduction to clear the edge of the step, and place the prosthetic foot beside the sound foot. The use of a handrail is permissible for this activity; however, the amputee should be able to negotiate stairs without any additional support.

  D. Descending stairs.

    1. Place the heel of the prosthetic foot on the edge of the stair.

    2. Shift weight over the prosthesis, maintaining the knee in full extension by pressing the amputation limb into extension.

3. When the normal foot is advanced in position to recover on the next step, the amputee flexes the hip and allows the prosthetic knee to bend (jack-knife).

4. Extend the prosthetic knee with sufficient force to swing the shin forward enough to be able to place the heel on the edge of the next lower step. Shift the body weight onto the prosthesis quickly so that the knee will not buckle and then continue the progression.

5. Develop a rhythmic pattern of progression. In certain cases, depending on such factors as age, amputation limb length, and musculature, and type of steps (narrow or slippery), a modified technique may be necessary. For example, one might need to continue leading with the prosthesis, one step at a time.

   Caution: Hesitation between the time the prosthetic heel hits the edge of the next lower step and shifting of the body weight forward will cause the knee to buckle.

E. Picking up an object.
   1. Place prosthetic foot behind the sound foot.
   2. Body weight remains on sound limb.
   3. Bend at waist, flexing hips and knees bilaterally. Grasp object. If the amputee is quite tall and uses considerable knee friction, it may be easier to use this technique:
      a. Place sound leg forward a normal step length.
      b. Keep prosthetic knee extended and slightly laterally rotated.
      c. Bend trunk and sound knee; grasp object.

F. Clearing obstacles—direct approach (for obstacles up to 4 inches high).
   1. Face obstacles squarely with feet about 3 inches away.
   2. Transfer weight to normal limb.
   3. Extend hip on prosthetic side, allowing the sole of the shoe to scrape the underlying surface, then use forceful hip flexion to whip the prosthesis over the obstacle. In going over obstacles higher than approximately 4 inches, the prosthetic hip may need to be abducted and medially rotated slightly to allow the prosthetic foot to clear the obstacle.
   4. When prosthetic foot touches the ground, transfer the body weight forward and press back strongly with amputation limb to maintain stability of the knee.
   5. Step over the obstacle with the sound leg and regain balance by stepping off with the normal leg into the normal gait pattern.

G. Clearing obstacles—side approach.
   1. For clearing higher obstacles, stand sideways with the prosthesis about 5 inches away from obstacle.
   2. Use forceful hip flexion to whip the prosthetic knee into extension and clear the obstacle. Allow the prosthetic foot to land slightly behind the sound foot.
   3. On heel contact, press back strongly with the amputation limb to maintain stability behind the sound foot.
   4. Bring sound leg over the obstacle, rotate the trunk toward the prosthetic leg, and regain balance.

H. Hop-skip for speed (simulated running).
   1. Step forward with sound limb.
   2. Shift weight to sound limb.

3. Hop forward on sound limb.
4. Swing prosthesis forward and shift body weight onto it, using it for momentary support.
5. Immediately transfer weight to sound leg and repeat sequence.

Assessment Forms

12 ≡

The objective of a functional training evaluation is the same as for any patient evaluation—to establish baseline data on the patient from which a treatment plan is developed. The examples of evaluation forms included in this section can be used for initial patient evaluations and for periodic reevaluation of patient progress. To understand fully the grading system for the evaluation forms, a careful review of each grading key is necessary. Some of the forms indicate specific time limitations for accomplishing the tasks; if a time period is not indicated, consideration should be given to this factor. Realistically, a patient should perform the tasks on the evaluation form independently because functional independence is being evaluated. However, patient safety must be maintained throughout the evaluation period. If the patient cannot perform an activity without creating a safety hazard or requires assistance to complete the activity, this should be noted on the evaluation form.

EXPLANATION OF EVALUATION OF PERSONAL INDEPENDENCE TEST*

I. Objectives to Present
   A. A graphic representation of functional ability with sufficient detail for the physical and occupational therapists.
   B. Details on patient status, prognosis, and effectiveness of appliances for program planning by the physicians and physical and occupational therapists.
   C. A method for patient motivation.
   D. General knowledge of the patient's functional status for the medical, nursing, and social service staffs.
   E. A guide to home and vocational planning.
   F. An additional measurement for overall study and classification of patients.
   G. A quick numerical reference for case histories and presentations when the entire test cannot, or need not, be used.
II. Description
   A. The test is limited to 50 activities that are broad in scope and by definition are representative of others that may not be included, such as brushing the teeth, which includes turning on faucet and putting paste or powder on brush.
   B. Divided into two general groups.
      1. Stationary activities: test items that can be performed without a large movement or transition of the body.
      2. Moving activities: test items that require transition or large movements of the body.

---

*Adapted from the Texas Institute for Rehabilitation and Research, Texas Medical Center, Physical Therapy Department, Houston, TX.

III. Grading
   A. Letter grades are used for testing muscles (See key in lower left hand corner for definition of grades.)
   B. Recording areas next to activities are colored up to and including the appropriate grade. If item cannot be performed, draw a single line down the left side of the first (trace) block to indicate the item has been tested.
      1. Red on first testing.
      2. Blue on second testing.
      3. Orange on third testing.
      4. Green on fourth testing.
      5. Red hatch marks on fifth testing.
      6. Blue hatch marks on sixth testing.
      7. Orange hatch marks on seventh testing.
      8. Green hatch marks on eighth testing.

IV. Apparatus and special conditions necessary for activities are listed in the column to the right. The letters corresponding to that specific item are written in the grade box in ink.

V. Numbering
   A. Each letter grade is assigned a number: N = 4, G = 4, F = 3, P = 2, T = 1, O = 0. Normal and good are assigned the same value (4) because the score is based on independent function and not on normalcy.
   B. Each item has been assigned a factor. The factors are based on the amount of time required for someone else to do the activity if the patient is unable to do it for himself or herself. These were obtained by doing a time study of patients who are now at home, by sections (communication, eating, hygiene, and so on) and then by further divisions according to items based partly on time, fitting it to the section, and slightly on importance. However, importance is relative and cannot be considered to any great extent.
   C. The grade value is multiplied by the item factor and placed in the appropriate column.
   D. Next, numbers are totaled for each side of the page and placed in the box at the bottom right hand corner of the first page of the form. These are added together for the total score. It should be realized that the items do not have equal value, and that in general, the items requiring the least expenditure of energy or muscle power have the greatest points. Persons with a score of 900 still require help 10 percent of their time and may be very limited (depending on the particular activities involved).
   E. "Activity not indicated" items are defined as those items not pertinent to that particular patient. For example, "Drive car" is not indicated for a child or for an adult who never learned to drive.

TEXAS INSTITUTE FOR REHABILITATION AND RESEARCH
TEXAS MEDICAL CENTER HOUSTON,TEXAS

STATIONARY ACTIVITIES		GRADE FOR ACTIVITY					APPARATUS USED FOR ACTIVITY	Factor	FACTOR TIMES GRADE VALUE				
		T (1)	P (2)	F (3)	G (4)	N (4)							
300 COMMUNICATION	Ability to signal						a. wheelchair (1)	10					
	Speak adequately						b. reclining chair (2)						
							c. crutches (3)	20					
	Write signature						r. cane (4)						
							d. braces (5)	5					
	Write or type 10 words per minute						e. corset (6)						
							f. sliding board (7)	15					
	Turn pages						g. handsplints (8)						
							h. feeders (9)	20					
	Complete phone call						j. slings (10)						
							k. lapboard (11)	5					
240 EATING	Eat with fingers						m. breathing aid (12)						
							n. adapted equip. (13)	10					
	Eat with fork or spoon						o. mouth stick (14)						
							s. positioner (15)	10					
	Drink from cup						SPECIAL CONDITIONS	10					
	Drink from glass						t. Modified environment (16)	10					
	Cut meat						(special height, weight, or size of standard equipment)	10					
	Move dishes						COMMENTS	10					
60 HYGIENE	Use handkerchief							2					
	Wash hands and face							4					
	Brush teeth							3					
	Comb hair							2					
	Shave or makeup							4					
60 MISC.	Put on and remove slings or feeders							3					
	Put on and remove splints							2					
	Sitting							10					

GRADING KEY

N — Normal performance
G — Independent performance for practical purposes
F — Performance possible but not practical (Lacks speed, safety or endurance)
P — Partial performance of activity (more than ½)
T — Partial performance of activity (less than ½)
O — Activity impossible
X — Activity not indicated (shave or makeup for a child)

Test Date					
Examiner Init. (OT)					
Stationary Activi. (660)					
Test Date					
Examiner Init. (PA)					
Moving Activi. (340)					
TOTAL SCORE (1000)					

☐ TEST 1   ☐ TEST 2   ☐ TEST 3   ☐ TEST 4
EVALUATION OF PERSONAL INDEPENDENCE
TIRR-OT-PT- (rev.) 3/65

MOVING ACTIVITIES		GRADE FOR ACTIVITY					APPARATUS USED FOR ACTIVITY	Factor	FACTOR TIMES GRADE VALUE				
		T (1)	P (2)	F (3)	G (4)	N (4)		Date					
40 BED	Turn to side						a. wheelchair (1) b. reclining chair (2)	3					
	Move across bed						c. crutches (3) d. braces (4)	3					
	Sit-up						r. cane (5) e. corset (6)	2					
	Get in & out of bed W.C./Walk						f. sliding board (7) g. handsplints (8)	2					
100 DRESSING	Put on and remove shoes and stockings						h. feeders (9) j. slings (10)	5					
	Put on and remove slacks or skirt						k. lapboard (11) m. breathing aid (12)	5					
	Put on and remove jacket						n. adapted equip. (13) o. mouth stick (14)	5					
	Put on and remove slipover garment						p. mechanical lift (17) q. car hand controls (18)	5					
	Put on and remove braces						s. positioner (15)	3					
	Put on and remove trunk support						SPECIAL CONDITIONS t. Modified environment (16)	2					
40 HYGIENE	Get on & off toilet W.C./Walk						(special height, weight, or size of standard equipment)	3					
	Get into & out of shower or bathtub W.C./Walk							2					
	Bathe self						COMMENTS	5					
160 LOCOMOTION	Travel 50 ft. smooth surface W.C./Walk							3					
	Travel 50 ft. rough surface W.C./Walk							2					
	Travel 200 yards smooth surface W.C./Walk							3					
	Travel up and down 10° grade W.C./Walk							2					
	Stand up from a chair							2					
	Sit down in a chair							2					
	Transfer from a wheel chair to a chair							2					
	Manage all usual door combinations W.C./Walk							3					
	Manage 6 steps with 7" risers							3					
	Manage curb & cross street c̄ traffic light W.C./Walk							2					
	Get down to and up from floor W.C./Walk							2					
	Get into and out of a car W.C./Walk							2					
	Put wheelchair into and out of a car							2					
	Drive car							4					
	Move 20 ft. without apparatus							2					
	Pick up object from the floor W.C./Walk							2					
	Walk sideways 20 ft.							2					

ACTIVITIES OF DAILY LIVING EVALUATION
Form reprinted by permission of Texas Rehabilitation Hospital
Gonzales Warm Springs Foundation, Gonzales, Texas

BED ACTIVITIES	Date					COMMENTS:
	Initial					
Roll to side						
Roll supine to prone						
Roll prone to supine						
Roll using bedrail or object to grab						
Come to sitting on edge of bed						
Come to sitting in middle of bed						
Manage pillows and blankets						
Reach object on bedside table						

DRESSING

Put on and remove: Orthosis					
Corset					
Prosthesis					
Lock and unlock braces					
Put on and remove: Pants					
Underwear					
Shoes					
Socks					
Hose					

BALANCE

Sitting on edge of mat: Unsupported					
Supporting self					
Able to lean: Right					
Left					
Forward					
Backward					
Head control—Normal or abnormal					

WHEELCHAIR ACTIVITIES

Propels wheelchair using:					
(a) Electric (b) Foot and hand					
(c) Both feet (d) Both hands					
Propels on smooth surfaces (yards)					
Propels: Up 20° incline					
Down 20° grade					
Across the grass					
Over rough roads or walks					
Up and down curbs (inches)					
Remove footrests and replace					
Swing away footrests and swing in					
Fold up footplates					
Lock and unlock brakes R/L					
Remove armrests R/L					

TRANSFERS AND MISCELLANEOUS

Get on and off mat					
Get in and out of bed					
Lift feet up onto mat or bed					
Get on and off toilet					

Chart No. _____ Name _____ Diagnosis _____

_____ Age _____ Onset _____

Page 2	Date					
	Initial					
						COMMENTS:
Able to manage clothes for toilet						
Use toilet paper						
Get in and out of bathtub						
Able to bathe self						
Wash hair						
Get into car: Driver side						
Passenger side						
Put wheelchair in and out of car						
Open, go through, and close common doors						
Pick up object off floor						
Get down to and up from floor: To W/C						
To standing						
To sofa or mat						
GAIT						
Stand up and sit down: From W/C						
From straight chair						
Stand in parallel bars						
Walk in parallel bars						
Walk on smooth surfaces (feet)						
Walk on carpet						
Walk on roads or sidewalks						
Walk on grass						
Walk up 20° ramp						
Walk down 20° ramp						
Walk sideways						
Walk backwards						
Go up and down stairs with rails						
Go up and down stairs without rails						
Go up and down curbs						
AMBULATION DEFICITS						
Loss of balance R L						
Hip drop R L						
Genu recurvation R L						
Toe drag R L						
Supination of foot R L						
Hip abduction R L						
Hip adduction R L						
Knee flexed R L						
R L						

Chart No. _____ Name _____ Diagnosis _____

_____ Age _____ Onset _____

Apparatus used for activity

1. Wheelchair
2. Reclining chair
3. Crutches
4. Cane
5. Braces
6. Corset
7. Sliding board

8. Hand splints
9. Feeders
10. Slings
11. Lapboard
12. Adapted equipment
13. Mouth stick
14. Modified environment
   (special height, weight, or size of standard equipment)

Grading Key

√   Independent in activity

S   Can perform activity, but needs supervision because activity is not safe or patient needs to be reminded what to do next.

A   Needs assistance because of undue fatigue or slowness. Able to do only part of activity.

O   Patient can perform no part of activity.

X   Not indicated for testing.

   (√) in blue, all other grades in red.

Comments:

Form reprinted by permission of Rancho Los Amigos Hospital, Physical Therapy Department, Downey, California.

FUNCTIONAL EVALUATION

I. BED ACTIVITIES (3 min. max. each)	Adm. Test	Disch. Test	Equipment Used & Specific Comments
1. Moves across bed			Adm.
2. Rolls supine to prone and return			
3. Sits up from supine			Disch.
4. Moves legs off and on to bed			
5. Sits with arms for support			
6. Sits without arms for support			
II. SITTING ACTIVITIES **A. WHEELCHAIR OPERATION (2-5 min. each)**			Adm.
1. Wheels chair 15 feet and returns			
2. Manages brakes, arms, footrests			Disch.
3. Approaches bed and table			
4. Wheels chair 75 feet and returns			
5. Opens standard door, wheels through, closes door and returns			
6. Wheels up and down 18-foot ramp (1 inch to 1 foot)			
7. Wheels up and down 6-inch curb			
B. SITTING TRANSFER (non-stand.) **(5 min. max. each way)**			Adm.
1. Transfers to and from bed			
2. Transfers to and from toilet			
3. Transfers to and from commode chair			Disch.
4. Transfers to and from tub			
5. Transfers to and from auto			
6. Transfers to and from shower			
7. Transfers to and from floor			

C. OTHER	Adm. Test	Disch. Test	Equipment Used & Specific Comments
1. Moves 30 feet on floor (crawls, scoots, drags body, etc.) (2 min. max.)			Adm.
2. Puts on and removes equipment needed for support and function in wheelchair (10 min.)			
3. Puts wheelchair in and out of auto (5 min.)			Disch.
4. W/C sitting tolerance (½ to 16 hr.)	hrs.	hrs.	
III. UPRIGHT ACTIVITIES (2 min. max. each way) A. STANDING			Adm.
1. Stands from and returns to wheelchair			
2. Gets into and out of bed			
3. Stands from and returns to straight chair			Disch.
4. Sits down on toilet and returns to standing			
5. Gets into and out of car			
6. Gets into and out of shower			
7. Gets into and out of tub			
8. Falls to floor and returns			
B. WALKING (2 min. max. each item)			Adm.
1. Walks forward 50 feet smooth surface			
2. Walks to R, L, and backward 5 feet			
3. Walks on rough terrain 20 feet			Disch.
4. Opens door, walks through, closes door, and returns			
5. Walks 10 feet with practical object (Specify object chosen for each patient)			
6. Walks forward 150 feet smooth surface (5 min. max.)			
7. Walks 30 feet in 30 seconds			

C. ELEVATION (2 min. max. each way)	Adm. Test	Disch. Test	Equipment Used & Specific Comments
1. Walks up and down 9-foot ramp (2 inches to 1 foot)			
2. Walks up and down 5 steps with rail (6-inch risers)			
3. Walks up and down 3 steps without rail			
4. Steps up and down 6-inch curb			
5. Steps up and down bus steps			
D. OTHER (2 min. max. each item)			
1. Picks up practical object from floor (Specify object chosen for each patient)			
2. Positions canes, crutches, or walkerette before and after use			
3. Puts on and removes equipment used for walking (10 min.)			
4. Locks and unlocks braces			

Adm. Test _____ Therapist _____
        (Mo.-Day-Year)

Disch. Test _____ Therapist _____
        (Mo.-Day-Year)

KEY TO GRADING

I Independent (Safe alone, time practical)
IS Indep. slow (Safe alone, time impractical)
S Supervised (Stand-by for direction & safety)
A Assisted (Practical with one person to assist)
U Unable (Requires assistance of more than one person)
— Not tested (Explain under specific comments)

ACTIVITIES OF DAILY LIVING EVALUATION
Form reprinted by permission of John Sealy Hospital
University of Texas Medical Branch, Galveston, Texas

Name _____ Diagnosis _____

_____ Tester _____

Key:

1 Performs independently
2 Performs with assistance
3 Unable to perform

4 Performance hazardous
5 Impractical performance speed
6 Not applicable

*Performs with apparatus

Date _____   Date _____

I. Mat Activities

A. Rolling

___ ___ ___ 1. Supine to prone
___ ___ ___ 2. Prone to supine
___ ___ ___ 3. Supine to rt. side
___ ___ ___ 4. Supine to lt. side

B. Changing bed position

___ ___ ___ 1. Moving toward rt. side of bed
___ ___ ___ 2. Moving toward lt. side of bed
___ ___ ___ 3. Moving toward foot of bed
___ ___ ___ 4. Moving toward head of bed
___ ___ ___ 5. Assumes sitting position
___ ___ ___ 6. Maintains sitting position with support
___ ___ ___ 7. Maintains sitting position without support

II. Transfer Activities

A. Wheelchair

___ ___ ___ 1. Bed to wheelchair
___ ___ ___ 2. Wheelchair to bed
___ ___ ___ 3. Wheelchair to toilet
___ ___ ___ 4. Toilet to wheelchair
___ ___ ___ 5. Wheelchair to toilet
___ ___ ___ 6. Bathtub to wheelchair
___ ___ ___ 7. Wheelchair to floor
___ ___ ___ 8. Floor to wheelchair
___ ___ ___ 9. Wheelchair to chair
___ ___ ___ 10. Chair to wheelchair

B. Stretcher

___ ___ ___ 1. Bed to stretcher
___ ___ ___ 2. Stretcher to bed
___ ___ ___ 3. Stretcher to wheelchair
___ ___ ___ 4. Wheelchair to stretcher

Use addressograph stamp below here

III. Wheelchair Activities

A. Management

L R L R L R
___ ___ ___ 1. Locks lt. and rt. sides
___ ___ ___ 2. Unlocks lt. and rt. sides
___ ___ ___ 3. Raises lt. and rt. foot pedals
___ ___ ___ 4. Lowers lt. and rt. foot pedals
___ ___ ___ 5. Raises lt. and rt. legrests
___ ___ ___ 6. Lowers lt. and rt. legrests
___ ___ ___ 7. Swings away lt. and rt. foot pedals
___ ___ ___ 8. Swings back lt. and rt. foot pedals
___ ___ ___ 9. Removes lt. and rt. foot pedals
___ ___ ___ 10. Replaces lt. and rt. foot pedals
___ ___ ___ 11. Removes lt. and rt. armrests
___ ___ ___ 12. Replaces lt. and rt. armrests

B. Propulsion

___ ___ ___ 1. Propels w/c forward 20 ft.
___ ___ ___ 2. Propels w/c forward 50 ft.
___ ___ ___ 3. Propels w/c backward 10 ft.
___ ___ ___ 4. Complete circle to left
___ ___ ___ 5. Complete circle to right
___ ___ ___ 6. Up incline
___ ___ ___ 7. Down incline
___ ___ ___ 8. Open, through, and close door
___ ___ ___ 9. Pick up test object from floor

The University of Texas Medical Branch Hospitals

Galveston, Texas

Date   Date

| | | | |

IV. Ambulation Activities
    A. Pre-Ambulatory
___ ___ ___   1. Wheelchair to standing
___ ___ ___   2. Standing to wheelchair
___ ___ ___   3. Chair to standing
___ ___ ___   4. Standing to chair
___ ___ ___   5. Bed to standing
___ ___ ___   6. Standing to bed
___ ___ ___   7. Toilet to standing
___ ___ ___   8. Standing to toilet
___ ___ ___   9. Standing to floor
___ ___ ___ 10. Floor to standing
    B. Level Surface
___ ___ ___   1. Forward 20 feet
___ ___ ___   2. Forward 50 feet
___ ___ ___   3. Backward 10 feet
___ ___ ___   4. Side step 5 feet to right
___ ___ ___   5. Side step 5 feet to left
___ ___ ___   6. Complete circle to right
___ ___ ___   7. Complete circle to left
    C. Rough Surface
___ ___ ___   1. Forward 20 feet
___ ___ ___   2. Backward 50 feet
___ ___ ___   3. Backward 10 feet
___ ___ ___   4. Side step 5 feet to right
___ ___ ___   5. Side step 5 feet to left
___ ___ ___   6. Complete circle to right
___ ___ ___   7. Complete circle to left
    D. Elevation
___ ___ ___   1. Up incline
___ ___ ___   2. Down incline
___ ___ ___   3. Ascend stairs with handrail
___ ___ ___   4. Descend stairs with handrail
___ ___ ___   5. Ascend stairs without handrail
___ ___ ___   6. Descend stairs without handrail
___ ___ ___   7. Up standard curb
___ ___ ___   8. Down standard curb
V. Dressing Activities
___ ___ ___   1. Dresses self
___ ___ ___   2. Undresses self
___ ___ ___   3. Puts on shoes
___ ___ ___   4. Takes off shoes
___ ___ ___   5. Laces and ties shoes
VI. Feeding
___ ___ ___   1. Eats with fork
___ ___ ___   2. Eats with spoon
___ ___ ___   3. Cuts with knife
___ ___ ___   4. Holds and drinks from glass
___ ___ ___   5. Holds and drinks from cup
___ ___ ___   6. Wipes mouth
VII. Personal Hygiene
    A. Toilet Activities
___ ___ ___   1. On and off bedpan
___ ___ ___   2. Bladder control
___ ___ ___   3. Bowel control
___ ___ ___   4. Toilet management

    B. Bathing Activities
___ ___ ___   1. Washes and dries body
___ ___ ___   2. Turns faucets on and off
___ ___ ___   3. Brushes teeth
___ ___ ___   4. Combs hair
___ ___ ___   5. Shaves
___ ___ ___   6. Applies makeup
VIII. Advanced Activities
___ ___ ___   1. Transfers to and from car
___ ___ ___   2. Folds and unfolds wheelchair
___ ___ ___   3. Rides and operates elevator
___ ___ ___   4. Climbs up and down bus steps
___ ___ ___   5. Signs own name
XI. Apparatus - check appropriate item
                Type:
___ ___ ___   1. Braces _____
___ ___ ___   2. Splints _____
___ ___ ___   3. Corset _____
___ ___ ___   4. Sling _____
___ ___ ___   5. Crutches _____
___ ___ ___   6. Cane _____
___ ___ ___   7. Walker _____
___ ___ ___   8. Wheelchair _____
___ ___ ___   9. Sliding Board
___ ___ ___ 10. Tub Seat
            11. Accessory Items
___ ___ ___
___ ___ ___
___ ___ ___
___ ___ ___
X. Comments:
_____
_____
_____
_____
_____
_____
_____
_____
_____

ABOVE-KNEE PROSTHETIC EVALUATION FORM*

Checkout for Above-Knee Prosthesis

_____ 1. Is the prosthesis as prescribed? Check original prescription. Are modifications justified?

Check With Patient Standing in Parallel Bars with Prosthesis on

_____ 2. Is the patient comfortable? (Observe and question amputee as to comfort).

_____ 3. Is the knee stable on weight-bearing? (Causes of knee instability include (a) hip flexion contracture, (b) knee joint set too anteriorly, (c) foot in too much dorsiflexion, (d) not enough initial flexion in prosthesis.)

_____ 4. Is the prosthesis the correct length? (Anterior superior iliac spines should be level when stump is in socket properly.)

_____ 5. Is the stump maintained within the socket?

_____ 6. Does the ischial tuberosity rest properly on the ischial seat? (Amputee bends forward from hips. Find ischial tuberosity and have amputee resume erect position. Amputee should be sitting on ischial seat.)

_____ 7. Is any flesh roll above the rim of the socket minimal? (Be sure stump is pulled into socket with a pull sock. There should be no medial roll.) Finger breadth clearance.

_____ 8. Is there adequate clearance between the inferior ischial and pubic rami and the medial brim of the socket? (Medial brim should be approximately 1/2 inch lower than the posterior brim.)

_____ 9. Is there freedom from discomfort in the anteromedial corner of the socket? (There should be accommodation for the adductor longus. Scarpas bulge should not cause discomfort.)

_____ 10. Does the lateral wall of the socket maintain firm and even contact with the stump? (Check to ensure there is no mediallateral instability inside the socket.)

_____ 11. Are the lateral and anterior attachments of the Silesian bandage correctly located? (Approximate lateral attachment 1/4-inch posterior and 1/4-inch superior to greater trochanter. Approximate anterior attachment, bisect socket into medial and lateral and find point at the level of ischial tuberosity. Attach one end of V 1/2 to 1 inch above this joint and other end 1/2 to 1 inch below this joint.)

_____ 12. Do the pelvic band and belt accurately fit the contours of the body? (Between iliac crests and greater trochanter. Should fit snugly.)

_____ 13. Is the pelvic joint correctly positioned? (The pelvic joint should be slightly superior to and slightly anterior to the greater trochanter.)

_____ 14. Is the valve conveniently located? (Valve should be on anteromedial wall and slightly below level of the stump.)

Check with Patient Sitting in a Firm Chair in Parallel Bars

_____ 15. Does the socket remain securely on the stump? (Pulling out may be caused by pelvic joint that is too anterior or by a high anterior wall.)

_____ 16. Does the prosthesis remain in good alignment? (The shin should remain perpendicular to the floor.)

_____ 17. Do the thigh and shank lengths correspond to those of the good leg? (A long above knee stump might necessitate a slight discrepancy).

---

*Form reprinted by permission of Simmons College Program in Physical Therapy, Boston, MA.

_____ 18. When the foot is off the floor, does the extension aid allow the knee to remain flexed? (Should allow a normal sitting posture.)

_____ 19. Can the patient remain seated without discomfort in the ischial region? (Thick posterior wall or one that has not been slanted downward toward inside of socket will cause a burning sensation.)

_____ 20. Can the patient bend forward without discomfort? (Keep the anterior wall as high as possible.)

_____ 21. Can the patient rise to a standing position without objectionable air noises? (Suction should not be lost with this activity, and it means socket adjustments are probably necessary.)

Note. 112 degree knee flexion is necessary to assume kneeling position.

Check with Patient Walking

_____ 22. Is the patient's performance in level walking satisfactory? (Should be safe, effective, and cosmetic.)

_____ 23. Does the patient go up and down stairs satisfactorily? (Check with and without rail.)

_____ 24. Does the patient go up and down ramps satisfactorily? (Check with and without rail.)

_____ 25. Can the patient kneel comfortably? (Kneel on prosthetic knee.)

Check After Walking

_____ 26. Does the ischial tuberosity maintain its position on the ischial seat? (Determines effectiveness of suspension.)

_____ 27. Is the amputee free from discomfort in the perineal region? (Ischial tuberosity slipping inside socket?)

_____ 28. Is the medial wall high enough to prevent an adductor tissue roll? (Do not cut down medial wall more than 1/2 inch lower than posterior wall. It may be possible to ream out inside.

_____ 29. Does the prosthesis operate quietly? (Determine point of origin of noise.)

_____ 30. Are size, color, and contour approximately the same as the sound limb? (Cosmetics may be somewhat sacrificed for function in certain cases.)

Check with Prosthesis Off

_____ 31. Is the patient's stump free from discoloration, abrasions, and irritations immediately after socket is removed? (Carefully inspect and try to determine cause and rectify. Do not allow patient to wear ill-fitting prosthesis.)

_____ 32. Is the socket quadrilateral in shape? (Occasionally plug fits are ordered.)

_____ 33. Is the socket set in initial flexion? (Use medial brim and posterior wall for determination.)

_____ 34. Is the brim of the socket properly flared to meet the patient's needs? (Fleshy amputee needs more flaring.)

_____ 35. Is the inside of the socket smoothly finished? (Check carefully for areas that might irritate or tear flesh or stump sock.)

_____ 36. Are the anterior and lateral walls approximately 2- to 3-inches higher than the posterior and medial walls? (High lateral wall gives lateral stability and high anterior wall keeps stump back in socket so that ischial tuberosity will not slip off ischial seat.)

_____ 37. Do hip, knee, and ankle joints operate freely? (Put all joints through full range of motion.)

_____ 38. Is the knee extension stop padded? (Bumper will be on thigh and/or shin piece.)

_____ 39. Is there proper clearance between the knee and shank pieces? (Put knee through full range of motion and determine if there is undesirable contact between shin and shank pieces.)

_____ 40. Do the posterior surfaces of thigh and shank match when the knee is fully flexed? (Contact should be even at all points.)

_____ 41. Does the knee flex to at least 100 degrees? (Necessary for kneeling and sitting.)

_____ 42. Is the artificial foot upholstered? (Cosmetic, plus prevents stockings from getting caught.)

_____ 43. Does the valve function properly? (Should allow air to escape but not to gain entrance.)

_____ 44. Is the extension aid provided with a means of adjustment? (Used not only for assisting knee extension but also for preventing excessive heel rise.)

BELOW-KNEE PROSTHETIC EVALUATION

The following is a compilation of the majority of problems possible for the below-knee amputee wearing a corsetless prosthesis. Changing the inset, outset, or anterior-posterior position of a foot cannot be accomplished on a finished prosthesis without rebuilding it. Alternate solutions should be tried before a recommendation is made for a major alteration. Changing the plantarflexion/dorsiflexion attitude of a solid ankle cushioned heel (SACH) foot is also something not readily accomplished, and alternate procedures exist that are beyond the scope of this listing. Actually, the decision regarding the solution to any prosthetic problem should rest with the prosthetist. The intent of this listing is merely to promote increased understanding on the part of the other members of the clinic team.

Problem	Cause	Solution
There is delayed, abrupt, and limited flexion after heel strike.	Heel wedge too soft; foot too anterior.	Stiffen heel wedge; move foot posterior.
Knee stays extended throughout stance phase.	Too much plantarflexion.	Dorsiflex foot.
Toe stays off floor after heel strike.	Heel wedge too stiff; foot too anterior; too much dorsiflexion.	Soften heel wedge; move foot posterior; dorsiflex foot.
"Hill climbing" sensation toward end of stance phase.	Foot too anterior; too much plantarflexion.	Move foot posterior; dorsiflex foot.
High pressure against patella throughout most of stance phase; heel is off the floor when standing.	Foot too plantarflexed.	Dorsiflex foot.
Knee too forcefully and rapidly flexed after heel strike; high pressure against anterodistal tibia at heel strike, and/or prolonged discomfort at this point.	Heel wedge too stiff; foot too posterior; foot too dorsiflexed.	Soften heel; move foot anterior; plantarflex foot.
Hips are level but prosthesis seems short.	Foot too posterior; foot too dorsiflexed.	Move foot anterior; plantarflex foot.
Drop-off at end of stance phase.	Foot too posterior.	Move foot anterior.

Continued

Toe off floor as patient stands, or knee flexed too much.	Foot too dorsiflexed.	Plantarflex foot.
Knee moves in ("knock-kneed") during stance phase; excessive pressure on distomedial limb and proximal-lateral surface of knee.	Foot too outset.	Inset foot.
Knee moves out excessively during stance phase (a varus moment at the knee should occur in stance phase but never excessive);pain on lateral distal limb.	Medial or lateral wall of socket too large; foot too inset.	Fit of socket should be checked; outset foot.
Abrasions: Head of fibula, Tibial tubercle, Tibial condyles, Anterodistal tibia, Hamstrings tendon.	Setting due to residual limb shrinkage. Piston action in swing phase. Excessive withdrawal in sitting. Socket not properly relieved or aligned. Poorly fitted sock.	Add socks; fit of socket must be checked.
Distal edema.	Corset laced too tightly; settling causes proximal constriction; posterior brim too low or high; anterior-posterior diameter of socket too small; lack of total contact.	Correct suspension. Foam fill-in distally. Socket changes.

HOME EVALUATION FORM*

I. Medical Issues   Comments
   A. Respiratory Care
      1. Suction? Yes/No
      2. Tracheostomy? Yes/No
      3. Frequent respiratory infection? Yes/No
      4. Oxygen? Yes/No
      5. Ventilator Yes/No
      6. Space for equipment in bedroom? Yes/No
      7. Space for equipment in living room? Yes/No
   B. Nutrition
      1. Current diet? _____
      2. Measuring cup? Yes/No
      3. Blenderizer? Yes/No
   C. Skin
      1. Pressure ulcer? Yes/No
      2. Open wound? Yes/No
      3. High risk for skin breakdown? Yes/No
      4. Type of mattress? _____

_____
Date

_____

*Form reprinted by permission of Greenery Rehabilitation and Skilled Nursing Center, Boston, MA.

Comments

    5. Type of chair and cushion? _____
D. Elimination
    1. Bladder: Independent/dependent
             self-catheterization? Yes/No
    2. Bowel
      a. toilet? Yes/No
      b. commode? Yes/No
      c. toilet seat padded? Yes/No
      d. commode type? _____
    3. Space for catheterization? Yes/No
    4. Distance from bedroom to bathroom? _____
E. Seizure
    1. History? Yes/No
    2. Types of seizure? _____
    3. bed siderail? Yes/No
    4. siderail pad? Yes/No
    5. Layout of furniture in bedroom? _____

    6. Layout of furniture in living room? _____

    7. Family/patient knowledge of emergency care? Yes/No
F. Safety
    1. Confused? Yes/No
    2. Agitated? Yes/No
    3. Impairment: Sensory? Yes/No
    4. Memory? Yes/No
    5. Bed alarm? Yes/No
    6. Door lock system? Yes/No
    7. Safety gate at living room or kitchen? Yes/No
    8. Breakable furniture in bedroom? Yes/No
    9. Breakable furniture in living room? Yes/No
    10. Heating system? _____
    11. Does family member have room next to patient's room? Yes/No
G.
    1. How did patient respond to home visit? _____

    2. What was patient and family interaction at home? _____

    3. Was family member able to manage? _____

    4. Teaching needs? _____
H. Community Resources
    1. Emergency Services? Yes/No
    2. M.D.? Yes/No

_____
Date

Comments

3. V.N.A.? Yes/No
4. Home health aid? Yes/No

II. Neighborhood Type
1. Residential/commercial/other? _____
2. Are the following accessible?
   a. Bank? Yes/No
   b. Laundry? Yes/No
   c. Medical services? Yes/No
   d. Food store? Yes/No
   e. Postoffice? Yes/No
   f. Social organization? Yes/No
3. Local EMS system?
4. Transportation available?
5. Independent/dependent in scheduling?
6. Ramps available? Yes/No
7. Curb cuts accessible? Yes/No
8. Curb height — technique to clear?

III. Dwelling
A. General
1. Does person live alone or with family? _____
2. Is housing, owned, rented, private home, apartment, condominium, other? _____
3. Is location of housing level or on a hill? _____
4. Is driveway level or inclined? _____
   Condition? _____
5. If person lives in an apartment, which floor does he or she live on? __
6. Number of levels of apartment? _____
7. Elevator in apartment accessible? Yes/No
8. If person lives in house, is house one family or two family? _____
9. Is house multilevel? Yes/No
10. Number of floors? _____
11. Consider the following miscellaneous items, and address as appropriate in comment section:
    Radiators, emergency numbers posted and accessible, phones, extension cords, outlets, lights, thermostats, curtains, basement, windows, shades, secure doors, fireplace, woodstove, informed police, fire departments, fuse box or circuit breakers, trash garbage disposal, mats, mailbox, plants, speed dialing phone, smoke detector, and emergency call system.
    Comments: _____
    _____
    _____
    _____

B. Access to dwelling
1. Entrances
   a. Most accessible entrance?
   b. Location?

_____
Date

Comments

  c. Terrain? (grass, gravel, pavement) _____

  d. Stairs at most accessible entrance

    (1) Number _____ railings r/l width?

    (2) Depth? _____

    (3) Height? _____

    (4) Lips:　Yes/No?

    (5) Surface _____

    (6) Back of stairs: Open/Closed?

  e. Emergency entrance

    (1) Location _____

    (2) Terrain (grass, gravel, pavement) _____

  f. Stairs of emergency entrance

    (1) Number _____

    (2) Railings r/l, width _____ depth _____

    (3) Height? _____

    (4) Lips　Yes/No?

    (5) Surface _____

    (6) Back of stairs?　Open/Closed?

  g. Doors

    (1) Width _____

    (2) Height _____

    (3) Door swing: Inward/Outward? Left/Right

    (4) Storm door present?　Yes/No

    (5) Door sill present?　Yes/No height? _____

    (6) Type of Door handle _____ Accessible?　Yes/No

    (7) Timing of door closure _____

    (8) Door lock-type _____ Accessible?　Yes/No

    (9) Foyer depth_____

  h. Living room

    (1) Door width _____

    (2) Threshold height _____

    (3) Type of floor covering _____ Any changes room to room?　Yes/No

    (4) Do furnishings allow room to maneuver in wheel-chair?　Yes/No ambulate?　Yes/No

    (5) Most accessible chair _____

    (6) Light switch accessible?　Yes/No

    (7) Can person open and close windows?　Yes/No

    (8) Can person manage television and radio?　Yes/No

    (9) Phone accessible?　Yes/No. Location? _____

    (10) Thermostat accessible　Yes/No

  i. Indoor Stairways

    (1) How many steps? _____ height of step? _____

    (2) Depth _____ rails　Right/Left

    (3) Lip on staircase?　Yes/No carpet?　Yes/No

    (4) Are back of stairs open or closed? _____

_____

Date

Comments
(5) Type of floor covering? _____ Is it safe? Yes/No
(6) Lighting accessible? Yes/No
j. Bedroom
    (1) Door width? _____ threshold? _____ height? _____
    (2) Type of bed? _____ height of bed? _____
    (3) Mattress _____
    (4) Closet accessible? Yes/No
    (5) Type of floor covering _____
    (6) Is maneuverability around bedroom feasible with present layout? Yes/No
    (7) Can person open and close closet door? Yes/No
    (8) Can person reach lights? Yes/No
    (9) Bureaus accessible? Yes/No
    (10) Can person open and close the drawers? Yes/No
    (11) Can person reach and store clothes? Yes/No
    (12) Mirror accessible? Yes/No
    (13) Is there a place for the person to dress in his or her room? Yes/No
    (14) Can person transfer wheelchair to bed and bed to wheelchair? Yes/No
    (15) Is night table within person's reach from bed? Yes/No. Is telephone on it? Yes/No
k. Kitchen
    (1) Door width _____
    (2) Threshold height _____
    (3) Can wheelchair fit under table? Yes/No
    (4) Appropriate chair available? Yes/No. Armrests available? Yes/No
    (5) Can person open refrigerator door and take food? Yes/No
    (6) Can person open freezer door and take food out? Yes/No
l. Sink
    (1) Can person be seated at sink? Yes/No
    (2) Can person turn faucets on and off? Yes/No
    (3) Can person reach bottom of basin? Yes/No
    (4) Are there any exposed pipes? Yes/No
    (5) Temperature of hot water? _____
m. Shelves and Cabinets
    (1) Can person open and close? Yes/No
    (2) Can person reach dishes, pots, silverware and food? Yes/No
n. Transport: Can person carry utensils and food from one part of the kitchen to another? Yes/No
o. Stove
    (1) Can person reach and manipulate controls? Yes/No
    (2) Can person light pilot on oven? Yes/No
    (3) Can person manage oven door? Yes/No
    (4) Can person place food in oven and remove? Yes/No

_____

Date

Comments

    (5) Can person manage broiler door? Yes/No

    (6) Can person put food in and remove? Yes/No

p. Microwave

    (1) Can person reach and operate dials? Yes/No

    (2) Can person manage door? Yes/No

    (3) Can person put food in and remove? Yes/No

    (4) What equipment is necessary for eating? _____

q. Bathroom

    (1) Threshold height? _____

    (2) Door width? _____

    (3) Top of the rim of the bathtub to the floor? _____

    (4) Length of tub on inside? _____

    (5) Width of tub on inside? _____

    (6) Height of toilet seat from floor? _____

    (7) Height of the sink? _____

    (8) Does the person use wheelchair, walker, cane, crutches, or no device in bathroom? _____

    (9) Is light switch accessible? Yes/No

  (10) What material is the bathroom walls made of? _____

  (11) If tile, how many inches does it extend from the floor beside the toilet? _____

  (12) Does person use toilet? Yes/No

  (13) Can person transfer independently to and from toilet? Yes/No

  (14) Does wheelchair wheel directly to toilet for transfers Yes/No

  (15) Are there bars or sturdy supports near toilet? Yes/No

  (16) Is there room for grab bars? Yes/No

  (17) Can person use sink? Yes/No

  (18) Is person able to reach and turn on faucets? Yes/No

  (19) Is there knee space beneath sink? Yes/No

  (20) Is person able to reach necessary articles? Yes/No

  (21) Mirror accessible? Yes/No

  (22) Lights accessible? Yes/No

  (23) Outlets accesible? Yes/No

r. Bathing

    (1) Does person take tub bath? Yes/No shower? Yes/No sponge bath? Yes/No

    (2) If tub, can person transfer safely without assistance? Yes/No

    (3) Bars or sturdy supports present beside tub? Yes/No

    (4) Is equipment necessary? Tub seat, hand spray attachment, tub rail, non skid strips, grab rails, other _____

    (5) Can person manage faucets and drain plug? Yes/No

    (6) Is tub built in? Yes/No on legs? Yes/No

    (7) If he or she uses separate shower stall, can person transfer independently and manage faucets? Yes/No

    (8) If person takes sponge bath, describe method.

_____

Date

Comments

s. Laundry
  (1) If person has no facilities, how is laundry done?
  (2) Location of facilities in home and description of facilities present?
  (3) Can person reach laundry area? Yes/No
  (4) Can person use washing machine and dryer? Yes/No
  (5) Can person load and empty laundry? Yes/No
  (6) Can person manage doors and controls? Yes/No
  (7) Is laundry cart available? Yes/No
  (8) Can person hang clothing on line? Yes/No
t. Ironing
  (1) Location? _____
  (2) Is ironing board kept open? Yes/No
  (3) If not kept open, can person set up and take down? Yes/No
  (4) Can person reach outlet? Yes/No
  (5) Can the person safely iron? Yes/No
  (6) Does iron automatically shut-off? Yes/No
u. Cleaning
  (1) Can person remove mop, broom, vacuum, and pail from storage? Yes/No
  (2) Can person use equipment? Yes/No
v. Emergency
  (1) Location of telephones in house. _____
  (2) Could person use fire escape or back door in a hurry if alone? Yes/No
  (3) Does person have neighbors, police, fire, and M.D. phone numbers? Yes/No
w. Shopping
  (1) Will person do own shopping? Yes/No
  (2) Is family member or friend available? Yes/No
  (3) Is delivery service available? Yes/No

_____

_____

_____

Signatures of examiners

Date: _____

LEVELS OF COGNITIVE AWARENESS

The Greenery has adapted a scale devised by researchers at the Rancho Los Amigos Medical Center, who studied a number of head-injured patients. Through their observations, they were able to classify behavior according to common traits and responses exhibited. A synopsis of their descriptors follows:

Levels of Cognitive Functioning*

1. *No response:* Patient appears to be in deep sleep and is completely unresponsive to any stimuli presented.

2. *Generalized response:* Patient reacts inconsistently and nonpurposefully to stimuli in a nonspecific manner. Responses are limited in nature and often are the same regardless of stimuli presented. Responses may be physiologic changes, gross body movements, and/or vocalization. Often, the earliest response is to deep pain. Responses are likely to be delayed.

3. *Localized response:* Patient reacts specifically but inconsistently to stimuli. Responses are directly related to the type of stimulus presented, as in turning head toward a sound or focusing on an object presented. The patient may withdraw an extremity and/or vocalize when presented with a painful stimulus. He or she may follow simple commands in an inconsistent, delayed manner, such as closing the eyes and squeezing or extending an extremity. Once external stimuli are removed, the patient may lie quietly. He or she may also show a vague awareness of self and body by responding to discomfort by pulling at the nasogastric tube or catheter or resisting restraints. The patient may also show a bias toward responding to some persons (especially family and friends).

4. *Confused-Agitated:* Patient is in a heightened state of activity with severely decreased ability to process information. These patients are detached from the present and respond primarily to their own internal confusion. Behavior is frequently bizarre and nonpurposeful, relative to their immediate environment. They may cry out or scream out of proportion to stimuli, even after removal; may show aggressive behavior; attempt to remove restraints or tubes; or crawl out of bed in a purposeful manner. They do not, however, discriminate among persons or objects and are unable to cooperate directly with treatment efforts. Verbalization is frequently incoherent and/or inappropriate to the environment. Confabulation may be present; patient may be euphoric or hostile. Thus, gross attention to environment is very short and selective attention is often nonexistent. Being unaware of present events, patient lacks short-term recall and may be reacting to past events. He or she is unable to perform self-care (feeding, dressing) without maximum assistance. If not disabled physically, patient may perform such motor activity as sitting, reaching, and ambulating, but as part of the agitated state, and not as a purposeful act or on request necessarily.

5. *Confused-Inappropriate-Nonagitated:* Patient appears alert and is able to respond to simple commands fairly consistently. However, with increased complexity of commands or lack of any external structure, responses are nonpurposeful, random, or, at best, fragmented toward any designed goal. Patients may show agitated behavior—not on an internal basis (as in level 4) but rather as a result of external stimuli and usually out of proportion to the stimulus. They have gross attention to the environment but are highly distractible and lack ability to focus attention to a specific task without frequent redirection back to it. With structure, these patients may be able to converse

---

*Adapted from Rancho Los Amigos Medical Center, Adult Head Trauma Service, Downey, CA.

on a social automatic level for short periods of time. Verbalization is often inappropriate; confabulation may be triggered by present events. The memory is severely impaired, with confusion of past and present in patient's reaction to ongoing activity. Patients lack initiation of functional tasks and often show inappropriate use of objects without external direction. They may be able to perform previously learned tasks when structured for them, but are unable to learn new information. These patients respond best to self, body, comfort, and often family members. They can usually perform self-care activities with assistance and may accomplish feeding with maximum supervision. Management on the unit is often a problem if the patient is physically mobile, as he or she may wander off, either randomly or with the vague intention of "going home."

6. *Confused-Appropriate:* Patient shows goal-directed behavior but is dependent on external input for direction. Response to discomfort is appropriate and he or she is able to tolerate unpleasant stimuli (as nasogastric tube) when need is explained. Patient follows simple instructions consistently and shows carry-over for tasks that have been relearned (as self-care). He or she is at least supervised with old learning and is at least maximally assisted for new learning with little or no carry-over. Responses may be incorrect owing to memory problems, but they are appropriate to the situation. Responses to immediate stimuli may be delayed and patient may show decreased ability to process information with little or no anticipation or prediction of events. Past memories show more depth and detail than recent memory. Patients may show beginning awareness of situation by realizing they do not know the an answer. They no longer wander but are inconsistently oriented to time and place. Selective attention to tasks may be impaired, especially with difficult tasks and in structured settings, but is now functional for common daily activities (30 minutes, with structure). Patient may show a vague recognition of some staff and may have increased awareness of self, family, and basic needs (such as foods), again in an appropriate manner, in contrast to level 4.

7. *Automatic-Appropriate:* Patient appears appropriate and oriented within facility and home settings, goes through daily routine automatically but frequently robotlike, with minimal to absent confusion, but has shallow recall of what he or she has been doing. There is increased awareness of self, body, family, foods, people, and interaction in the environment. Patient has superficial awareness but lacks insight into his or her condition, demonstrates decreased judgment and problem-solving abilities, and lacks realistic planning for the future. He or she shows carry-over for new learning, but at a decreased rate. The patient requires at least minimal supervision for learning and for safety purposes and is independent in self-care activities, with supervised at-home and community skills for safety. With structure, patient is able to initiate tasks such as social or recreational activities in which there is now interest. Judgment remains impaired, such that patient cannot drive a car. Prevocational or avocational evaluation and counseling may be indicated.

8. *Purposeful and appropriate:* Patient is alert and oriented, is able to recall and integrate past and recent events, and is aware of and responsive to the culture. These individuals show carry-over for new learning if acceptable to them and their life role, and need no supervision once activities are learned. Within their physical capabilities, they are independent in home and community skills, including driving. Vocational rehabilitation's main objective is to

determine ability to return as a contributor to society (perhaps in relation to premorbid abilities, in abstract reasoning, tolerance for stress, judgment in emergencies, or unusual circumstances). The social, emotional, and intellectual capacities may continue to be at a decreased level for the patient, while remaining functional in society.

It is not unusual for patients to maintain one level for long periods of time. It is especially difficult for families to adjust to their loved one as they progress through various stags. Behaviors may be exhibited that would not have been displayed prior to injury. The interdisciplinary team is aware of these behavior patterns, and members of the staff are available to discuss appropriate coping techniques with family members. The process is a long, difficult one—a fact that our staff is well aware of and receptive to. At the discretion of the interdisciplinary team, various treatments and/or techniques may be used to help patients best cope with their dysfunction, their environment, and their program. These can include behavioral, pharmacologic, or cognitive-based approaches. It is important to keep in mind that the "personality" changes are a manifestation of the nature of the patient's injury. Although a fairly reliable scale with which to measure progress, these changes can possibly hinder further rehabilitation, in which case they should be addressed.

WHEELCHAIR COMPARISONS*

 EVERYDAY CHAIRS

MANUFACTURER	ACTION TECHNOLOGY*	ACTIVEAID, INC.	DAMACO	DUPREE WHEELCHAIR SERVICES, INC.	EAGLE SPORTSCHAIRS	ELITE WHEELCHAIR PRODUCTS
Model	Action AC	Active II Infinity PS	Enabler	Pro-Lite	Hurricane II	Elite DG
WEIGHT WITH WHEELS	14-23 lb	30 lb	27 lb	12 lb	16 lb	16-18 lb
CUSTOM-BUILT	Yes/no	Yes	Yes	Yes	Yes	Yes
FRAME: Composition	Advanced composite aluminum	Stainless steel	Aluminum	Chrome-moly	4130 chrome-moly tubing	4130 chrome-moly
No. of colors available	8	5 + custom	9	Unlimited	Unlimited	Choice
Folding/modular	No/yes	Yes/yes	Yes/yes	No/no	No/no	No/no
Antitip casters	No	Yes	Yes	No	No	Optional
Widths available	15'', 16'', 17'', 18''	14-24''	12-20''	Custom	10-20''	10-20''
ARMREST TYPES AVAILABLE	1	3	5	Custom	4	5
BACK: Folding/locking	Yes/yes	Yes/yes	Yes/no	No/no	Yes/optional	Yes/yes
Adjustable angle range	8° back - 10° forward	3-9°	3-12° (optional)	—	Unlimited (optional)	—
Adjustable height range	10-14'', 12-16'', 14-18''	10-18''	14-19'', 20'' optional	—	Unlimited (optional)	8-16'', 12-19''
UPHOLSTERY: Type of fabric	Nylon	Nylon, Dacron	Cordura	Nylon Parapak	Nylon, pack cloth	Nylon
No. of colors available	1	1	3	10	6	12
Seat-depth range	15'', 16'', 17'', 18''	15-20''	11-20''	Custom	Unlimited	10-20''
Adjustable tension	Yes	Yes	No	Yes	Yes	Yes
CUSHION STANDARD	Yes	Yes	Optional	Optional	Optional	Optional
Height	2''	2-3''	2-4''	Custom	1'', 2'', 3'', 4''	1-4''
Composition	Foam	Foam	Foam	Foam	Temper foam	Foam
BRAKES STANDARD	Optional	Yes	Yes	Optional	Optional	Optional
Extension handles available	Yes	Yes	Yes	Yes	Yes	Yes
Mount	Low & high	Mid	Low & high	Low, mid, & high	Low, mid, & high	Low & high
CASTERS: Quick-release	Yes	No	No	No	No	No
Adjustable	—	Yes	Yes	No	No	No
5''/8''	5''	Both	Both	—	Both	Both
Rubber/polyurethane	—	Both	Rubber	—	Polyurethane	Both
Other	5'' solid, 6'' solid or pneumatic	8'' pneumatic	5'' & 8'' polyurethane	Wide variety	—	8'' air
FOOTRESTS STANDARD	Rigid single unit, adjustable	Flip-up, swing-away, adjustable	Swing-away, adjustable	Rigid single unit	Rigid single unit, adjustable	Rigid single unit, adjustable
HANDRIMS: Projections available	Optional	Optional	Optional	Optional	Optional	Optional
Coated	Optional	Optional	Optional	Optional	Optional	Optional
Size	20⅝''	¾-⅞''	20'', 22'', 24''	Varies	21'', 22'', 23''	18'', 21'', 23''
Other	—	Variable diameters	—	—	—	—
MAIN WHEELS: Quick-release	Yes	Yes	Yes	Yes	Yes	Yes
No. of axle positions	—	3 vertical; infinite horizontal	4	1	2	Multiple
Camber/angle	0°, 2°, 4°, 8°	Adjustable	Yes	Custom	2-12° or double-camber tube	Customer choice
Mag wheels available	Optional	Standard/optional	Standard	Optional	Optional	Standard/optional
WARRANTY	Lifetime - chassis	5 yrs - frame; 1 yr - other	Lifetime - side frames & crossbraces	Lifetime - frame	5 yrs - frame; 1 yr - upholstery	Lifetime - frame; 1 yr - other
DELIVERY TIME	2 wks	3 wks	1-4 wks	4-6 wks	3-4 wks	2-4 wks

*A division of Invacare Corp.

*Copyright © 1990, Paralyzed Veterans of America. By permission of Sports 'N' Spokes 15(6):32–34, 1991.

ENDURO BY WHEEL RING INC.	ETAC USA	EVEREST & JENNINGS	FORTRESS	INVACARE CORP.	IRON HORSE PRODUCTIONS, INC.	K-CHAIR
Enduro 2	Swede Elite	Profile	Custom	9000	The Iron Horse	F-100
20.4 lb	19.3-21 lb	26 lb	29 lb	29 lb	45 lb	27 lb
Yes	No	Yes	Yes	No	No	Yes
Titanium	Titanium & aluminum	Aluminum	Aluminum	Steel	304 18-gauge stainless steel	Aluminum
6	5	10 + 8 custom	22	5	1	2
No/yes	Yes/yes	Yes/yes	Yes/yes	Yes/no	Yes/yes	Yes/yes
Yes	No	Optional	Yes	Yes	No	No
13-19''	14'', 15'', 16'', 17'', 18''	14-20''	13-20''	14-20''	16-25'', 18-27''	16-18''
3	2	5	4	9	1	2
Yes/yes	Yes/yes	No/no	Yes/yes	No/no	No/no	No/no
to 10°	+3°, 0°, −3°, −5°, −10°	0-8°	0-10°	—	—	—
to 21''	12-16''	10-20''	13-15'', 15-17'', 17-19''	14-18''	15-17''	13½-19½''
Nylon	100% polyester	Nylon Parapak	Dacron	Nylon	Polypropylene	Nylon
10	1	5	13	8	1	1
13-19''	14-18''	15-18''	13-18''	16-20''	15-17''	16-18''
No	Yes	Yes	Yes	Yes	No	Yes
Yes	Optional	Optional	Optional	Optional	No	Optional
½'', 1''	2''	2'', 3''	2-4''	2'', 3''	—	1-3''
Medium-density foam	100% polyester foam	Foam	Foam	Foam	—	Foam
Yes	Yes	Yes	Yes	Yes	Yes	Yes
—	Yes	Yes	Yes	Yes	Yes	Yes
High	Mid	High	Low & high	High	High	Low & high
No	No	No	Yes	No	No	No
Yes	Yes	Yes	Yes	No	No	Yes
Both	5''	Both	Both	8''	Both	Both
Polyurethane	Polyurethane	Polyurethane	Both	Rubber	Polyurethane	Both
6'', 8'' pneumatic	6'' rubber, 6'' polyurethane	6'' foam-filled, 2¾'' roller blades	5'' polyurethane, 8'' pneumatic	6'' & 8'' pneumatic, 6'' polyurethane	8'' pneumatic	—
Rigid single unit, adjustable	Rigid single unit	Flip-up, swing-away, adjustable	Flip-up, swing-away, adjustable	Elevating, swing-away, hemi-height, adjustable	Flip-up, adjustable	Flip-up, adjustable, swing-away, hemi-height
Optional	Optional	Optional	Optional	Optional	Standard	Optional
Optional	Optional	Optional	Optional	Optional	Standard	Optional
20'', 22'', 24''	20'', 22'', 24''	21'', 23''	Multiple	¾'' aluminum	22''	21''
—	Cellular rubber, spoke-mounted	Anodized standard	—	—	Stainless steel	—
Yes	Yes	Yes	Yes	Yes	Yes	No
5	11	Multiple	Multiple	1	1	3
Yes	3° standard	0°, 4°, 6°, 8°	0-10°	—	Weight-initiated	4°
Yes	—	Standard	Optional	Standard	No	Standard
1 yr - frame	Lifetime - main frame	Lifetime - frame	Lifetime - side frames & crossbraces	1 yr - materials & workmanship	Lifetime - frame; 1 yr - components	Lifetime - frame
2-3 wks	4-6 wks	2-4 wks	3-4 wks	3-6 wks	5-10 days	5 working days

KUSCHALL OF AMERICA	MAGIC IN MOTION	QUICKIE DESIGNS/ SUNRISE MEDICAL	REDMAN WHEELCHAIRS INC.	SOPUR WEST INC.	TOP END WHEELCHAIR SPORTS, INC.	WHEELSPORT INTERNATIONAL
Champion 1000	Shadow One Everyday	Quickie 2	Cheyenne	Easy	Terminator Everyday	Volant
27 lb	19-21 lb	29¾ lb	29 lb	29 lb	16-22 lb	25 lb
Yes	Yes	Yes	Yes	Yes	Yes	No
Aluminum	Chrome-moly	Aircraft aluminum	Chrome-moly	Aluminum	Chrome-moly	Aluminum
17	Unlimited	13	5	16	Custom	3
Yes/yes	No/no	Yes/yes	Yes/—	Yes/—	No/—	Yes/yes
Yes	No	No	No	Yes	No	No
14-20"	Unlimited	12-20"	16-30"	12½-20"	Custom	16", 18"
2	Custom	2	2	9	2	2
No/no	Yes/yes	No/no	No/no	No/yes	Yes/yes	No/no
—	2-9°	8° (fixed back angle also avail.)	—	0-20° reclined	0-4°	No
12-16", 15-19"	11-14", 14-17"	8½-19"	—	Yes	Custom	16-19"
Nylon	Pack cloth, nylon	Nylon	Naugahyde, Dacron	Nylon or waterproof (plastic-coated)	Nylon	Naugahyde, Dacron
2	3	1	5	14	1	1
14-20"	13-18"	10-18"	16"	13-18½"	Custom	16"
Yes	No	Yes	No	Yes	Yes	No
Yes	Yes	Yes	Optional	Yes	Optional	Optional
2"	2-4"	2", 3", 4"	1-4"	1-2", 2", 3"	2-4"	2", 3", 4"
Foam	T-foam	Foam	Foam	Foam (soft, med, or hard)	Foam	Foam
Yes	Yes	Yes	Yes	Yes	Optional	Yes
Yes	No	Yes	Yes	Yes	—	Yes
Low & mid	Low, mid, & high	Low & high	Low, mid, & high	Mid	Low, mid, & high	Low & high
No	No	No	No	No	No	No
Yes	No	Yes	No	Yes	No	Yes
Both	Both	Both	Both	Both	Both	Both
Polyurethane	Both	Polyurethane	Polyurethane	Both	Polyurethane	Both
5" soft roll	—	6" polyurethane & pneumatic, 8" pneumatic	—	Pneumatic	—	7½" polyurethane, pneumatic
Flip-up, rigid single unit, swing-away, hemi-height, adj	Rigid single unit, adjustable	Flip-up, swing-away, hemi-height, adjustable	Flip-up, swing-away, adjustable	Flip-up, rigid single unit, swing-away, adjustable	Rigid single unit, adjustable	Flip-up, swing-away, hemi-height, adjustable
Optional	Optional	Optional	Optional	Optional	Optional	Optional
Optional	Optional	Optional	Optional	Optional	Optional	Optional
20", 22", 24"	21-23"	20-26"	½-1"	24", 26"	18-22"	21"
—	Any size optional	Vertical oblique 6, 8, 10, or 12 projections	—	Anodized, stainless, painted, & quad push rims available	—	—
Yes	Yes	Yes	Yes	Yes	Yes	Optional
36	Unlimited	Multiple	1	20	Adjustable	4
0-4°	3°, 6°, 9°, 12°	Set at 2°	—	Adjustable	Custom	
Standard	No	Standard	Optional	Optional	Optional	Standard
Lifetime - frames, cross members, axles; 1 yr - rest	Lifetime - frame	Lifetime	5 yrs - frame; 90 days - parts	Lifetime - frame	5 yrs	Lifetime - frame & braces
4 wks	4-6 wks	2-3 wks	2-4 wks	4-6 wks	4-6 wks	2 wks

Bibliography

Adams, RD, and Victor, M: Principles of Neurology, McGraw-Hill, New York, 1981.

American Academy of Orthopaedic Surgeons: Atlas of Orthotic. ed 2. CV Mosby, St Louis, 1985.

American Academy of Orthopaedic Surgeons: Atlas of Prosthetic. CV Mosby, St Louis, 1981.

Apts, D, and Blankenship, PK: Back facts for the American Back School, FPR, Ashland, KY, 1981.

Arnett, RW: Acquisition of skill. Br Med Bull 27:266, 1971.

Bach-y-Ria, P: Central nervous system lesions: Sprouting and unmasking in rehabilitation. Arch Phys Med Rehabil 62:413, 1981.

Banerjee, SN (ed): Rehabilitation Management of Amputees. Williams & Wilkins, Baltimore, 1982.

Basmajian, JV: Therapeutic Exercise, ed 3. Williams & Wilkins, Baltimore, 1978.

Beavis, A: Cervical orthoses. Prosthet Orthot Int 13:6, 1989.

Bishop, B: Basic Neurophysiology. Medical Examination Publishing, Garden City, NY, 1982, pp 346–358.

Bobath, B: The application of physiological principles to stroke rehabilitation. Practitioner 223:793, 1979.

Bobath, B: The problem of spasticity in the treatment of patients with lesions of the upper motor neurone. Western Cerebral Palsy Centre, Cerebral Palsy Unit, Harperbury Hospital, London, 1978.

Bobath, B: Treatment of Adult Hemiplegia. The Bobath Centre, London, 1976.

Bond, MR: Assessments of the psychosocial outcome. In Ciba Foundation Symposium 34: Outcomes of Severe Damage to the Central Nervous System. Elsevier, New York, 1975, pp 141–157.

Booth, BJ, Doyle, M, and Montgomery, J: Serial casting for the management of spasticity in the head-injured adult. Phys Ther 63:12, 1983, p 1960–1966.

Calvin, W, and Ojemann, G: Inside the Brain, New American Library Mentor Book, New York, 1980.

Carpenter, MB: Human Neuroanatomy, ed 7, Williams & Wilkins, Baltimore, 1976.

Cicenia, E, Hoberman, M, and Dervitz, H: Safety: A factor in functional training of the disabled child.

Cicenia, E, et al: Parallel bar activities in physical therapy and rehabilitation medicine. Am J Phys Med 34:591, 1955.

Curtis, B, Jacobson, S, and Marcus, E: An Introduction to the Neurosciences. WB Saunders, Philadelphia, 1972.

Corcoron, P: Energy expenditure during ambulation. In Downey, D: Physiological Basis of Rehabilitation Medicine. WB Saunders, Philadelphia, 1971.

Edelstein, JE: Prosthetic feet: State of the art. Phys Ther 68:1874, 1988.

Engstrom, B and Van de Ven, C: Physiotherapy for amputees: The Roehampton Approach. Churchill Livingstone, Edinburgh, 1983.

Fisher, B: Effect of trunk control and alignment and limb function. J Head Trauma Rehabil 2(2):72, 1987.

Gram, M: Using the parapodium: A manual of training techniques. Eterna, New York, 1984.

Hallet, M: Physiology and pathophysiology of voluntary movement. In Tyler, HR and Dawson, D (eds): Current Neurology. Vol 2. Houghton Mifflin, Boston, 1979, pp 351–356.

Hirschberg, G, Lewis, L, and Vaughan, P: Rehabilitation, ed 2. JB Lippincott, Philadelphia, 1976.

Hoberman, M and Cicenia, E: Rehabilitation techniques with braces and crutches. I. Occupational therapy and rehabilitation. Am J Phys Med 30(4):203, 1951.

Hoberman, M and Cicenia, E: Rehabilitation techniques with braces and crutches. II. Occupational therapy and rehabilitation. Am J Phys Med 30(6):377, 1951.

Hoberman, M and Cicenia, E: Rehabilitation techniques with braces and crutches. IV. Methods of falling and of getting down and up from the floor. Am J Phys Med 31(1):21, 1952.

Hoberman, M and Cicenia, E: Rehabilitation techniques with braces and crutches. V. Travel techniques. Am J Phys Med 31(2):82, 1952.

Hoberman, M and Cicenia, E: Rehabilitation techniques with braces and crutches. VI. Techniques with forearm crutches. Am J Phys Med 31(5):373, 1952.

Hoberman, M, et al: The use of lead-up functional exercise to supplement mat work: Exercise without apparatus or equipment. Phys Ther Rev 31:1, 1951.

Humm, W: Rehabilitation of the Lower Limb Amputee, ed 2. Williams & Wilkins, Baltimore, 1964.

Kottke, FJ, Stillwell, GK, and Lehmann, JF: Krusen's Handbook of Physical Medicine and Rehabilitation, ed 3. WB Saunders, Philadelphia, 1982, pp 921–935.

Karacoloff, LA: Lower Extremity Amputation: A guide to Functional Outcomes in Physical Therapy Management. Aspen, Rockville, MD, 1985.

Kostuik, JP (ed): Amputation Surgery and Rehabilitation: The Toronto Experience. Churchill Livingstone, New York, 1981.

Krebs, DE, Edelstein, JE, and Fishman, S: Comparison of plastic/metal and leather/metal knee-ankle-foot orthoses. Am J Phys Med Rehabil 67:175, 1988.

Landau, WM: Spasticity: The fable of a neurological demon and the emperor's new therapy. Arch Neurol 31:217, 1974.

Lawton, EB: Activities of Daily Living for Physical Rehabilitation. McGraw-Hill, New York, 1963.

Lehmann, J, et al: Plastic ankle-foot orthoses: Evaluation of function. Arch Phys Med Rehabil 64:402, 1983.

Licht, S: Stroke and Its Rehabilitation. Waverly Press, Baltimore, 1975.

Lockard, MA: Foot orthoses. Phys Ther 68:1866, 1988.

Lower Extremity Prosthetics. Orthotics and Prosthetics Center, Northwestern University Medical School, Chicago, 1976.

Malkmus, D: Integrating cognitive strategies into the physical therapy setting. Phys Ther 63:12, 1983, pp 1952–1959.

Manella, K: Comparing the effectiveness of elastic bandages and shrinker socks for lower extremity amputees. Phys Ther 61:334, 1981.

McCall, RE and Schmidt, WT: Clinical experience with the reciprocal gait orthosis in myelodysplasia. J Pediatr Orthoped 6:157, 1986.

McHugh, B and Campbell, J: Below-knee orthoses. Physiotherapy 73:380, 1987.

Mensch, G and Ellis, PM: Physical Therapy Management of Lower Extremity Amputations. Aspen, Rockville, MD, 1986.

Montgomery, J: Overview of head injuries. Phys Ther 63:12, 1983 p 1945.

Moore, WS and Malone, JM: Lower Extremity Amputation. WB Saunders, Philadelphia, 1989.

Mountcastle, VB: The view from within: Pathways to the study of perception. Johns Hopkins Med J 136:109, 1975.

Murdock, G and Donovan, RG (eds): Amputation Surgery and Lower Limb Prosthetics. Blackwell, Oxford, 1988.

Netter, F: The Ciba Collection of Medical Illustrations. Vol 1: Nervous System, Part I, Anatomy and Physiology. Ciba, Summit, NJ, 1983, p 128.

Pronsati, MP: Fashionable can be functional. Adv Phys Ther 1(11):5, 8, 1990.

Redford, JB (ed): Orthotics Etcetera, ed 3. Williams & Wilkins: Baltimore, 1986.

Rinehart, MA: Considerations for functional training in adults after head injury. Phys Ther 63:12, 1983 pp 1975–1982.

Robbins, SL, Contran, RF, and Vinay, K: Pathologic Basis of Disease. WB Saunders, Philadelphia, 1984.

Scully, R, and Barnes, M (ed): Physical Therapy. JB Lippincott, Philadelphia, 1990, pp 1059–1062.

Rose, GK: Orthotics: Principles and Practice. Heinemann, London, 1986.

Rubin, G, Fischer, E, and Dixon, M: Prescription of above-knee and below-knee prostheses. Prosthet Orthot Int 10:117, 1986.

Sahrmann, SA and Norton, BJ: The relationship of voluntary movement to spasticity in the upper motor neuron syndrome. Ann Neurol 2:460, 1977.

Sanders, GT: Lower Limb Amputations: A Guide to Rehabilitation. FA Davis, Philadelphia, 1986.

Shands, AR and Raney, RB: Handbook of Orthopedic Surgery, ed 7, CV Mosby, St Louis, 1967, pp 286–295.

Sypert, GW: External spinal orthotics. Neurosurgery 20:642, 1987.

Williams, PL and Warwick, R: Functional Neuroanatomy of Man, WB Saunders, Philadelphia, 1975, pp 1047–1064.

Winstein, CJ: Current concepts in motor learning applied to assessment and treatment. Presentation, Hyannis, MA, 1988.

INDEX

An F following a page number indicates a figure; a T following a page number indicates a table.